Ellyn Satter's

Child of Mine

ALSO BY ELLYN SATTER

Your Child's Weight: Helping without Harming

Secrets of Feeding a Healthy Family: How to Eat, How to Feed Children, How to Cook

Child of Mine: Feeding with Love and Good Sense

How to Get Your Kid to Eat: But Not Too Much

Feeding with Love and Good Sense: The First Two Years

Feeding with Love and Good Sense: 18 Months through 6 Years

Feeding with Love and Good Sense: 6 through 13 Years

Feeding with Love and Good Sense: 12 through 18 Years

Feeding Yourself with Love and Good Sense

Feeding in Primary Care Pregnancy through Preschool: Easy-to-read Reproducible Masters

Feeding with Love and Good Sense II DVD

Feeding with Love and Good Sense I DVD

Ellyn Satter's

Child of Mine

Nurturing a Confident and Joyful Eater

Ellyn Satter, MS, MSSW

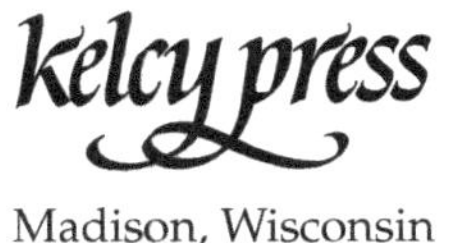

Madison, Wisconsin

Kelcy Press
4226 Mandan Crescent
Madison, WI 53711-3062

Satter, Ellyn
Ellyn Satter's Child of Mine: Nurturing a Confident and Joyful Eater/Ellyn Satter

ISBN 9780990897545 (print)
ISBN 9780990897552 (ePub)

Library of Congress Cataloging-in-Publication Data
Satter, Ellyn.
Ellyn Satter's Child of Mine: nurturing a confident and joyful eater/Ellyn Satter
Includes bibliographic references and index
Parenting. 2. Child rearing. 3. Nutrition. 4. Child development
HQ768
649.3

Printed in the U.S.
Cover and interior design: Happenstance Type-O-Rama

Books, discounted bulk purchases and PDFs of Kelcy Press books are available at
https://www.ellynsatterinstitute.org/

Ellyn Satter's Child of Mine is distributed to the trade by
Publishers Group West
819 Bancroft Way
Berkeley, CA 94710

DEDICATED

To our children and grandchildren
with love and gratitude.
It is so good to be a part of all this!

CONTENTS

PREFACE

This book is written *to* parents, to encourage you to trust your natural instincts with feeding your child. It is also written *for* professionals who work with you, who need evidence to be able to support you in doing well with feeding. As I write, I am also speaking on behalf of my professional colleagues in the Ellyn Satter Institute (ESI), a nonprofit organization that supports and furthers the Satter trust models of feeding and eating. ESI provides resources, education, and training for professionals and the public to help them reimagine and reshape anxiety-infused relationships with food into joyful journeys of healthful well-being.

Feeding well isn't it just about raising a confident and joyful *eater*. It is about raising a confident and joyful *person*. Feeding well is about loving, knowing, and respecting your child, responding to their needs, and feeling successful with them. Because you and your child spend most of your early years with feeding, the feeding relationship gives your child powerful messages: I see you, I value you, I respect you, I am willing to go to some trouble to work things out with you. Feeding well satisfies your needs, as well. You need to feel you can give your child what they need to make them happy.

Ellyn Satter's Child of Mine helps make the world a loving and accepting place for children by emphasizing feeding based on the Satter Division of Responsibility in Feeding (sDOR). Parents do the *what, when,* and *where* of *feeding* and trust their child to do the *how much* and *whether* of *eating* the food that they, the parents, provide. Following sDOR, taking appropriate leadership on the one hand and giving your child autonomy on the other, gives your child security and a sense of self-acceptance.

My ESI colleagues and I are all too painfully aware that there is much in our culture that interferes with such accepting and responsive feeding. Parents are supposed to raise a child who is lean and healthy, and they are bombarded with advice about what and how much their child should eat and how they should grow. Professionals are expected to *give* that advice. Book titles make alarming demands such as "disease-proof your child," and "prevent disease before it starts." The message everywhere is the same: get children to eat certain foods, avoid others, and weigh within certain limits.

FOLLOWING sDOR IS GOOD PARENTING

Following sDOR is the gold standard of feeding because it lets you meet your needs to nurture and your child's needs to *be* nurtured. You don't have to try to get your child to eat and grow in certain ways. In fact, I beg you not to because it will make you all miserable and likely accomplish the opposite of what you want for your child. Being controlling with feeding tends to make children finicky, prone to weight acceleration or weight faltering, and be so poorly behaved around food that parents are tempted to give up on family meals. Underlying it all, such controlling feeding is likely to make your child feel bad about themself because they won't be able to eat and grow to please you.

What you can do instead, and this is critically important, is establish a positive feeding relationship. Some fear that sDOR is too simple to be effective. It is simple to say, not so simple to enact. sDOR is providing family meals every day for 18 years or however long your child lives at home. It is overlooking your child's eating a little of this and a little of that and not a single vegetable. It is trusting that as long as you hang in there with pleasant and reliable family meals, your child will eat what and as much as they need. It is trusting that as your child matures, they will learn to enjoy more and more foods and eventually get around to eating most of what you eat. It can take *years*, and that is a *lot* of trust and a *lot* of hanging in there.

Following sDOR presents you with nuances. Can you encourage a child to eat certain food? Insist they leave the meal when they misbehave? *Let* them leave when they have eaten only bread? It comes down to *intent*. If your intent is to enhance the feeding relationship, it is consistent with sDOR. If the intent is to get your child to eat and/or grow in certain ways, it is inconsistent with sDOR.

Following sDOR means raising your child to be Eating Competent. That means they enjoy food, eating, and family meals; are comfortable being around unfamiliar food; and go by their feelings of hunger and fullness to know how much to eat. Children whose parents follow sDOR do better nutritionally,[1] even though sDOR says nothing at all about what children should eat. sDOR allows raising children to be Eating Competent, and that supports their wellness throughout life. Eating Competent grown-ups have the same or lower BMIs; are more active; sleep better;

are less stressed, depressed, and anxious; and have fewer symptoms of eating disorders.[2]

sDOR makes your child the priority

My advice may be a bit of a mind-bender for you because it is poles apart from what is current. That is because sDOR makes your *child* the priority: their feeling relaxed and positive about eating and their body, and their growing in the way that is right for them. Prevailing practice—the control paradigm—makes the *outcome* the priority: getting your child to eat and grow in certain ways.

You can tell whether you are on the right track—the *trusting* track—by considering feeding from your child's point of view. Is your baby relaxed and comfortable with breast- or bottle-feeding? Is your older baby comfortable with eating—or not eating—solid food? Are they engaged in trying to figure it all out? Does your toddler or preschooler enjoy family meals? Are they able to be around new food without getting upset? Does your child of any age grow consistently? That is, do they generally follow along a particular growth curve?

If you are able to answer yes to all these questions, feeding is going well and you are being trusting. If not, something is leading you to be controlling, and you need to get to the bottom of it. And you can—with the guidance on these pages. You can learn about your child's capabilities with eating and increasingly trust and be guided by those capabilities. When you change your ways with feeding, your child will change their ways with eating.

Consider nutrition politics

I review a good bit of research evidence to support my advice in *Ellyn Satter's Child of Mine*. You may or may not want to read it—skim it or ignore it. You will soon have the best evidence of all in that your child will show you that the advice *works*. Your health and nutrition professional advisors need to hear about your success, but they also need the research evidence to reassure them that it is okay to follow this advice. It is no small thing to ask of them, because it means they will have to go against their standards of practice. Allow me to elaborate.

For both adults and children, "healthy eating pattern" policies and guidelines are today's background music against which food selection advice plays out. Those policies and guidelines are regularly reestablished by government agencies and passed on as standards of practice to professional organizations such as the American Academy of Pediatrics and the Academy of Nutrition and Dietetics. Agencies that directly support child nutrition and feeding, such as the WIC program and university extension programs, are mandated to teach "healthy eating pattern" guidelines for parents and children.

Which puts health professionals in a bind—the same bind I experienced early in my career. Do we do as we are told by policy makers and professional organizations and agencies? Or do we allow ourselves to be guided by experience to act on behalf of our patients? After that, there is another bind: Many learn from experience that what they are doing doesn't work, but they don't know what to do instead. I spent several years in my early career wading through what-not-to-do and arriving at what-to-do instead. That's what *Ellyn Satter's Child of Mine* is all about.

Consider the hot potato

Today's nutrition and growth policies and standards amount to pressure on feeding. Pressure, the same as a hot potato, gets tossed down the line from policy makers to health professionals to parents until it ends up in the lap of the person least able to cope with it: your child. Health professionals who resist standards of practice hang on to that hot potato rather than tossing it to you. That takes courage and the willingness to endure pain. Ironically, it takes less courage and causes less pain to go along with the status quo—to resort to pressure and toss the potato on down the line.

A BIRDS-EYE VIEW OF FEEDING

I love feeding stories, and in *Ellyn Satter's Child of Mine* I tell many stories about parents, babies, and older children. Stories capture in a few words what it takes paragraphs to explain. Stories about when things go wrong with feeding tell you why you are doing things right. The few words in these vignettes introduce you to the possibilities of being trusting with feeding.

Consider the parents of a preemie who were able to relax and follow their baby's lead with feeding when they learned about sDOR. They had been struggling to follow NICU advice to feed him so many ounces every two hours, and it was making them all miserable. Consider the mother, who was able to stop panicking and ignore health professionals' advice to get her small baby to eat more when she realized she had to trust him—that pressuring him to eat spoiled feeding and made him eat less. Consider Sebastian, who at six months was totally *not* interested in solid food. His mother hung in there with sDOR for months while Sebastian messed about with the food on his high-chair tray. Then one day he picked it up and ate it. Consider the mother of twin toddlers who found her boys ate better when she started following sDOR and stopped scouring the kitchen to find something they would eat. Consider 5-year-old Sophie, who only came willingly to meals after her parents stopped trying to get her to eat vegetables. Consider 12-year-old Noah, the very selective eater, whose parents followed sDOR and were secretly astonished when they asked for the broccoli. Consider the Minnesota parents who only let themselves enjoy meals with their children when the food was "healthy and home-cooked."

These vignettes forecast the messages in *Ellyn Satter's Child of Mine.* The first message is that feeding goes well when it is built on trust. You do your bit by having regular meals that you, yourself, enjoy—and then you trust your child to determine whether and how much to eat at those meals. Part I, Undertand Trust with Feeding and Eating, provides backup and support for doing just that. The second message is that even when you follow sDOR, there is much to learn: following your child's cues, interpreting their behavior, feeding so they can eat well. The first year offers a particularly steep learning curve, and Part II, How to Feed: The Early Months, walks you through that learning. The third message is that sDOR is the gift that keeps on giving. Part III, How to Feed: The Toddler and Preschooler, still gives much to learn but it doesn't seem quite so challenging when your child is no longer so small.

The vignettes also demonstrate that following sDOR can mean doing the exact opposite of what seems right: trusting that a tiny baby will let you know when they are hungry and how much they need to eat; trusting that a six-month-old will get around to eating solid food, even though they couldn't seem less interested; trusting that a toddler will eat better once you stop catering to them; trusting that your child will get around to eating the vegetables you eat—even if it takes *years*; trusting that the food you can manage is all right for your family—even when it is on someone's "bad food" list. Trusting a child in those situations is downright nerve-wracking, especially when you factor in today's constant background of controlling advice. At first it may be easier on the nerves to go along with prevailing advice and try to force the outcome you want, but you and your child will pay for it in the long run.

A PARADIGM SHIFT

The theme of this book is that feeding and parenting with trust is critical for your child nutritionally, essential to their capabilities with eating, and fundamental to their social and emotional development. Making the shift from trying to get your child to eat *what* and *how much* to following sDOR is that radical change I talked about earlier. A shift from control to trust is a *paradigm shift*: a change to a fundamentally different way of perceiving, thinking, doing, and being. It is a paradigm shift to go to child-competence thinking from child-deficit thinking: from believing that children have to be controlled to get them to eat and grow in certain ways to believing that children can be trusted with eating and growing. That's big. It was a paradigm shift to go from believing the earth is flat to believing it is round; so was believing the earth revolves around the sun rather than vice versa. Paradigm shifts are major, and prevailing paradigms are protected—either consciously or by habit. It is *hard* to give up principles that have guided your life!

With control paradigm thinking, you strive for a particular outcome; with trust paradigm thinking, you depend on the process and let yourself be surprised by the outcome. Many try to resolve contradictions between paradigms by trying to do both: Nutrition and health professionals often mechanically repeat sDOR and still say what and how much. If you have been following sDOR and also trying to impose *what* and *how much* on your child, you have no doubt discovered that you have to choose. Either the earth is flat or it is round. Either you are trusting or controlling. Following sDOR leaves no leeway for trying to produce a certain outcome with what and how much your child eats. "Healthy eating pattern" guidelines, which prioritize eating nutrient-dense foods and achieving certain BMIs, leave no leeway for trusting children to eat what and as much as they need. It is still control paradigm even if guidelines come packaged with sDOR or some derivative of it, such as "responsive feeding."

Remember: Even if your health professional and/or educator advises you to follow sDOR, it is control paradigm if they also advise you to get your child to eat more or less, higher- or lower-calorie food, grow faster or more slowly. Ask yourself: Is this advice intended to try to get the child to eat certain food, eat more or less, or grow in a certain way? If so, it is control paradigm, no matter its claims.

Learning to depend on trust

It isn't easy to act in ways that are contrary to the prevailing paradigm, and it isn't easy to ignore expectations that you will get your child to eat and grow in certain ways. Instead, you have to depend on trust. As illustrated by the vignettes I just shared with you, trust means to believe in your child's ability. To begin with, your trust might be a leap of faith, but it will build over time. For you to be able to trust your child, they have to have the chance to be *trustworthy.* While you wait for them to surprise you with how well they can do, reassure yourself that your trust is well founded. Your child was born *wanting* to eat, knowing *how much* to eat, and able to *grow* in the way that is right for them. Given the support of pleasant and reliable family meals and sit-down snacks, children's naturally erratic eating allows them to eat the variety of food they need to have a nutritionally adequate diet.

The way you feed your child—your being trusting rather than controlling—determines their lifetime eating attitudes and behaviors. Consider what you want for your child. Do you want them to feel relaxed and positive about eating and accepting of and loyal to their body? That would be the trust paradigm, the basis for this book. Or do you want them to worry about good-food/bad-food, stress about how much to eat, anguish over the bathroom scale, and feel bad about their body? That would be the prevailing control paradigm.

Your being trusting with feeding can have far-reaching consequences. Let me give you an example. Being able to read your baby's sleep cycles and respond to their hunger cues prevents issues with crying, feeding, and sleeping. Conversely, trying to get baby to eat or grow in certain ways contributes to problems with crying, eating, and sleeping. Unsolved early problems in those areas correlate with cognitive and behavioral issues later in life.[3]

Evidence supporting the trust paradigm

Beyond the sDOR and Eating Competence evidence,[1,2] this book reviews a lot of evidence supporting trusting children's capabilities with eating and growing. As I said before, you can skim it or skip it. The evidence will be most useful for you if you are unsure whether or not to follow sDOR and raise your child to be Eating Competent. The nutrition and health professionals who work with you are taking a risk in following the trust paradigm, and the research will reassure them.

Older research demonstrated child capabilities and supported the conviction that parents and professionals can help best by looking for and enhancing those capabilities. Current research is mostly control paradigm: It tries to get children to eat and grow in certain ways. Or it tries to identify presumed flaws in children's eating attitudes and behaviors that keep them from eating and growing in prescribed ways. Research with "responsive feeding" is particularly challenging to interpret. I use the term *responsive* to describe sDOR-consistent feeding: warm and accepting leadership that is tuned in and supportive of the child's independence and individuality. "Responsive feeding" can be a whole different matter because it most often describes guidelines, research, or programming that includes tactics to get children to eat and/or grow in certain ways. The control tactics are likely to be subtle, but they are there and sooner or later children react to them. Clearly, terminology can mislead you. You can determine whether an intervention is trusting or controlling by examining the goal. Does it try to get the child to eat certain food or grow in certain ways? If so, it is controlling.

Goal-directed research doesn't stand up to scrutiny because it fails to take the basics into account: family dynamics, children's natural capability and behavior with eating, and/or children's natural patterns of growth. Child "obesity" interventions are widespread and heavily funded. Even highly ambitious programs show minor and unsustainable weight changes, changes that are more often than not reported as being highly successful. Most professional journals protect the prevailing paradigm by favoring articles that do child-deficit thinking: believing that children have to be controlled to get them to eat and grow in certain ways. To get published, researchers may resist the child-competence conclusions of their own data and give child-deficit interpretations. The research discussed in the Chapter 4 section, "Parents are reluctant to accept diagnosis," page 122, offers a particularly vivid example. By the way, I put "obesity" in quotes because I do not agree with prevailing thought that high body weight is a disease in and of itself.

In *Ellyn Satter's Child of Mine*, I sort through both the old and new research and identify the strengths and flaws. There is a *lot* of child-deficit research and there are a lot of media blasts to broadcast their conclusions. Supporting the child-trusting point of view in the midst of today's controlling children-have-to-be-made-to-eat-and-grow-right mindset feels like whistling in a hurricane.

But here we are, whistling.

MY PARADIGM SHIFT

I made my own paradigm shift when I was practicing as an outpatient dietitian in a group medical practice. My patients were having problems I couldn't resolve using my conventional methods; in fact, my methods were *causing* their problems. The modified diets I had learned in my training to use for medical nutritional therapy were making them miserable. Very few could adhere, and adherence didn't address their medical maladies. Those who couldn't adhere were on and off their diets, enjoying their eating and then feeling guilty, adhering and feeling deprived. They had lost their ease and comfort with food and their medical maladies worsened.

While I soft-pedaled the dieting advice with children and gave only general food-management guidance, my advice was still controlling, and it still produced the negatives I saw in adults. There was more. Once I had my family therapy training, I could see that trying to manage what and how much a child ate was a surefire way of creating family conflict. Parents become police officers rather than being loving and nurturing. Children continually begged for and sneaked food. Siblings became spying tattletales who resented the fallout from their brother's or sister's diet. You may think that today's children are no longer put on diets, but you would be wrong. National nutrition policy is just that: a diet for everyone. Attempts to impose ***what*** and ***how much*** are carefully clothed, but the end result is still control.

sDOR is a paradigm shift from control to trust, and it came to me suddenly in the midst of a charged counseling session. A mother was infuriated by my general food management guidance: "I am already doing that and it isn't working! How am I to get my fat child to eat less and my thin child to eat more?" "You don't have to," I responded. Blurted, actually. "How they grow is up to them. You just need to do your jobs with feeding." Even though it was my own brainchild, sDOR seemed drastic but it worked, and the child-capability research at the time supported it.

I taught sDOR to others and my colleagues and I found over and over that it worked. Children ate and grew well when parents followed sDOR. Children ate and grew poorly when parents crossed the lines of sDOR: when parents failed to do their jobs with feeding and/or tried to do their child's jobs with eating. But were we suffering from group self-delusion? Again, we needed research: full-fledged scientific inquiry testing parent and child outcomes when parents followed sDOR.

I have told the story elsewhere of the research that was conducted by my colleague Dr. Barbara Lohse,[4] so I will just give you the spoilers. We successfully developed a questionnaire, sDOR.2-6y. The questionnaire worked, and children of parents who scored high had lower nutrition risk. *Lower nutritional risk* is a *very* big deal in the nutrition and health community, and it is a very big deal for you. The prevailing paradigm insists that children must be made to follow a "healthy eating pattern" in order to do well nutritionally. Here was hard evidence freeing parents—freeing *you*—from that expectation. Instead, parents could do their jobs with feeding, then trust their children to eat what and as much as they needed.[1] It is that hard evidence—and my shared clinical experience—that supports my advice in *Ellyn Satter's Child of Mine*.

There was more. Parents who scored high on sDOR.2-6y were more likely to be Eating Competent and were less likely to try to eat less or different food than they really wanted. Trusting their own eating appeared to let parents trust their child's eating: They were less likely to interfere with their child's eating using restriction and/or pressure. The research also confirmed our clinical impressions that following sDOR appeared to make family life more harmonious: Parents who followed sDOR slept better, were less stressed, were less depressed and anxious, and felt more able to manage their lives.

Was higher parent quality of life the cause or result of following sDOR? Probably both. Following sDOR sorts out control issues and supports authoritative parenting. Doing better with parenting allows both parents and child to feel and do better.

Practicing nutritional judo

In following sDOR, you are raising your child to be Eating Competent. Being Eating Competent supports you in following sDOR: In order to be able to trust your child's eating, you need to be able to trust your own. Let's pick up the story where I left off, with my making my patients miserable with my controlling advice.

I can't get my patients to eat my way, I reasoned, so why not ask them about doing it their way? What did they want with eating? At first, they told me how much they wanted to adhere to my wonderful diet. With a little encouragement, they were able to get past what they *wanted* to want—or they thought *I* wanted them to want—and told me what they *really* wanted: To eat as much as they wanted of food they enjoyed and to share that food with those they loved.

My dietitian training emerged, this time as a positive force. My physiology background told me that they were talking about cooperating with their bodies' homeostasis. They were describing their biological need to eat enough to sustain life and living, their emotional need for enjoyable food that satisfied their appetite, and their social need to nurture their children and others they loved by sharing food that was precious to them. The other way—the controlling way—struggled against those biological, psychological, and social needs and systematically tried to ignore and overrule hunger and appetite.

I was like a phoenix rising from the ashes. All right, I reasoned, why not practice nutritional judo? Why not go *with* people's energy to eat what and as much as they want rather than struggling *against* it? At that critical juncture, a patient I will call Marjorie walked into my office, collapsed into a chair, and burst into tears. "Dr. so-and-so [who was notorious for harping on weight] told me that if I don't lose weight, I will die. But I just can't do it anymore. I can't stick to a diet and if I lose weight, I gain it all back and more besides." "Why don't we go at this in a different way?" I asked her. "Clearly another diet won't work. Instead, why don't we explore what happens when you eat normally?" "How do I do that?" she wondered. "I don't know," I said, "but let's see if we can figure it out together." We were both in recovery.

The first step was for Marjorie to have regular meals. "How would I do this if I were a normal eater?" she asked herself, then answered, "I would have food I enjoyed." That went fine, but she complained about eating too much. "Maybe or maybe not," I responded. "Your ideas of *how much* come from dieting. Let's keep on and see what happens." Once again, she asked herself, "How would I do this if I were a normal eater?" "I would eat as much as I want," she answered. And she did. Giving herself permission was the key, and her eating became positive and orderly. Over the weeks we felt our way together on our adventure to arrive at a positive and workable definition of normal eating. You may have seen the little article that came out of our work, "What is normal eating?" Do a web search. It shows up on refrigerator doors, bulletin boards, and in other people's articles, books, and presentations. Search until you find the most-recent copyright.

Even though Marjorie was eating as much as she wanted and eating food that she had previously allowed herself only when she was falling off her diets, her weight stabilized and even went down a little. Not only that, but her blood pressure and blood lipids improved, although her doctor had trouble seeing beyond his weight stigma to acknowledging those significant improvements in her wellness. Looking back, based on considerable evidence about the health consequences of yo-yo dieting, I wonder if her blood pressure and blood lipid problems grew out of her up-and-down weight rather than her high weight per se.

I continued to learn from many patients after Marjorie and eventually formalized that early nutritional judo work as the Satter Eating Competence Model (ecSatter). I wrote and rewrote a paper and pencil questionnaire and found that patients who scored high had positive and stable eating and their health conditions improved. The key for them was to feed themselves faithfully and give themselves permission to eat. (Read more about that in Chapter 5, Discover the Joy of Eating.) But those were my clinical impressions, and it is way too easy to fall in love with one's own brainchild and ignore anything that contradicts it.

RESEARCH FOUNDATION FOR ecSATTER

That didn't stop me from talking in my presentations about how well Eating Competence worked. Then one day in Kansas, nutrition professor

Barbara Lohse, RD, PhD, was in my audience. Dr. Lohse is an experienced and exacting researcher: She sets up well-controlled studies and publishes each study in its entirety in a single article. "Can you prove it?" she asked, and I knew she was talking about honest-to-goodness nailed-down research. "Only clinically," I admitted. She offered to subject ecSatter and my paper-and-pencil questionnaire to a research trial and I was thrilled. I *should* have been scared, because what I had been working on for 20 years was about to be given the acid test.

The questionnaire—and what it demonstrated—worked beyond my wildest dreams! Since then, ecSatter has been tested by many researchers and my questionnaire, ecSI 2.0, has been translated for usage in many countries. It gains credibility with each trial. To help you understand the implications of ecSatter, below are some even-thoughs. You can track down the research supporting these even-thoughs on the Ellyn Satter Institute website.[2]

- Even though ecSatter says nothing at all about eating "healthy" food and avoiding "unhealthy" food, and instead gives strong permission to eat preferred food, people who are Eating Competent do better nutritionally *and* enjoy their fruits and vegetables.
- Even though ecSatter encourages using fat, salt, and sugar to make food taste good, people who are Eating Competent do better medically: They have lower blood pressures and better blood lipids. They even have better oral health.
- Even though ecSatter does not encourage trying in any way to lose weight and instead encourages trusting hunger and appetite to guide how much to eat, people who are Eating Competent have the same or lower BMIs as the general population.
- Even though ecSatter offers no guidance on budgeting or food resource management, people who are Eating Competent do better with managing their food money.
- Even though ecSatter says nothing about activity, people who are Eating Competent are more active.
- Even though ecSatter says nothing about feeding children, Eating Competent parents do better with following sDOR and raising children to have lower nutritional risk.

There you have it: The foundation on which *Ellyn Satter's Child of Mine* is built—and the foundation for your feeding relationship. Raising your child to be Eating Competent allows them to be joyful and confident with eating throughout life.

NAVIGATING THIS BOOK

Despite my best efforts, this is a long book. Bring it down to size by reading it your way. Get the main points by examining the figures. Start with Part I if knowing the *why* of my advice is important and interesting for you. Or skip Part I and dive right into the *How to Feed* advice in Part II or Part III. Cross-references to Part I will help fill in any blanks in your understanding. The last five chapters are particularly heavy in chapter cross-references. I find the cross-referencing a bit aggravating, and you might feel the same way. The equally aggravating alternative is repeating the basic information over and over.

Part I. Understand Trust with Feeding and Eating

This part is about—well—trust: Trust in you to take good care of yourself and your child with eating. The title of Chapter 1 says it all: Feed Your Child with Love and Trust. It lays out the basics of following sDOR, tells you why it makes sense nutritionally and with respect to parenting, and gives evidence. Chapter 2, Raise Your Child to Know What to Eat, and Chapter 3, Your Child Knows How Much to Eat, outlines child eating capabilities in detail and tells you what those capabilities mean with respect to feeding. Chapter 4, Your Child Knows How to Grow, tells you that trusting your child's growth is a celebration and what you have to guard against in keeping that celebration going for you and your child. Chapter 5, Discover the Joy of Eating, applies trust to you and your relationship with food and tells you how trusting yourself with eating lets you trust your child with feeding. That chapter also addresses being positive and relaxed about eating during pregnancy.

Part II. How to Feed: The Early Months

Based on the principles laid out in Part I, Parts II and III get into the stage-by-stage nitty-gritty of feeding. Part II addresses feeding from birth until your child joins you in eating family meals. Although the time is short—generally from birth until about 12 to 15 months, and perhaps only until 7 or 8 months for rapidly developing children—the complexity is great. Chapters in this section help you understand, and as much as you can, get in sync with your baby around feeding. Chapter 6, Your Feeding Decision: Breastfeeding or Formula-Feeding, is a shame-free run-down on what to consider as you make your decision about whether to breastfeed or formula-feed from the bottle. There is much to learn about your baby. Chapter 7, Understanding Your Newborn, gives you essential information about helping your baby achieve and maintain homestasis:

eat and sleep well and be relatively calm and predictable. Chapters 8, 9, and 10 address breastfeeding, formula-feeding, and starting solid foods. Each has a lot of detail, and it is easy to get bogged down in it. It can be tedious—until you need it! I have tried to relieve the tedium and convey the detail with stories about parents and children. I am counting on you to take the detail for what it is—important, but not as important as having a positive feeding relationship. You can get confused about the details, but if your attitude toward your baby is accepting and supportive, things will turn out just fine: You and your baby will find your way.

Part III. How to Feed: The Toddler and Preschooler

This section makes up only about the last fourth of *Ellyn Satter's Child of Mine* because it builds on everything that has gone before. It is just as important. You still feed older children based on information coming from them, but interpreting that information is less straightforward than for younger children. Your toddler feels strongly about having their own way and you need to know when—and when not to—respect that. When your child was a baby, you fed them on demand to keep them content and comfortable. Feeding on demand won't keep your toddler content and comfortable. In fact, it will turn them into a little tyrant. Your toddler needs structure and limits, and they will become more and more extreme in their demands until you provide that leadership. sDOR provides structure and leadership.

Having established their identity as a toddler, the preschooler, still again, is different: They are more compliant, and they want to please you. Unlike the toddler, your preschooler may not make a fuss if you get controlling and manage their *how much* and *whether* of eating. But it *will* make them unhappy and they *will feel like they can't please you.* Intruding on their *whether* and *how much* will also teach them to eat based on what you want them to eat rather than on their own sensations of hunger and appetite. You won't always be around, and depending on you for that most basic of functions will handicap them when they get older.

Food-related issues

I have been as gentle and strategic as I know how about giving you food selection information. I don't want you to feel that I have given you permission to eat the food you enjoy only to take it away. I have found that folks have been so programmed by "healthy eating pattern" messages that talking about food, even in the most positive ways, can trigger negative messages. That is especially true if for a long time you have been pressured—and tried and failed—to eat certain foods or weigh a certain amount. If something I say scares you, remember: I am not taking away permission. It is still all right to eat what you enjoy and as much as you want.

You don't need conventional nutrition guidance in order to be healthy. Instead, you need routine plus trust: For your child following sDOR; for you being Eating Competent by feeding yourself faithfully and giving yourself permission to eat. Both you and your child need meals and the Chapter 2 section, "Master family meals," page 56, shows you how to successfully establish the meal habit. I also warn you: "When you think meals, do not get hung up on 'healthy home-cooked'… Instead, think possible, practical, and enjoyable. If you currently aren't having regular meals, start by eating what you eat now and build in structure. …" That section observes, "You will find yourself considering food groups." However, this is not to enslave you. Use food groups if they help, ignore them if they don't. It's natural to think of food groups when you plan meals, and it needn't get in the way of your eating foods you enjoy.

Not until Chapter 10, Feeding Your Older Baby and Almost-Toddler, do we discuss food selection in any detail, but it is not paired with shoulds and oughts. The starting-solid-foods message is that your child is growing up to eat the food you eat so why not start right away by adapting the texture of family food? Parents want to know in detail, "Is this food okay? How about this?" So much food is demonized in today's world that I am trying to neutralize that. I am saying, "It is okay to feed your baby this and that as well." My food lists are divided into basic food groups—they are handy for that. Again, there is no "feed this, not that;" they are just lists.

In the Chapter 11 Section, "Celebrate food," page 395, I give you permission. I discuss nutrition and food selection from the perspective of "why it is okay to eat this." Enjoy bread, cereal, rice and pasta; enjoy meat, poultry, fish, dry beans, eggs, and nuts; enjoy fruits and vegetables, and so on. Included in the "enjoys" are enjoy sweets and enjoy fats and oils. There could be a lot of triggers here for you: Let me know what those triggers are at ellyn@ellynsatterinstitute.org. I might be able to get rid of them.

The Chapter 12 section, "Nutrition-related stuff," page 445, addresses topics such as activity; letting your child eat sugar; Halloween candy; letting your child eat fat; and food and behavior. Again, your shoulds and oughts might be activated. Take a deep breath: You don't have to throw away your trust in your child and in yourself. Instead, think *possible*, *practical*, and *enjoyable*.

MY EARLIER BOOKS

Ellyn Satter's Child of Mine is different from my other books in that it builds on recent evidence to be absolutely clear about the critical importance of raising children to be Eating Competent. My earlier books are place-markers of my journey to this point. My first book, *Child of Mine: Feeding with Love and Good Sense*, was mostly about nutrition with a few feeding stories thrown in. The second edition had more about feeding dynamics and I talked about being competent with eating, but I had yet to formalize the Satter Eating Competence Model and apply it to feeding.

My second book, *How to Get Your Kid to Eat*, now old and close to being out of print, was about the feeding relationship. It's still good but if you read it, ignore what I said in Chapter 14, Helping All You Can to Keep Your Child from Being Fat. I talked about sDOR but I hadn't completely let go of being controlling. I straddled paradigms, and that is worse than doing one or the other, because it is so confusing for parents—and for children.

My third book, *Secrets of Feeding a Healthy Family: How to Eat, How to Feed Children, How to Cook*, introduced my readers to the Satter Eating Competence Model and told readers how to free themselves to enjoy eating. My fourth book, *Your Child's Weight: Helping without Harming*, was written to combat today's terrible advice about child weight by showing parents how to feed well, parent well, raise children to be Eating Competent, and let children grow up to have bodies that are right for them. *Secrets* and *Your Child's Weight* are still available and are standbys in the nutrition and parenting world.

While I am at it, allow me to tell you that Kelcy Press has published five 40-page booklets about feeding and eating: *The Feeding with Love and Good Sense* series. Those are great as an introduction to positive feeding and eating. They tell the whole story in brief for those who don't have the time or inclination to do much reading. I have published feeding videos as well. Do a web search for *Feeding with Love and Good Sense Booklets* or *Feeding with Love and Good Sense Videos.* I have told stories from those videos in several places and reassure you that although footage is old, the feeding stories are as fresh and pertinent as ever.

THE SHOULDERS I STAND ON

Writing *Ellyn Satter's Child of Mine* book has been a celebration of collaboration and history. I wrote and revised (and revised and revised) and gave it all I had. Then I sent it around to my colleagues at ESI and elsewhere whom I respect and who were willing to give their scrutiny and contribute their expertise. I thank them for their generosity. Think of them as you read.

Peggy Crum, MA, RDN, and Eve Reed, Paediatric Dietitian (Eve is Australian, which explains the spelling), both Ellyn Satter Institute faculty members, were early content reviewers. They evaluated the manuscript's overall organization, content, and message to make sure it was clear, concise, and engaging. They also made sure that I didn't say or imply anything that is contradictory to the Satter models. Peggy and Eve know whereof they speak, having worked in the child health and wellness world throughout their careers.

New parents Kristen Schweers, MS, RD, also an Ellyn Satter Institute faculty member, nutritionist Michaela Trautman, PhD, and her husband Dan read the new-baby chapters, shared their experience, and clued me in on today's happenings for good or ill in the new-parent world.

Other members of the Ellyn Satter Institute read and commented as their time allowed. Kerry Regnier, MPH, RDN, LDN, who administers a pediatric practice and works daily with parents, reviewed early drafts until too many other life demands accumulated. Alexia Beauregard, MS, RDN, CSP, LD, who specializes in food allergies, restricted diets, and eating and feeding disturbances, loaned her expertise to the sections on feeding children with food allergies. Rebeca Hernández, MS, LD, who had a wonderfully light touch with nutrition counseling, helped me to be as careful as possible that what I say to parents doesn't decode as being critical.

My Ellyn Satter Institute colleagues have been with me throughout this journey. You can find their names on the ESI website; here, I am citing the ones who read the whole shebang. Cristen Harris, PhD, RDN, CD, CEDS, CSSD, ACSM-CEP, FAND, helped enormously with gender-inclusive thinking and language and loaned her considerable expertise on neurodiversity. She read the whole book despite her many demands as a professor at UW Seattle. Peggy Crum, MA, RDN, brought her communication expertise to bear in giving her stamp of approval to the excellent organization she had advised me to follow in the first place. Peggy is a wizard at tracking down correct usage, patching up awkward wording, and catching me when I wander into the weeds. My colleague Anne Blocker, MS, RDN, CSSD, LD, CD, CDCES, shared the language she has refined after years of explaining the Satter models to her many audiences.

My dear friend Harriet Brown, professor of journalism at Syracuse University New York, edited *Ellyn Satter's Child of Mine* from start to finish. I am in awe of her virtuosity, and we all can be grateful to her for her contributions to this book's readability. Harriet is the author of the excellent and insightful *Brave Girl Eating: A Family's Struggle with Anorexia*. My granddaughter Marin Herlinger did proof-reading and so much more. Marin has an eagle eye for lack of clarity, grammatical errors, and typos as well as making sure I said *they* and *them* rather drifting back into *he* and *she.* My friend and colleague Joni Trautman, Kelcy Press operations manager, has been a varied, steady and ongoing presence. My children and grandchildren gave the deciding vote to the book cover and my son-in-law James Secord proposed a subtitle that worked far better than my own.

Even more shoulders

Reviewers of previous editions and previous colleagues have left their mark as well, and I would like to acknowledge them: Ines Anchondo, Edie Applegate, Christine Berman, Susan Clark, Pam Estes, Jane Fowler, Gretchen Hanna, Joanne Tatum Hattner, Betty Lucas, Patty Morse, Paulette Sharkey, Barbara Turner, Karen Webber, and Donald Williams. Who am I missing? Those colleagues represent agencies, populations, and areas of expertise that are important to children. I also credit Marsha Dunn Klein, occupational therapist, and Suzanne Evans Morris, speech pathologist, both of whom address acquisition of oral feeding skills.

The topic of feeding dynamics hooked my early audiences, and it hooked me. Understanding feeding dynamics made me stray outside the confines of nutrition and dietetics, get a master's in clinical social work, and practice as a family therapist. In my formative 1986 article on the feeding relationship,[5] I depended on the observations of Mary Ainsworth, a psychologist who is well known for her work with infant attachment; Hilde Bruch, Maria Palazzoli, and Salvadore Minuchin, all clinicians who worked with adolescents who had eating disorders; nutritionist Ernesto Pollitt and physician Peter Wright, both of whom pioneered observations of the impact of parent-child feeding dynamics on growth; physician Clara Davis, public health nutritionist Virginia Beal, and child development specialists Arnold Gesell and Frances Ilg, all of whom did extensive observational research identifying children's innate capabilities with eating.

The selected references in *Ellyn Satter's Child of Mine* read like a who's who of the feeding dynamics world. I found especially empowering the sharing and insights on child psychosocial development and feeding of Irene Chatoor, child psychiatrist at Children's Hospital Medical Center in Washington, D.C. I also depended on the early research of Dr. Leanne Birch, then at Illinois State University Urbana-Champaign. Leanne's studies demonstrated children's considerable capabilities with eating. I held my breath as I read her studies to discover that her laboratory evidence and my clinical findings were the same.

The topic of the feeding relationship has now become mainstream. The Satter Division of Responsibility in Feeding (sDOR) is widely recognized and used, if not always accurately, and is endorsed as best practice in feeding by prominent child nutrition and pediatric agencies. That's a pretty fast turnaround for such a major change in thinking and practice, and I credit dietitians for leading the way. I think particularly of Charlie Slaughter, public health nutritionist with the Oregon WIC program, who immediately recognized the possibilities for enhancing quality of life for parents and the nutritionists who serve them.

Charlie—and many others—took considerable leadership and as a result, programs devoted to child nutrition include considerations of the feeding relationship as a routine part of their service and educational mission. I am thinking of professionals in agencies that directly support child nutrition and feeding, including the WIC program (Special Supplemental Nutrition Program for Women, Infants, and Children); CACFP (the Child and Adult Care Food Program); the School Nutrition Program; University Extension (especially through the Expanded Foods and Nutrition Education Program and the SNAP-ed); Head Start, the federally-funded, state-sponsored and variously named early childhood programs for children with functional needs; and the myriad state, locally- and privately-funded parent education and support programs.

It is with sweet sadness that I remember the talented and splendid Karen Foget, who contributed so much to the attractiveness and accessibility of *Ellyn Satter's Child of Mine* and many of my other materials.

I would also like to honor my long-standing association with publisher David Bull, who was fond of saying my *Child of Mine* book proposal "came in through the transom." Dave liked my writing because it was entertaining and informative without being preachy, and I liked Bull Publishing for its commitment to accurate and responsible nutrition and health information. Unlike larger publishers, Bull Publishing kept *Child of Mine* on their list while it—and I—found our niche in the child care and parenting world. Dave and his wife, Mary Lou, became my respected friends over the years, as did many of the other authors of the Bull Publishing family. Dave's death in 1994 was a considerable loss to us all.

Finally, I would like to honor you, the parents and professionals who read this book. People who love children and go to bat for them are simply my very favorite people.

REFERENCES

1. Lohse B, Mitchell DC. Valid and reliable measure of adherence to Satter Division of Responsibility in Feeding. *J Nutr Educ Behav.* 2021;53:211–222.
2. Satter Eating Competence Model (ecSatter): Evidence-based research. *https://www.needscenter.org/resources/satter-eating-competence-model-ecsatter/*
3. Jaekel J. Associations of crying, sleeping, and feeding problems in early childhood and perceived social support with emotional disorders in adulthood. *BMC Psychiatry.* 2023. doi:10.1186/s12888-023-04854-1
4. Satter E. Webinar: Introducing sDOR.2-6y: development and validation. Ellyn Satter Institute. *https://www.ellynsatterinstitute.org/product/introducing-sdor-2-6ytm/*
5. Satter E. The feeding relationship. *J Am Diet Assoc.* 1986;86:352–356.

PART I

Understand Trust with Feeding and Eating

CHAPTER 1

Feed Your Child with Love and Trust

As I write *Ellyn Satter's Child of Mine*, my hope is exactly what it says in the subtitle—for you to raise your child to be a confident and joyful eater. At the same time, you will be raising them to be a confident and joyful *person*. Feeding is truly parenting. When feeding goes well, you and your child feel good about yourselves and about your time together sharing food. When feeding goes poorly, it affects everything else in your lives. You *can* feed well, and in the process discover the joy of feeding and the joy of eating and thereby enhance your joy of being a parent.

By *you*, I mean parents of either gender. One of you will likely take primary responsibility for your child with the other playing a supportive role, but not necessarily. If you are a single parent, do your best to recruit someone you trust to play that supportive role. However you work it out, I honor you for doing your level best to parent this lovable, mystifying, and at times maddening small person who has just moved into your home.

ATTITUDES AND BEHAVIORS, NOT *WHAT* AND *HOW MUCH*

According to my conversations, reading, and browsing, parents today want their child to have a diet that is nutritious and balanced, includes a variety of fruits and vegetables, limits added sugars and "junk" foods, and keeps their child's weight from being too high or too low. *Ellyn Satter's Child of Mine* tells you how to accomplish those goals, but likely not in the way you expect. Instead of telling you what and/or how much your child should eat and what they should weigh, I emphasize raising your child to have positive eating attitudes and behaviors: to enjoy food, eating, and family meals; be comfortable around unfamiliar food; and eat as much or as little as they need to grow in the way that is right for them. Having the achievable goal of raising your child to have positive eating attitudes and behaviors helps you approach feeding in an enjoyable, confident, and relaxed way. It frees you from the maddening and impossible expectation of getting your child to eat certain foods and grow in certain ways. It also frees your child to be all they can be in terms of their security and self-esteem.

You may worry that setting aside the whats and how-muches is an alarming about-face in nutrition and feeding—and it is. I made that about-face long ago in my dietetics practice after I discovered that teaching my patients the whats and how-muches simply didn't work: The few who could stick to their diet were handicapped by their food dos and don'ts, and their medical conditions didn't improve. The rest were frustrated with trying and failing to adhere and lost their pleasure and confidence with eating. As I told you in the Preface, what I came up with instead, the Satter Eating Competence Model (ecSatter),[1] works. More and more studies show that adults who are Eating Competent, as measured by the validated ecSI 2.0,[2] have higher-quality diets than the general population, as well as lower body mass indexes (BMIs), superior metabolic profiles, and more positive quality-of-life indicators.[3] In the same way, raising your child to be Eating Competent allows them to be well-nourished and grow predictably.

Being Eating Competent is natural for children

Your child was born *wanting* to eat, knowing *how much* to eat, and able to *grow* in the way that is right for them. Your task is to preserve those powerful eating attitudes and behaviors by being wise and positive with feeding: by following the Satter Division of Responsibility in Feeding (sDOR). You do the *what*, *when*, and *where* of *feeding* and let your child do the *how much* and *whether* of *eating*. Research with sDOR.2-6y, the inventory for measuring parent adherence to sDOR, shows that children do better nutritionally when parents follow sDOR. The same research shows that parents who follow sDOR do not pressure or encourage their children to eat certain amounts or types of food. Parents simply provide children with repeated neutral exposure to the foods that they themselves enjoy. A positive feeding relationship carries benefits for parents as well: Parents who follow sDOR have higher quality of life indicators with respect to sleep, stress, and psychosocial functioning.[4]

Even if your child is ill and/or needs particular help with maintaining their nutritional status, they have the drive to eat and grow up with eating and can have positive eating attitudes and behaviors. Children with unusual challenges need more skillful support, but they can feel and do well with eating in the ways that we will be discussing.

Figure 1.1 outlines children's eating competence. To summarize, a child who is a Competent Eater will:

- Feel good about food and eating.
- Enjoy family meals (and behave so you enjoy having them there).
- Be comfortable with unfamiliar food (even if they don't eat it).
- Eat as much or as little as they want and need to grow in the way that is right for them.

FIGURE 1.1: CHILDREN'S EATING COMPETENCE

When parents follow sDOR, children retain their positive eating attitudes and their inborn ability with internal regulation. They gradually develop food acceptance and food context skills.

Eating attitudes

- Enjoys eating.
- Feels positive about enjoying eating.
- Is relaxed at meals and snacks and feels good about being there.

Food context

- Goes along with the structure of meals and snacks.
- Participates comfortably in family meals.
- Does their part to contribute to enjoyable family meals.
- Can comfortably eat in other places besides home.

Food acceptance

- Picks and chooses from the food that is at the meal.
- Stays calm in the presence of unfamiliar or not-yet-enjoyed food.
- Says "yes, please" and "no, thank you."

Internal regulation

- Eats as much as they are hungry for.
- Is relaxed about getting enough to eat.
- Enjoys their body and is relaxed about weight.
- Can forget about eating between meal and snack times.

Give up on *getting* your child to eat and grow

Following sDOR and letting your child have positive eating attitudes and behaviors and grow in the way that is right for them are achievable goals; *getting* your child to eat certain amounts and types of food and grow in particular ways are *not* achievable goals. *Get* is a control word that comes loaded with pressure and persuasion. Giving up on trying to control your child's eating and growth will not impair their wellness. In fact, the opposite is true. Children of parents who adhere to sDOR have lower nutritional risk:[4] Children eat what they need to have a nutritionally adequate diet. Clinical observations show that they also eat as much as they need to grow consistently.

Giving up on trying to control what and how much your child eats and how they grow is a big ask, because those are the current goals of almost everybody, professionals and non-professionals alike. Those goals persist despite the fact that generations of parents and professionals have found that trying to achieve them leads to frustrating and destructive struggles around feeding. No matter how creatively professionals teach, how hard parents try to adhere, or how desperately children want to please their parents, children simply can't eat certain foods or certain amounts of food. And neither can anybody else. It is simply not realistic to go through life depriving yourself of food or forcing your body to weigh what it doesn't want to weigh.

Based on the ecSatter research I just discussed, you do not have to sacrifice your own eating enjoyment to be responsible with feeding yourself or your child. You do not have to restrict your diet, force yourself to eat all and only "healthy" food, or sneak around to eat food you have been told your child shouldn't have. You simply follow sDOR and translate sDOR into feeding yourself: Feed yourself faithfully and give yourself permission to eat (more about that in Chapter 5). You simply do your jobs with feeding yourself and your child, then trust yourself and your child to eat whether and as much as each of you needs.

In this chapter

This chapter outlines how to feed based on *trust*: trust in yourself to follow the sDOR, and trust in your child to determine whether they eat and how much they need from what you provide. It introduces the ecSatter principles and research and outlines the implications of Eating Competence for you and your child. It emphasizes the importance of family meals and of making meals enjoyable and manageable.

Since the advice I give you is so much different from what you usually hear, I discuss professional articles: I give you the evidence. The professionals who work with you particularly depend on this evidence for support in giving trust-paradigm feeding advice. This chapter cites a *lot* of evidence; other chapters, not so much. I think the research discussions are interesting, but if you don't, you can safely skip them until or unless you need them. Much of the evidence in this chapter is made up of older studies investigating what happens when children are trusted with eating. Most current research is done from the control perspective, that of exploring what happens when you try to get children to eat and grow in certain ways. I point out the flaws in those studies to reassure you that being controlling is neither supported by the evidence nor good for you and your child. Again, the evidence is important for both parents and professionals to help resist the influence of today's control-based nutrition guidance.

FOLLOW THE SATTER DIVISION OF RESPONSIBILITY IN FEEDING

Your following the sDOR supports your child in being a Competent Eater: in having positive eating attitudes and behaviors. Being a Competent Eater, in turn, supports them in eating what and as much as they need to be healthy and grow well.

sDOR plays out in different ways at different ages and stages. The version that is most familiar to parents and professionals is the one cited earlier, which applies to toddlers through adolescents:

Parents do the *what, when,* and *where* of *feeding*.

Children do the *whether* and *how much* of *eating*.

As you can see from Figure 1.2 on the next page, sDOR is somewhat different for younger children.

Parents keep the demand-fed infant in charge of everything but the *what*—breastmilk, formula, or a combination—and only gradually take over the *when* and *where* during the older baby's transition to eating family food. The principle for all stages is the same: Parents provide the food, children eat it—or not. sDOR guides you in supporting your child's eating without taking over and in giving your child independence without neglecting them.

FIGURE 1.2: THE SATTER DIVISION OF RESPONSIBILITY IN FEEDING

Children are born Eating Competent: They *want* to eat, know *how much* to eat, and can *grow* in the way that is right for them. Following sDOR preserves those powerful eating attitudes and behaviors and supports children in participating in family meals and learning to eat a variety of food.

sDOR for infants

- The parent is responsible for what.
- The child is responsible for how much (and everything else).

Parents choose breast- or formula-feeding. Then they feed smoothly, paying attention to the baby's cues about timing, tempo, frequency, and amounts.

sDOR for babies making the transition to family food

- Parents are still responsible for what, and are becoming responsible for when and where.
- The child is still and always responsible for *how much* and *whether.*

Parents offer and progress solids based on what the child can *do,* not on how *old* they are. Routine changes from demand feeding to family meals and sit-down snacks.

sDOR for toddlers through adolescents

- Parents are responsible for what, when, and where.
- The child is responsible for *how much* and *whether.*

Parents do their feeding jobs:

- Choose and prepare the food.
- Provide regular meals and snacks.
- Make eating times pleasant.
- Provide their child with repeated neutral exposure to the food they eat.
- Avoid letting children have food or beverages (except for water) between meal and snack times.

Parents trust children to do their eating jobs:

- Children will eat.
- They will eat the amount they need.
- They will learn to eat the food their parents eat.
- They will grow predictably.
- They will learn to behave well at mealtime.

sDOR CHANGES THE PARADIGM

The fundamentally important point about emphasizing positive eating attitudes and behaviors rather than what or how much to eat is easy to read past and also a mind-bender, so bear with me while I belabor it. Consider the definition of *paradigm*: a way of looking at something, of thinking and doing. A *paradigm shift* is a change to a completely different way of thinking and doing. Establishing sDOR and raising your child to have positive eating attitudes and behaviors rather than eat-this-don't-eat-that is a paradigm shift. The conventional "healthy eating pattern" advice that we hear most, growing out of the US Dietary Guidelines,[5] is *control paradigm* thinking and doing. For adults, it emphasizes what and how much to eat and what to weigh; for children, it does all that and says to get children to grow within certain limits. In contrast, *Ellyn Satter's Child of Mine* is *trust paradigm* thinking and doing. It emphasizes having a loving and supportive feeding relationship so that your child can have positive eating attitudes and behaviors. Growing out of that positive relationship, it trusts that your child will be well nourished and grow predictably.

The trust paradigm makes all the difference between success and failure with feeding and eating because it defines outcome goals with eating and feeding in the way that they can be achieved. It is an achievable goal to do your jobs with the *what*, *when*, and *where* of feeding. It is an achievable goal, once you have done your feeding jobs, to trust your child to eat *whether* and *how much* they want from what you provide and grow in the way that is right for them. It is an achievable goal, based on sDOR, to let your child have the Eating Competent attitudes and behaviors summarized in Figure 1.1, page 5.

In contrast, getting ourselves and our children to eat certain foods and weigh certain amounts are not achievable goals. After over 50 years of trying to eat and weigh according to the Dietary Guidelines, we score only about 60 out of 100 percent on the Healthy Eating Index, a measure of the degree to which we follow the "healthy eating pattern."[5] That "healthy eating pattern" is intended to prevent "obesity," but as a nation we are getting fatter and fatter.[6] Some people are just fatter than others and that is normal. But accelerating fatness means something is out of whack: Most times, that *something* is restrained eating and yo-yo dieting.

The trust paradigm works

The eating order that goes along with Eating Competence carries nutritional benefits: Adults who are Eating Competent do well nutritionally, are healthier, weigh the same or less as the general population, and have better quality of life.[3] As noted earlier in the chapter, children whose parents follow sDOR have lower nutritional risk. Not only that, but trusting children is easier on parents: Research and experience show that parents who follow sDOR have lower stress, anxiety, and depression and even sleep better.[4]

Emphasizing children's Eating Competence works with children's naturally erratic ways with eating; trying to get them to eat certain amounts and types of food does not. Children eat a lot one day and hardly anything the next; what they eat one day, they ignore the next; they tire of even their favorite food and eat something else. They eat bread for weeks and then ignore it and eat rice—or even vegetables!

In the face of all that variability, imagine cultivating your child's Eating Competence by hanging in there with the *what*, *when*, and *where* of feeding. Now imagine trying to get your child to eat certain foods and avoid others. Boggles the mind, doesn't it? No child ever ate according to a formula, and Healthy Eating Index scores show that even adults have trouble adhering to the "healthy eating pattern."

Competent Eating changes as your child grows

Babies are born knowing how to suckle, but beyond the early months, eating is a set of skills and attitudes that children learn over time from their trusted adults. It isn't like breathing, where the child does it automatically. It's more like learning to move on purpose—to roll over, crawl, and then walk. By the time your child is six or seven years old—the age where we leave off with *Ellyn Satter's Child of Mine*—your child can be well on their way to being a grownup Competent Eater. Competent Eating is ecSatter[1] (see Figure 1.1) and, like sDOR, is trust paradigm.

Like everything else about children's attitudes and behaviors, their doing well with eating grows out of their relationship with you. That's where sDOR comes in: your reliably doing the *what*, *when*, and *where* of feeding. After that, you have to let go. Pleasant family meals and your child's eating comfort and enjoyment are the goals of sDOR; the hoped-for-but-can't-make-it-happen bonus is your child's gradually developing a longer and longer list of foods they enjoy. The give-up-on-it dream is getting your child to grow in a certain way.

We all have dreams and ambitions for our children—what we would like them to be and do. With respect to your child's eating and growth, some ambitions are reasonable, and others are not. Having your children grow up to be a Competent Eater is reasonable; having your child eat certain food and grow in certain ways is *not* reasonable, and trying to make it happen will create the opposite of what you intend. Chapters 2, 3, and 4 address the specifics of what you can do to support your child's growing up to be Eating Competent. They will eat and grow in *their* way, and they will be well nourished. Again, children who are Competent Eaters—those whose parents follow sDOR—have lower nutrition risk[4] and grow well.

Blueprints Are All Around

Parents and professionals are given blueprints for children's eating and growth. Standard, control-paradigm nutrition advice is to follow a "healthy eating pattern:"[5] Keep your child's weight within certain limits by getting them to eat lots of fruits and vegetables, whole grains, low-fat dairy and meat, and few if any sweets and chips.[7] Despite the fact that this advice has been routinely and unblushingly delivered for the last several decades, there is no evidence that it delivers the promised outcomes. It is difficult advice to follow, and very few people can do it, either for themselves or their children.[5] Moreover, food and beverage selection make no difference to whether or not children get fatter than nature intended them to be.[8] In short, following the "healthy eating pattern" appears to be doubtfully effective and achievable for very few people. Getting children to weigh within certain limits is certainly *not* an achievable goal.

On the other hand, following sDOR and letting children have bodies that are right for them *are* achievable goals.

sDOR is built on trust

sDOR *works* because it is built on trust—your child's trust in you to understand what they want and provide them with what they need. Trust goes both ways. For your part, you must trust your child to do their part with eating and growing. Following sDOR allows you to set boundaries with feeding and give your child freedom within those boundaries. Given today's rigid ideas about food selection and weight, giving such freedom may feel dangerous to you, like your child will gorge on everything that is wrong for them. That's where the trust in children's capabilities comes in, and this book will support you in building that trust.

The analogy in Figure 1.3, from Ellyn Satter Institute faculty member Peggy Crum, might help you understand the concept of boundaries. As Peggy visualizes it, trust depends on everyone's staying in their own lane—each of you sticking to your jobs and not interfering with the other's jobs. If either of you strays into the other's lane and tries to do their job, there will be crashes! You will get crashes, for instance, if you, for whatever reason, try to get your child to eat more, less, or different food

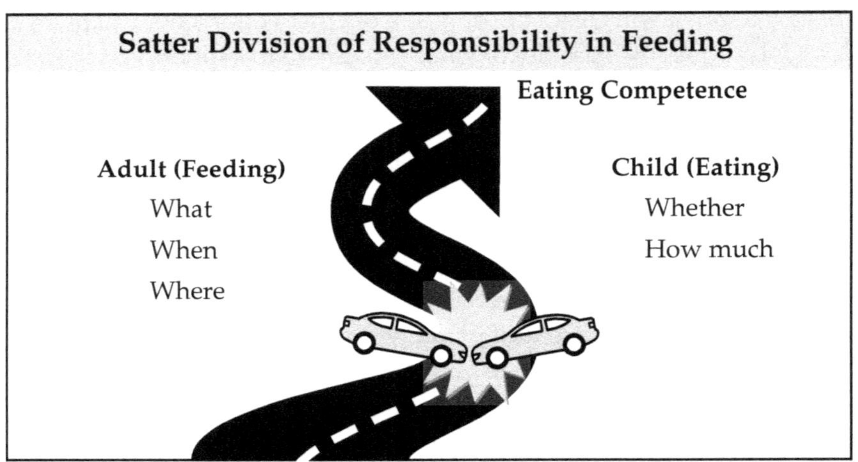

FIGURE 1.3: TRUST IS A TWO-WAY STREET

from what they want. You will also get crashes if you let your child do your jobs of *what, when,* and *where:* if you, for instance, feed your toddler whenever and whatever they want rather than having family meals and sit-down snacks.

As your child matures, their lane gets wider, but only after they demonstrate they are capable of respecting the boundaries. A child can be allowed to make their own snack after they show they can and will eat their snack right after school and at the table, choose food that you agree on, and for the most part not munch along in front of the TV or over homework.

You might be thinking that this approach could apply not just to eating but to sleeping and toileting and walking alone. It does; there are many other examples.

sDOR is *simple* but not *easy*

The rewards for both children and parents from following sDOR are enormous, but following it takes endurance, steady nerves, and a leap of faith. Managing the *what, when,* and *where* of *feeding* day after day, year after year, is a tall order, but it is straightforward. Trusting your child to manage the *how much* and *whether* of *eating* is an even taller order, and not nearly as straightforward.

Trusting your child means not only letting go of your expectations but also ignoring others' convictions about what and how much your child should eat. "My family criticizes me for letting my children 'get away' with not eating what's on their plates," wrote a young mother of a toddler and preschooler. "But I have persisted with sDOR. My children's eating habits are so good my coworkers comment." "My health professional told me my toddler was 'obese' and that I had to slim her down," commented another. "But she has always grown at the 90th percentile. Trying to change that would have me trying to control her eating. I simply can't stand the idea of making her so unhappy. I have continued following sDOR, and my daughter is still growing along the 90th percentile. That's just the way she is. She is healthy and strong."

Trusting your child means keeping your courage when others lose theirs. Says the mother of a 10-year-old,

> *I exclusively breastfed my first baby and it was hard—he barely hit the second weight percentile. The doctors did all sorts of tests and there was nothing wrong with him, but they still urged me to get him to eat more. I tried everything I could think of, but he fought me and took in less. So I would back off and follow my son's lead with feeding, reassuring myself that developmentally he was right on track. I would make peace with his being thin, but after every weight check I went into panic mode. Then I discovered sDOR. I kept my nerve and stopped panicking about his eating and growth, although I still worried. He is still thin, but his eating is great.*

Trusting your child—and yourself—means being able to recover when a crash happens. Sophie's parents were so determined to get their five-year-old daughter to eat vegetables that they reasoned, insisted, rewarded, and even punished her. In turn, Sophie argued, bargained, delayed, and had tantrums. Meals were long struggles that left everyone exhausted and not liking each other very much. To Sophie's parents, sDOR sounded totally nuts, but they were desperate enough to try it for a week. They explained to Sophie that the rules had changed and that she didn't have to eat anything she didn't want to. They passed her the serving bowls and reassured her that she didn't have to eat if she didn't want to, even if she put some on her plate. After that, except for reassuring Sophie when she asked, "I don't have to eat that, right?" they were careful not to talk about food and eating.

It was a revelation. Within a few days, Sophie was coming willingly to the table and the struggles had stopped. For the first time, Sophie's parents enjoyed having her at family meals. That gave them the courage to go on, even though it was difficult for them to ignore the fact that she wasn't eating any new foods. A dietary calculation showed that Sophie's nutrition was just fine, but her parents had to remind themselves that it takes children time to recover from feeding struggles and that some children don't start to experiment with new food until they are approaching adolescence or even later.

Parents can resist interference

Some parents instinctively follow sDOR; others cross the lines of sDOR, get into trouble, and get out again by following sDOR. A mother described mealtimes with her two toddlers, who gleefully refused food after food that she presented to them on their high-chair trays. She was reluctant to change, reasoning, "If their eating is this bad when I cater to them, what would it be like if I lighten up?" In desperation, she gave sDOR a one-week trial. She put a single meal on the table, sat down, and shared it with them. She was amazed at how well they ate. She commented, "I feel better knowing I did my jobs and let them do theirs. And they certainly seem happier." She was happier as well.

FOLLOWING sDOR TEACHES PARENTING

sDOR is authoritative parenting, the gold standard. Authoritative parenting sorts out control issues. Authoritative parents are warm and responsive. They are open, accepting, and supportive of their child's independence and individuality. With infants, they choose food, then give autonomy with all the rest: how much, how often, how fast, how enthusiastically (Figure 7.3, page 188). With toddlers and older children, they sort out their feeding jobs from their child's eating jobs (Figure 11.2, page 355). They say, essentially, "It is time to eat. Here is what we have. You may eat it or not. Another eating time is coming soon."

Gentle parenting and attachment parenting are partly authoritative parenting, partly permissive, particularly with respect to feeding. Dr. Sears's attachment parenting books, for instance, recommend putting food out for toddlers and letting them munch along all day. Depending on your point of view, that is either permissive or neglectful.

Structure may seem rigid to you, but it is reassuring for your child. Structure provides boundaries and routine, which allow children to do better in all things. Structure lets your child feel trusting and confident that they will be fed. Your child is a captive audience who can't provide for themself. Despite all your reassurances, without your going through the motions of providing family meals and sit-down snacks at more or less predictable times, they can't be certain they will be fed.

Providing positive structure, then giving your child autonomy with eating, is in contrast to *authoritarian* parenting, which uses structure as a way to control the child's eating. Authoritarian parenting is all expectations and no autonomy. It essentially says, "Here is your food. Eat it."

Other patterns of parenting are permissive and neglectful. In both, parents give over to the child their jobs of *what*, *when*, and *where*. Permissive parenting provides neither structure nor expectations, is all autonomy, and says, essentially, "What would you like? When would you like it?" While suspending expectations seems kind, in reality it is frightening. Children need boundaries and predictability.

Neglectful parents provide neither structure nor responsiveness, expecting their children to provide for themselves. Children become afraid of going hungry, horde food, and eat as much as they can when they can get it.

Authoritative parenting is best for children

The authoritative principles of sDOR apply to parenting in general, as established in classical research by UC Berkeley developmental psychologist Diana Baumrind. Starting when the children were preschoolers, Dr. Baumrind observed almost 150 toddlers and preschoolers at school and in their homes through school age to late adolescence. Dr. Baumrind found that authoritative parents were warm, accepted and supported their child's independence and individuality, and at the same time provided structure and clear expectations. Their children were likely to be self-reliant, self-controlled, inquisitive, curious, and content. In contrast, children of authoritarian parents—the ones with all expectations and little or no responsiveness—tended to be relatively discontent, withdrawn, and distrustful. Children of permissive parents, who were all responsiveness and no expectations, also did less well: They were cautious, fearful, and dependent on grownups to manage their behavior and tell them what to do.[9] Baumrind didn't find any neglectful parents in her study population.

I talk about Baumrind's research in more detail in the Chapter 12 section "Parenting Preschoolers" (page 424).

CONSIDER YOUR EATING COMPETENCE

sDOR translates into routine plus trust and works for adults as well as it does for children. For you, sDOR translates into feeding yourself faithfully and giving yourself permission to eat. As a shorthand, I call sDOR for adults *Becoming Eating Competent* and abbreviate it sBEC: Satter Becoming Eating Competent. (I put my name on the Satter models and applications to protect them against others' changing their meaning and thereby spoiling them.) sBEC—feeding yourself faithfully and giving yourself permission to eat—means making time to eat, paying attention while you do it, and eating as much as you want of food you enjoy. As for children, *routine plus trust* supports dietary excellence for adults.

Eating Competence supports wellness

Chapter 5, "Discover the Joy of Eating," discusses Eating Competence in detail. In brief, following ecSatter—letting ourselves eat as much as we want of the food we enjoy—leads to dietary variety,[10] and dietary variety is key to nutritional excellence and wellness. Variety also helps with respect to protecting ourselves against dietary components that are not so good for us. Even "native and actual" foods can contain toxins, such as the goitrogen in uncooked vegetables from the cabbage family. You protect your thyroid gland by eating coleslaw or raw broccoli only every so often, not all the time. Coleslaw and broccoli are good for you, but you can get too much of a good thing.

The same folks who set standards for children's eating set standards for adults' eating: Eat this, don't eat that; weigh this, not that. It is so much a part of our thinking and behavior with respect to food and health that it seems normal. It's not. Normal is trusting your body and going along with your hunger, appetite, and satiety, not trying to outwit and ignore them. To recognize controlling thinking with respect to your eating, consider the opposite: Eating Competence. Research on Eating Competence demonstrates that people do well nutritionally when they regularly and consistently provide themselves with enjoyable and tasty meals and snacks and let themselves eat what and as much as they want at those predictable times.[3]

While many fear that giving permission to eat preferred foods in satisfying amounts will promote gluttony, in practice quite the opposite occurs. Eating becomes more moderate, but don't let that scare you. Moderate in the conventional food world means "don't eat so much; don't eat the food you like." Moderate in the Eating Competence context means consistently eating well, no big extremes of eating a lot and then compensating, no ricocheting between avoiding favorite foods and then eating them like there is no tomorrow. Foods that are no longer forbidden become ordinary foods that can be consumed matter-of-factly without extremes of avoidance or excess. Large portion sizes become less appealing in the context of regular and reliable meals and snacks where you can eat as much as you want of food you enjoy. Rather than having to force healthful foods down because they are good for you, you can enjoy them because you don't *have* to eat them.

Resist fear of food

You will do best with eating as well as feeding when you take a positive interest in food. That takes you into the realm of *how* you feed yourself and your child rather than getting tripped up on the *what*. Focusing on the *how* supports you in providing consistently for yourself and your family despite food and health craziness. At the same time, your child will learn from your eating attitudes and behaviors and be far better served by taking a positive interest in food than by being afraid of it. From the sDOR point of view, there are no bad foods and no bad diets.

Consider the media. Despite considerable evidence to the contrary,[3] many insist we are having a health crisis and that it is essential to worry about what and how much to eat. Health journalist David Katz is typical: "Our native intuitions about eating only really work in a world where native and actual foods prevail. In a world where engineered Frankenfoods prevail, those intuitions are far less reliable."[11] Clearly Katz doesn't know anything about Eating Competence, which demonstrates that people who feed themselves faithfully and give themselves permission to eat will gradually increase their dietary variety with all types of food, provided they are foods they enjoy.[10]

Not only is such name-calling and disrespect of other people's food downright impolite, it casts doubt on what most of us depend on to get ourselves and our families fed. Ultra-processed foods are currently the target of nutritional hand-wringing. These foods—frozen and canned meals, commercial enriched and whole-grain breads and crackers, ready-to-eat breakfast cereals, flavored yogurt, cakes, hot dogs, sweet and savory snacks, chicken nuggets, pizza, French fries, and ice cream—are staples in our food supply and contribute to our nutritional well-being. The same thinking applies to these foods as to any other food: Variety allows you to get the nutrients you need and protects against harmful effects from excess.

Many gain visibility from badmouthing food: In the same blogged interview I just quoted, David Katz stated, "Of course, there are 'bad' foods. More ominously, there are 'bad' dietary intake patterns that have resulted in diet being the single leading predictor of premature death in the U.S. and much of the modern world."[11] Such all-too-common, easy-to-make but impossible-to-substantiate claims are far better at attracting attention and making folks scared of food than they are at reflecting actual health data.

Why you don't have to be afraid of food

There are many who predict compromised health and even early death from eating the "wrong" food and/or failure to eat the "right" food.

The data does not support such claims. In reality, people who die young from heart disease tend to suffer from genetic conditions that make them vulnerable. Other than for that small and highly unusual group, data from the National Center for Health Statistics indicate that the leading cause of death for infants through age 34 years is accident followed by intentional self-harm. It is only in the later years that heart disease and cancer become leading causes of death. Because most people die when they are old, and because almost everyone develops heart and other cardiovascular disease if they live long enough, those are hardly premature deaths. These data are all online,[12] and if you wish, you can peruse all 163 pages, just like I did!

Does poor diet cause degenerative disease: Does eating French fries clog your arteries and give you cancer? Again, many claims, poor substantiation. "Bad" foods and "bad" dietary patterns are generally presumed to be those high in the wrong kind of fat and low in fruits, vegetables, and whole grains. However, as I said earlier, many randomized trials showed no support for recommendations to increase fruits and vegetables and restrict or modify dietary fat.[13, 14] Large-scale research found no decrease in diabetes, cardiovascular disease, cancer,[15] or early death[15, 16] from following the "healthy eating pattern." Folks on Dietary Guidelines–based regimens have no less heart disease or cancer.[17-19] They also aren't any thinner.[20]

Contrast those findings from the ones I told you about in the section "Attitudes and behaviors, not what and how much," (page 3). Adults who are Eating Competent have better diets, lower BMIs, superior metabolic profiles, and more positive quality-of-life indicators. Raising your child to be Eating Competent allows them to reap those benefits.

YOU NEED MEALS

Following sDOR and being Eating Competent does not mean throwing open the refrigerator door and having a food free-for-all. It means that you have certain feeding and eating jobs, and once you do those jobs, you do not have to control what or how much you and your child eat, how much you weigh, or how your child grows.

The cornerstone of both sDOR and Eating Competence is family meals: when you sit down together and share the same food. When you think *meals*, do not get hung up on "healthy home-cooked," as in broiled chicken breasts and steamed broccoli served on a beautifully set table. Instead, think *possible, practical, familiar,* and *enjoyable.* If you currently aren't having regular meals, start by eating what you eat now and build in structure. Fast-food, order-in, carry-out, delicatessen, and frozen meals eaten on a blanket on the floor are just as important as home-cooked meals eaten at a table. Whatever you have to eat is worthwhile: It is *food*. Dignify your food by observing the family meal ritual. A family meal is sitting together, facing each other, and sharing the same food.

Keep more-or-less predictable times

Family meals at more or less predictable times are essential for feeding your child and for feeding yourself. I say "more or less" predictable times because being flexible works better than being rigid on the one hand or random on the other.[21] You can bring your baby to the table on your lap or in an infant seat from the time they are born. Some start eating soft family foods at family meals as early as seven months; others take twice as long or even longer. Most are likely to be ready to join you in eating family meals by the time they are a year old.

I absolutely will not pick on you about what to have at family meals. I advise caution with respect to browsing for "nutritious" meal suggestions that are likely to send you on guilt trips. However, I must insist: For children, family meals and structured sit-down snacks between mealtimes are a must. I realize this may come as a shock to you, since today's increasingly common pattern is eating on the run—grabbing a pizza or salad, or carrying along a fancy coffee or smoothie.

People who have regular meals and snacks tend to do better nutritionally than those who show a random pattern. You may feel you beat the odds: that you do well and get the nutrients you need when you eat on the run. That may be true. However, a random eating pattern does not work for children. Children thrive on structure. To feel secure, they need to know when the next meal or snack is coming and that their important grownups will remember to feed them.

Have family meals *you* enjoy

Remember that the oddest family meal is better than no meal at all and, in fact, is likely to have some nutritional value. In the words of my Ellyn Satter Institute colleague Jennifer Harris, "No meal is perfect. Eat together anyway." Families tend to reserve the family-meal ritual for "healthy home-cooked" food, and each family member eats on their own when they have fast food, order in, have carry-out meals, or eat other food they consider unhealthy.[22] Treat your food with reverence, whatever it is. It is *food*, it sustains life, and it deserves respect.

Yes, I am REALLY telling you: EAT.WHAT.YOU.ENJOY. Keep that permission in mind as you read anything I tell you about nutrition and food selection. Given pervasive attitudes about food and eating, you may decode almost anything I say as: *Eat this; don't eat that.* I do not intend that. This book and all my current work are based on the concept of Eating Competence—a kinder, gentler, remarkably effective way of caring for yourself nutritionally.

Eat and enjoy your cultural foods and celebrate your culture with food and eating. Your customs guide you well. Every culture has food traditions that have stood the test of time in letting people survive and thrive. Your cultural foods are every bit as good as American food and, if you are a recent immigrant, your diet may be more varied than the usual American diet. As your child gets older, they will want to "Americanize" what you eat, and you can do that at the same time as you hang on to your traditions. An occasional fast-food meal goes a long way toward honoring your child's need to fit in with the other kids.

Be prepared for the long haul

Possible, practical, familiar, and *enjoyable* are absolutely essential, because you will be at this a long time. To hang in there with a decades-long commitment of providing meals day after day, year after year, you must find them richly rewarding to plan, prepare, and eat. When you start where you are and persist in having family meals, your meals will be enjoyable at the same time as you naturally increase the variety of food you prepare and enjoy.[10] You will, that is, as long as you take your time and don't put pressure on yourself to increase your mealtime fare—or on other family members to eat it.

FOLLOWING sDOR PREVENTS FEEDING PROBLEMS

Following sDOR prevents feeding problems, even in ill children or children with functional needs. Up to 70 percent of children with medical conditions have feeding problems.[23] As discussed in the Chapter 7 section, "Babies who require tube-feeding," page 212, often a child's vulnerabilities start the ball rolling in the wrong direction. You get advice that doesn't help and even makes matters worse, and before too long you are stuck: Feeding is consistently unrewarding and the problem goes on and on. The solution is following sDOR, but it can feel so risky to stop doing what you are doing to get your child to eat that you may need help to work your way out of the feeding deadlock. It is so important to address problems early. The Chapter 12 section, "Understand established feeding problems," page 428, describes what happens when parents cross sDOR as their child grows up: Problems start early and become more and more pronounced as parents compensate at each stage for previous errors in feeding.

sDOR works with children who seem vulnerable

Some children trigger their parents' often-unconscious food pushiness, overprotection, or restriction. Consider especially large or small children, those who are especially cautious or enthusiastic about eating, or those who are neurodiverse or who have some kind of syndrome. Traditional NICU practice dictates that once babies are able to suckle, they are to be awakened every two hours—or less—to eat a certain number of ounces. Parents are sent home with those instructions. However, professionals who work in those units are slowly freeing themselves from such controlling feeding practices. Research on cue-based feeding shows tiny premature infants are capable of eating on demand.[24]

Health policy contributes to feeding distortion by declaring children whose BMI is above the 85th percentile to be "overweight," and those whose BMI is above the 95th percentile to be "obese." The same distortions happen with smaller children: Those who grow below the 15th percentile are declared "underweight," and those who grow below the 5th percentile characterized as possibly having "failure to thrive."

Even without such health policy interference, parents' natural tendency is to try, often unconsciously, to moderate their child's extremes. Consider an Edinburgh, Scotland, study with normal, healthy but relatively small infants. Some, not all, formula-feeding parents tried to get their babies to eat more than they did voluntarily, and their babies grew less well. Breastfeeding neutralized that natural and understandable tendency to compensate for babies' small size. Breastfeeding mothers went by their baby's feeding cues, and their infants grew well. So did bottle-fed infants whose parents went by their feeding cues. Average-sized breast- and formula-fed babies were fed similarly and grew equally well.[25] It is more difficult, but not impossible, to be controlling when you are breastfeeding than when you are bottle-feeding.

sDOR works for children with medical conditions

Unusual, fragile, or ill children scare everyone, professionals included. Scared people get pushy, and pushed children eat poorly. It takes more nerve and feeding know-how to support and trust such vulnerable children than it does to be interfering.

Babies with medical conditions are entitled to eat orally to the best of their ability. A responsively fed baby—a baby fed according to sDOR—is able to eat as much as they need when their growth follows a particular percentile, even if it is below the fifth or the third percentile. A responsively fed baby who can't eat enough to support consistent growth is likely to require supplemental tube feeding.

While some babies with medical conditions require partial or total tube-feeding, they and their parents can have a positive feeding relationship. They can enjoy warmth, closeness, and getting on the same wavelength during feeding. Babies have trouble eating when they have chin, lip, or palate abnormalities; neurodevelopmental issues, such as difficulty coordinating sucking, swallowing, and breathing; low or high muscle tone; a gastrointestinal disorder, such as esophageal atresia; or a serious heart condition. Developmental disorders such as Down syndrome can be accompanied by these other complications.

Children with medical conditions such as cystic fibrosis or diabetes know how much they need to eat, and parents can follow sDOR in feeding them, as described in the Chapter 12 section, "Solving children's feeding problems." Rather than parents' being expected to control what and how much children eat, medication compensates for children's metabolic limitations and lets children eat pretty much normally. Children with developmental disabilities, such as Down syndrome and Russell-Silver syndrome, are often characterized as being incapable of regulating their food intake. It is simply not true.

sDOR helps prevent eating disorders

Doing an excellent job with feeding and raising your child to be a Competent Eater will protect them from having an eating disorder later on. It won't *guarantee* that they don't develop an eating disorder, because there are so many negative influences on eating, body self-esteem, and emotional well-being. However, your child's fundamental Eating Competence—and your own—will make it a lot easier to treat that disorder if it occurs. Most of the eating disorder world uses Family-Based Treatment, where parents are expected to manage their child's eating. Stated in terms of the Satter models, parents administer both parts of sDOR: not only their own *what*, *when*, and *where* but their child's *how much* and *whether*. As the child gets better, parents gradually turn the *whether* and *how much* back over to them.

My professional colleagues at the Ellyn Satter Institute who work with adolescent eating disorders find treatment goes best and is most likely to be successful when parents are Eating Competent. Do a search for eating disorders on the Ellyn Satter Institute website (https://www.ellynsatterinstitute.org/). There are a number of webinars addressing the Eating Competence approach to Family-Based Treatment for eating disorders.

To do all you can to keep your child from having an eating disorder, understand and accept your child's eating attitudes and behaviors—even when they are extreme—and follow sDOR.

You can restore sDOR

I could go on, but you get the idea. There are many pitfalls and much interference that can lead you to cross the lines of sDOR, and crossing those lines causes problems with feeding. Even if you know better than to go along with destructive advice, it is difficult to ignore what you are told from professionals, family, or friends. It happens. Even if you go along with poor advice, paying attention to your child lets you self-correct. You observe that feeding is going poorly, you go back to following sDOR, and your child goes back to doing well with eating. Kids are resilient and change rapidly when you do.

If you aren't enjoying feeding and if the same problems keep coming up again and again despite your best efforts to solve them, get help. The time and money will be well spent and prevent years and years of stress and ill health. Look for a professional who is thoroughly versed in feeding dynamics and sDOR. The Ellyn Satter Institute has many resources to help you.

sDOR FREES YOU FROM THE NUMBERS

I have just told you *how* to feed. Now I will explain *why*. Knowing the evidence—or knowing it is here so you can go back to it—helps you hold steady with feeding. Because of today's considerable interference with feeding, I spend a good bit of this chapter reviewing the evidence supporting sDOR. In other chapters, I try to keep the evidence to a minimum. You may not need it, but your health professionals and other advisors could use some support in backing you up.

When you follow sDOR, you don't have to be tied to the numbers. While family meals and snacks are essential, numbers that tell you what your child *should* eat get in the way of trusting them: how many fruits and vegetables or how little fat, sugar, red meat, or salt.

Given a positive eating and feeding environment, I trust you, and I trust your child, to do well with eating, nutrition, and health. Period. No monitoring or counting. No trying to get you or them to eat vegetables. While this all sounds alarmingly permissive, I know whereof I speak. I understand nutrition principles, and I am committed to good nutrition for both you and your child. I have both bachelor's and master's degrees in nutrition and completed a one-year dietetic internship at a major university hospital. Throughout my career, I have kept careful track of the goings-on in nutrition.

Source of nutrition dos and don'ts

The numbers originate with "healthy eating pattern" recommendations made every five years by the U.S. Departments of Health and Human Services (HHS) and Agriculture (USDA) and published as the Dietary Guidelines.[5] Professional organizations such as the American Academy of Pediatrics follow the recommendations and incorporate them in their position statements, and pediatricians pass Academy recommendations on to you. The media and advertisers amplify and further catastrophize the guidelines for their own purposes, and that is another way they reach you.

Nutrition policy says, essentially, eat "right," or you will be unhealthy and so will your child. The Dietary Guidelines use "nutrition quality" as a yardstick, and research sounds the alarm that infants and toddlers eat poorly.[26] That judgment is based on recommendations that young children should (not my word) eat over *two cups* a day of fruits and vegetables, two ounces of lean protein foods, three adult servings of breads and cereals, and two cups low-fat milk or other dairy foods. That is more than *six times* as many fruits and vegetables and twice as many high-protein foods as your child needs to get a nutritionally *adequate* diet, and far more than they are likely to eat. If you track your child's food intake on an app, those are the numbers being applied, and those numbers could make you miserable.

Avoidance of degenerative disease through diet is a *wish*, not a guarantee. It is also a moving target: Theories come and go about how to eat to prevent disease, and it hasn't been proven that eating inflated amounts of fruits and vegetables and avoiding certain kinds of fat does the trick. In fact, research shows the opposite: As I said earlier, folks on Dietary Guidelines–based "healthy eating pattern" regimens have no less heart disease or cancer.[17-19] They also aren't any thinner.[20] While eating a varied diet contributes to overall health, it isn't worth distorting your diet and making yourself miserable about eating in order to chase highly elusive long-term disease avoidance.

Nutritional *adequacy* is realistic

Based on the same data analyzed by the nutritional quality folks and using nutritional adequacy as the yardstick, others say the nutritional status of infants and young children is just fine.[27] The difference is the yardstick. Nutritional *adequacy* is the amounts children *really* need in order to get enough nutrients; nutritional *quality* is the *wished-for* amounts. By the nutritional adequacy standard, young children need five *child-size* servings of fruits and vegetables a day. A serving is a tablespoon per year of the child's age, or five tablespoons total—just over a quarter cup of fruits and vegetables, not over two cups.

Even those smaller, more realistic numbers are likely to worry you because on many days your child won't eat even the minimums. You are not alone. In their concern about doing the best for their child, parents take *any* numbers to heart and apply them literally. It is the impossible dream. As I said earlier: No child ever ate according to a formula. Trying to get children to eat even modest amounts or types of food spoils eating for them, spoils your feeding relationship, and makes their eating worse, not better.

Depend on routine plus trust

It turns out that you don't need either set of number: nutrition quality or nutritional adequacy. You only need routine plus trust. The routine is providing regular and reliable meals and snacks. The trust is letting your child eat whether and as much as they want of the food you provide at those regular eating times. In other words, you need to follow sDOR. That simple formula—routine plus trust—works because of the way children *are*. They are driven to grow up with eating, the same as with every other part of their life. They assume they will eat the food *you* enjoy, and they do, sooner or later—even *years* later, provided you haven't been promoting it in the meantime. Combining children's drive to grow up with their naturally erratic eating adds up to children's eating enough variety to get the nutrients they need. They do it in their own remarkably effective, hit-or-miss fashion.

EVIDENCE THAT YOUR CHILD IS CAPABLE WITH EATING

sDOR is built on trust that children are capable: the assumption that children do well with respect to nutrition and growth when they are trusted to eat what and as much as they want from what parents provide. This is in contrast to the child-deficit thinking that prevails in the nutrition and health world. Based on child-deficit thinking, even when parents do well with feeding, children must be enticed in some way to eat their vegetables, must have their food portioned out to keep them from overeating, and must have their overall food intake managed to get them to weigh between the 15th and 85th percentiles on growth charts. Health policy makers characterize growth outside of that BMI range as "overweight," "obese," "underweight," or even "failure to thrive." The Chapter 4 section "More About BMI Cutoffs," (page 120), discusses why such guidelines make no sense and why you can safely ignore them. The important consideration is your child's consistent growth at *any* percentile level.

Your child's growth is only concerning when it accelerates or falters—when it suddenly and considerably shifts up or down. Even growth-shifting has to do with the feeding relationship: Children's accelerating or faltering growth doesn't come out of thin air. Something in the environment causes it, and that cause starts, ends, or both with a distortion in the feeding relationship. See the Chapter 4 section, "Identify growth acceleration or faltering," page 114.

Why is it important to distinguish between child-capable and child-deficit thinking—consistent growth at any level versus BMI cutoffs? Because in following sDOR and trusting your child's capabilities, you will be swimming against the tide: You will be believing and doing the opposite of what most other people believe and do. As a consequence, you will get advice and even pressure from professionals, friends, and family to conform to their child-deficit thinking. They may feel that your child needs to be made to eat their vegetables or that your thin child should eat more or that your fat child should eat less. To withstand that pressure, you need evidence.

The Clara Davis studies

Some of the earliest research on child feeding was reported in 1928 by physician Clara Davis of New York's Mount Sinai Hospital. At the time, pediatricians dictated precisely the types and frequencies of foods for children from age seven months up, and the belief was that the transition from suckling to adult food had to be made over three or four years. Furthermore, based on the assumption that infants didn't know how much they needed to eat, amounts were dictated as well. Not surprisingly, 50 to 90 percent of pediatrician visits were about food refusal. Davis described such pediatricians as "science infatuated," and insisted that babies knew best. She tested her assumptions with a series of feeding experiments with 15 six- to-twelve-month-old infants. Adults, who were instructed to remain entirely neutral, provided babies trays at regular times with a variety of nutritious food—33 foods in all—and sat down with them while they ate. The babies mouthed utensils, dishes, doilies, and the tray itself to identify what was food and what wasn't.[28]

At first the babies put food in their mouths and spit it out again. After the first few meals, they promptly recognized and chose the food they wanted to eat, no matter where it was located on the tray. It was impossible to predict what a child would eat at a given meal, and the 15 infants ate 15 different diets. Over the six months to a year of the study, the babies ate nutritionally adequate diets and were entirely healthy. They developed food preferences and then abruptly abandoned them. They had what Davis called "waves" of eating, where they consumed eight to ten eggs, three or four bananas, or five to seven potatoes in a single meal. Milk consumption ranged from 11 to 48 ounces. They ate salt and cried and sputtered but didn't spit it out and ate more. An infant with rickets voluntarily consumed strong-tasting cod liver oil—a rich source of vitamin D—and abruptly stopped consuming it when the rickets was healed.[28] Dr. Davis's study is often misquoted and used to rationalize letting children freely graze for food, but essentially the researchers maintained a division of responsibility in feeding. They chose a variety of food for the infants, offered it at regular times, then let children pick and choose and eat as much or as little as they wanted from what the adults made available.

Clinical diet calculations

In my decades-long clinical dietetics career, I have found the same thing as Dr. Davis did, but in a different way. I have done many dietary calculations of the food intake of seemingly poorly eating young children, and my colleagues have as well. We have found that over a week or two most children's food intake was nutritionally adequate, even though for a given meal or day their eating was bizarre and even alarming. They ate tastes of this, fingerfuls of that, an adult-sized serving or more or nothing at all of something else—some days a lot and other days hardly anything. I said "most" children did well nutritionally. Some children's diets were nutritionally deficient. Those were the children whose well-intended parents didn't expect their child to join in with family meals and instead allowed them to eat or drink on the run. Generally, those parents struggled to get their child to eat certain foods.

RESEARCH EVIDENCE SUPPORTING sDOR

Growing out of these observations and building on my clinical frustration at not being able to give parents useful guidance, my subconscious gifted me with sDOR. It was an epiphany that changed everything: Could it really be true that children could be trusted to eat what and as much as they needed when parents did their jobs with feeding? sDOR seemed logical and I hoped so. My observations showed me that sDOR worked clinically, but I knew how easy it is for any of us to be infatuated with our own ideas.

Clinical and research evidence for children's eating capability

I held my breath while I read the then-emerging research on children's eating behavior, studies that have stood the test of time and become classics. The evidence confirmed sDOR: Provided adults gave children appropriate support and didn't interfere with their eating, children knew how much they needed to eat,[29, 30] gradually accepted new food,[28, 31-33] and grew consistently[34] in ways that reflected their genetic endowment.[35, 36] My audiences complain that these are old studies, but they proved their point and have not been disproven. Newer studies aren't as useful in understanding children's eating because they examine how to *get* children to eat in the way *researchers* want them to eat. Whenever the word *get* enters, pressure enters right along with it, and sDOR goes out the window.

Many other professionals as well as parents have found the concept of sDOR to be valuable. Since my first journal article in 1986,[37] sDOR has come to be regarded as best practice in feeding in public health, early childhood education, dietetics, and medicine. It took another 40 years before we had concrete evidence of children's eating capabilities in the context of sDOR from honest-to-goodness controlled observation. It is hard for me to even write that down—how time flies and how *could* it have taken so long? But I know. It took that long because it was difficult and complicated to measure the relationship between parent and child.

Research with sDOR.2-6y

To have direct evidence that sDOR works—to prove it—we had to be able to measure whether parents were following sDOR and what impact that had on their child's eating. To measure sDOR adherence, my research partner, Dr. Barbara Lohse, and I developed a paper-and-pencil inventory, sDOR.2-6y—a test, in other words. We started with almost 40 statements, read them to parents, and asked them to put the statements in their own words. Leadership statements—parent *what, when,* and *where* items—included "My family eats meals about the same times every day." Autonomy statements—child *how much* and *whether*—included "If I think my child hasn't had enough, I try to get him or her to eat a few more bites." That last statement is reverse scored, meaning when you follow sDOR you do *not* try to get your child to eat a few more bites.[38] That process of arriving at a shared understanding with parents narrowed the list down to the 15-statement inventory we used for the next step in testing.

To determine whether the inventory really tested what we wanted it to test, we had parents fill it out before and after we video-recorded what they did with feeding their child at a family meal. Parents actually did on the video what they *said* they did on sDOR.2-6y. That process brought us down to the 12 items that we could consistently observe and compare.[39]

Finally, we did validation, which means we compared parent responses on the 12-item sDOR.2-6y with their responses on other already validated inventories—tests—to determine characteristics of those who got high or low scores. What we found in that step was revealing and even sensational: When parents followed sDOR, children had lower nutritional risk.[4] *The key to children's nutritional excellence was routine plus trust.*

Children's nutrition is better when parents follow sDOR

The validation testing confirmed the research bridge between the child's eating, parents' eating, and parents' following sDOR. Parents who scored high on sDOR.2-6y were also likely to be Eating Competent and do less restricting and pressuring with their child's eating. High-scoring parents had better quality-of-life indicators: less stress, better sleep, and more positive psychological and social functioning.[4] When feeding goes better, you feel better all over! Parents who indicated on sDOR.2-6y that they were comfortable with providing meals generally had meals about the same times, had better diets,[21] and had lower mood and anxiety disorders.[4] I talk about parent Eating Competence in Chapter 5, Discover the Joy of Eating.

WHAT TO EXPECT FROM THIS BOOK

Ellyn Satter's Child of Mine is a book to begin reading before your baby is born and to go back to again and again as your child moves through the ages and stages of the first six or seven years. Sometimes you will read for information and other times for reassurance. I hope sometimes you will read for entertainment. I find writing about little ones to be immensely entertaining!

For an overview of *Ellyn Satter's Child of Mine*, don't forget to read the Preface. It gives you the main message and tells you why this book's radical perspective about food and nutrition is so important for you. Take a look at the table of contents and examine the figures in each chapter.

Part I is background. It explains and gives evidence for Eating Competence and sDOR and applies it to what and how much your child eats and how they grow and to your eating. Each of the "How to Feed" chapters applies the information in Part I by applying a stage-related sDOR, addressing common feeding issues, and solving feeding problems. Each chapter gives details about child development, parenting, and nutrition and has considerable cross-referencing to sections in other chapters. You may find that as I do, both helpful and aggravating. The alternative is a much longer book! *Ellyn Satter's Child of Mine* is evidence-based, and I discuss that evidence in more or less detail in each chapter. You may appreciate the evidence, or you may find it tedious. You don't have to read it if you don't want to. The evidence will be helpful for you if you find your trust faltering in feeding yourself or your child.

sDOR seems simple, but following it demands steady nerves and a leap of faith. To follow sDOR, you have the delightful task of coping with your child's eccentricities. You also have the far less delightful task of ignoring messages that urge you to manage what and how much your child eats and what they weigh. You may find yourself faltering; reviewing the evidence will help you get back on track.

DON'T FORGET TO ENJOY!

Children whose parents follow sDOR thrive within the structure of family meals and snacks and gradually learn to eat the food their parents eat. Adults who are Eating Competent provide themselves with regular, reliable, and enjoyable meals; have relaxed, positive, and orderly eating attitudes and behaviors; and do well nutritionally.

Rather than getting bogged down with your sense of responsibility or carried away by your ambitions for your child's eating and/or size, remind yourself why you decided to have a child in the first place. I hope a major reason is for the sheer joy of it. It is a grand privilege to have a front-row seat for someone else's life. If you can keep your ego out of it and let your child surprise you, they will provide the leavening for your concern about doing the right thing as a parent. Certainly, do your homework, but then set the homework aside and pick up your sense of wonder and your sense of humor. It is a grand adventure to have and raise a child. Relax and enjoy it.

REFERENCES

1. Satter E. Eating Competence: definition and evidence for the Satter Eating Competence Model. *J Nutr Educ Behav*. 2007;39:S142–S153.
2. Krall JS. Validation of a measure of the Satter Eating Competence model with low-income females. *Int J Behav Nutr Phys Act*. 2011;8. doi:10.1186/1479-5868-8-26 PMC3094263,
3. Satter Eating Competence Model (ecSatter): Evidence-based research. *https://www.needscenter.org/resources/satter-eating-competence-model-ecsatter/*
4. Lohse B. Valid and reliable measure of adherence to Satter Division of Responsibility in Feeding. *J Nutr Educ Behav*. 2021;53:211–222.
5. U.S. Department of Health and Human Services. *Dietary Guidelines for Americans. 8th Edition*. 2020.
6. Fryar CD. Prevalence of overweight, obesity, and severe obesity among adults aged 20 and over: United States, 1960–1962 through 2015–2016. *https://www.cdc.gov/nchs/data/hestat/obesity_adult_11_12/obesity_adult_11_12.htm*
7. Barlow SE. Obesity Evaluation and Treatment: Expert Committee Recommendations. *Pediatrics*. 1998;102:e29.
8. Kininmonth AR. The relationship between the home environment and child adiposity: a systematic review. *Int J Behav Nutr Phys Act*. 2021;18. doi:10.1186/s12966-020-01073-9
9. Baumrind D. Current patterns of parental authority. *Developmental Psychology Monograph*. 1971;4:1–103.
10. Satter E. Hierarchy of food needs. *J Nutr Educ Behav*. 2007;39:S187–S188.
11. Wharton R. A theory from the 1980s could be the key to solving picky eating. *Food52* blog. September 12, 2021. *https://food52.com/blog/26521-ellyn-satter-method-for-feeding-children-explained*
12. National Center for Health Statistics. LCWK1 Deaths, percent of total deaths, and death rates for the 15 leading causes of death in 5-year age groups, by race and sex: United States, 2002. *https://www.cdc.gov/nchs/data/dvs/lcwk1_2002.pdf*
13. Harcombe Z. Evidence from prospective cohort studies did not support the introduction of dietary fat guidelines in 1977 and 1983: a systematic review. *Br J Sports Med*. 2017;51:1737–1742.
14. Chowdhury R. Association of dietary, circulating, and supplement fatty acids with coronary risk: a systematic review and meta-analysis. *Ann Intern Med*. 2014;160:398–406.
15. McCullough ML. Adherence to the Dietary Guidelines for Americans and risk of major chronic disease in women. *Am J Clin Nutr*. 2000;72:1214–1222.
16. Ebrahim S. Multiple risk factor interventions for primary prevention of coronary heart disease. *Cochrane Database Syst Rev*. 2011. doi:10.1002/14651858.CD001561.pub3
17. Prentice RL. Low-fat dietary pattern and risk of invasive breast cancer: the Women's Health Initiative randomized controlled dietary modification trial. *JAMA*. 2006;295:629–642.
18. Howard BV. Low-fat dietary pattern and risk of cardiovascular disease: the Women's Health Initiative randomized controlled dietary modification trial. *JAMA*. 2006;295:655–666.
19. Beresford SAA. Low-fat dietary pattern and risk of colorectal cancer: the Women's Health Initiative randomized controlled dietary modification trial. *JAMA*. 2006;295:643–654.
20. Howard BV. Low-fat dietary pattern and weight change over 7 years: the Women's Health Initiative dietary modification trial. *JAMA*. 2006;295:39–49.
21. Lohse B. A definition of "regular meals" driven by dietary quality supports a pragmatic schedule. *Nutrients*. 2020;12. doi:10.3390/nu12092667

22. Berge JM. Perspectives about family meals from single-headed and dual-headed households: a qualitative analysis. *Journal of the Academy of Nutrition and Dietetics*. 2013;113:1632–1639.
23. Silverman AH. Feeding and vomiting problems in pediatric populations. In: Roberts MC, Steele RC, eds. *Handbook of Pediatric Psychology*. Guilford Publications; 2017:402–416.
24. Carrierfenster K. Getting to Full Feeds Faster in the Nicu Utilizing Cue-based Feeding. *Pediatrics*. 2018;141(1 MeetingAbstract):522.
25. Crow RA. Maternal behavior during breast- and bottle-feeding. *J Behav Med*. 1980;3:259–277.
26. Dwyer JT. The Feeding Infants and Toddlers Study (FITS) 2016: Moving forward. *The Journal of Nutrition*. 2018;148(suppl_3):1575S–1580S.
27. Bailey RL. Total usual nutrient intakes of US children (under 48 months): findings from the Feeding Infants and Toddlers Study (FITS) 2016. *J Nutr*. 2018;148:1557S–1566S.
28. Davis CM. Self selection of diet by newly weaned infants: An experimental study. *Am J Dis Child*. 1928;36:651–679.
29. Fomon SJ. Influence of formula concentration on caloric intake and growth of normal infants. *Acta Paediatr Scand*. 1975;64:172–181.
30. Birch LL. Caloric compensation and sensory specific satiety: Evidence for self regulation of food intake by young children. *Appetite*. 1986;7:323–331.
31. Birch LL. Appetite and eating behavior in children. *Pediatr Clin North Am*. 1995;42:931–953.
32. Addessi E. Specific social influences on the acceptance of novel foods in 2-5-year-old children. *Appetite*. 2005;45:264–271.
33. Beal VA. Dietary intake of individuals followed through infancy and childhood. *American Journal of Public Health*. 1961;51:1107–1117.
34. Tanner JM. Normal growth and techniques of growth assessment. *Clin Endocrinol Metab*. 1986;15:411–451.
35. Garn SM. Trends in fatness and the origins of obesity. *Pediatrics*. 1976;57:443–456.
36. Whitaker KL. The intergenerational transmission of thinness. *Arch Pediatr Adolesc Med*. 2011;165:900–905.
37. Satter EM. The feeding relationship. *J Am Diet Assoc*. 1986;86:352–356.
38. Lohse B. Development of a tool to assess adherence to a model of the division of responsibility in feeding young children: using response mapping to capacitate validation measures. *Child Obes*. 2014;10:153–168.
39. Lohse B. Use of an observational comparative strategy demonstrated construct validity of a measure to assess adherence to the Satter Division of Responsibility in Feeding. *Journal of the Academy of Nutrition and Dietetics*. 2021;121:1143–1156.e6.

CHAPTER 2

Raise Your Child to Know What to Eat

"Trust your child to know what to eat" is a title that demands some explanation! You may have visions of throwing open the refrigerator door or giving your child free access to the grocery store. At the other extreme, you may think of giving your child a smartphone and showing them how to track their fruits and vegetables and consult good-food-bad-food lists to decide what to eat. Not to worry. There is a good bit that is in the middle, and that is what *Ellyn Satter's Child of Mine* and the Satter Division of Responsibility in Feeding (sDOR) are all about.

sDOR says you do the *what*, *when*, and *where* of *feeding*; your child does the *how much* and *whether* of *eating*. When you follow sDOR and provide relaxed and positive family meals, your child doesn't have to know what foods to eat. You don't have to keep track of which foods your child eats. You just need to do your part with feeding, then trust your child to do their part with the *whether* (and *how much*) of eating. Even when they have a short list of foods that they eat, you can take your child to another family's home for dinner because they know how to politely turn down food they are not interested in eating.

CHILDREN'S PICKY EATING IS NORMAL

It is natural for children to be selective about what they will eat. They tend to have relatively short lists of foods they enjoy, may be uninterested in trying new food, and/or don't consistently eat food they have eaten before. A study in London of almost 5,000 toddler through preadolescent identical twins found that genetics explained 75 percent or more or their food fussiness. Children's food selectivity tended to increase until age 7 years, then decline after that.[1] Over half of parents see their child as not being picky at any age, and less than 5 percent of parents see their child as being picky at every age.[2] Some children are in their teens or even older before they begin to add on to their short list of enjoyable food.[1,3]

Not to worry. As Chapter 1 said, provided parents follow sDOR, even the most bizarre-looking diets add up to nutritional adequacy. Following sDOR gives children food-acceptance skills: They feel good about food and are able to participate comfortably in meals. Those food-acceptance skills allow them to eat a greater and greater variety of food as they grow up. They learn to eat new food through repeated neutral exposure. *Repeated exposure* is letting your child see the food and watch you eat and enjoy it, again and again, as the food shows up on family menus. *Neutral* means *no pressure*: not persuading your child to eat or rewarding them for eating but, instead, being clear with them that they don't have to eat anything they don't want to eat.

It's all about acceptance

To your child, accepting your child's natural pickiness is the same as accepting *them* and makes all the difference in terms of your feeding relationship. Accepting your child's natural pickiness protects their food-acceptance skills. You don't have to try to *get* your child to eat, but you do have to be patient and let your child find their own way with eating a variety of food—however slowly. In fact, it can take years. On the other hand, if you worry about what your child eats and try to get them to eat a greater variety of food, they will lose their food-acceptance skills. Their pickiness is likely to get stuck.

This box demonstrates how Eating Competence works.

EATING COMPETENCE AND *WHAT* YOUR CHILD EATS

Family meals + food-acceptance skills =
your child's eating a variety and therefore having good nutrition

By *family meals*, I mean the package: sit-down meals + sit-down snacks. I also mean sitting together and sharing the same food: not "perfect" food—just *food*.

Be wary of interference

Interference comes in the form of conventional, control-paradigm ways of getting children to eat certain, generally "healthy" food. Those pressuring ways include encouragement, rewards, reasoning, praise, I could go on. Those ways don't work and make children feel bad. No matter how hard they try or how much they want to please you, children simply can't eat food they find unappealing. Those pressuring methods might work for a while, but not in the long run, and they are costly in terms of the children's feelings.

Interference with food selection is expecting yourself and your child to eat "good-for-you" food and avoid "bad-for-you" foods whether you want to or not. Interference with food selection is hard to detect because it is so much a part of our lives that it seems like the way things "should" be. It isn't. The control paradigm expects you to ignore or overcome your biological, physiological, and psychosocial processes: hunger, appetite, satiety, and the need for sociability and pleasure.

In contrast, the trust paradigm is natural because it cooperates with your biopsychosocial drives to eat as much as you want of food you enjoy. You are in tune with your appetite and need for pleasure when you have rewarding family meals made up of food you enjoy, and you eat what tastes good at the time you eat it. You are in tune with your hunger and satiety when you instinctively eat more or less food and as much as you want of higher- or lower-calorie food. You are in tune with your emotional and social needs when you nurture yourself, your child, and others you love with food you enjoy that is meaningful for you.

Following the trust paradigm—doing what comes naturally—preserves the Eating Competence of both you and your child and lets you all eat the food you need to be healthy.

IN THIS CHAPTER

This chapter talks about practical, doable ways to do your jobs with feeding. Equally importantly, it helps you understand and trust how your child goes about doing their jobs with eating. Then it talks about solving feeding problems. This chapter also talks about *why*. It helps you protect yourself against interference by sorting out the Satter trust-based messages from the mainstream control-based messages. It winds up by helping you consider your choices for the long haul with raising your child with eating.

FOLLOW THE SATTER DIVISION OF RESPONSIBILITY IN FEEDING

Supporting your child's food-acceptance skills depends on your following the Satter Division of Responsibility in Feeding (sDOR). Here is the sDOR version that applies to toddlers through adolescents:

Parents do the *what*, *when*, and *where* of *feeding*.

Children do the *whether* and *how much* of *eating*.

While sDOR is different for babies and transitional children—those gradually learning to eat family food—the principle for all stages is that parents provide the food and children eat it—or not. sDOR guides you in knowing what to do and not do with feeding—and knowing when you have done it.

Because it is so important and because you may need the reassurance, I repeat this from Chapter 1: sDOR works with children of all sizes and temperaments, degrees of enthusiasm about eating, and eccentric ways with eating. It works with neurodiverse children, children who have medical conditions such as diabetes and cystic fibrosis, and children who have syndromes such as Down syndrome and Russell-Silver syndrome.

Figure 1.2, "The Satter Division of Responsibility in Feeding," page 8, outlines sDOR in more detail. Briefly, your jobs with respect to *what* are to manage meals and snacks, make those times pleasant for all concerned, and show your child what they have to learn with respect to enjoying a variety of food. Oh yes, and to reassure your child they don't have to eat anything they don't want to eat. Your job is *not* to get your child to eat. Your child's job is to eat the food when they are ready.

Figure 2.1 describes how sDOR plays out: what helps and what hinders with respect to children's learning to eat a variety of food.

Feed your child with love and trust

Following sDOR supports your child's powerful need to be understood. Conversely, understanding and accepting your child's unique ways will support you in holding steady with sDOR: to keep on feeding well no matter how tempted you are to do a bit of tweaking. To help you trust your child with eating and therefore hang in there with sDOR, see feeding from your child's point of view. They want to grow up with eating, and they are doing the very best they can to eat in ways that please you. At the same time, your food is all strange and new to them and they are skeptical of unfamiliar food. They are more sensitive than we can possibly imagine to how food tastes, smells, and feels. Eventually that sensitivity

FIGURE 2.1: SUPPORTING CHILDREN'S FOOD-ACCEPTANCE SKILLS

Children's food-acceptance skills allow them—sooner or later—to learn to enjoy a variety of food.	
WHAT HELPS	**WHAT HINDERS**
Eating with the family.	Focusing on *what* the child eats.
Pleasant family meals and sit-down snacks.	Limiting menus to "healthy" food.
Parents' having food they enjoy at mealtime.	Adults enthusing or being negative about food.
Trusted adults eating/enjoying the same food.	Parents using good-food-bad-food language.
Being allowed to eat/not eat.	Limiting menus to food the child readily accepts.
Not having to eat, taste, smell, or even *look*.	Positive pressure (rewarding, persuading).
Menus that are considerate without catering.	Negative pressure (criticizing, punishing).
Regular opportunities to eat "forbidden food."	Not including familiar food.
Knowing how to politely spit out food.	Avoiding high-fat, high-sugar food.

gets toned down, but it does take time, and you have to trust that over time your child will become comfortable eating more and more foods.

Although your child's developing a greater number of foods they enjoy is the can't-force-it bonus, you play an important role in supporting your child in achieving that bonus. You give them repeated neutral exposure: You provide the food at pleasant family meals, and you give them an out. You tell them once, then act it out the rest of the time, that they don't have to eat anything they don't want. After that, your mere presence at mealtime lets your child do and dare more with learning to enjoy a variety of food than they would otherwise.

In contrast to neutral exposure, trying to get your child to eat certain foods and grow in certain ways turns your presence into something negative rather than positive. It interferes with your child's autonomy with eating, spoils their food-acceptance skills, and makes them eat less well, not better.

FOOD-ACCEPTANCE SKILLS

When you follow sDOR, your child naturally develops the Eating Competent attitudes and behaviors described in Figure 1.1. As outlined in

Chapter 1, a child's being Eating Competent doesn't mean they enthusiastically eat everything that is put before them, including vegetables. Instead, it means they feel good about food and eating and join in comfortably with family meals and sit-down snacks. Their positive eating attitudes and behaviors let them eat what and as much as they need to be healthy and grow in the way that is right for them.

Let's single out the key attitudes and behaviors that have to do with your child's learning to eat a variety of food—their food-acceptance skills. Here is what those skills look like:

Joins in comfortably in family meals.

Feels positive about food.

Can be around unfamiliar food without getting upset.

Says "yes, please," and "no, thank you" to mealtime food.

I hope you can say that your child feels good about food and eating and does their part to contribute to enjoyable family meals. If not, ask yourself why not, and keep reading. Somewhere in this chapter you will find the answer.

After you start following sDOR, meals rapidly become more enjoyable—within days or weeks. Use that to keep you going. Achieving the hoped-for-but-can't-force-it bonus of your child's eating a greater variety of food takes longer. It can even take *years*. Trying to speed up achieving that bonus slows it down or makes it impossible . . . and makes meals unpleasant.

Food acceptance from a late-bloomer's perspective

Consider this story from a grown-up child—let's call her Andrea—who was a very late bloomer with respect to eating a variety of food:

> *If I had been a child today, I most likely would have been diagnosed with ARFID or something like it. I ate maybe five safe foods, absolutely zero meat, and if my food touched on a plate that was it. My parents practiced what we now call sDOR. They didn't pressure me or shame me and were gentle with my food issues. I slowly but surely started trying new things (though for about two years in my teens I ate nothing but rice, beans, and maybe three vegetables and fruits, and drank milk). By my early twenties, my food could finally touch and by my late twenties, I mixed rice and beans. Now in my forties, I'm* almost *an adventurous eater.*

Andrea's story is extreme, but it makes a number of points. The most important point is that Andrea's parents' gentleness with her food issues allowed her to develop positive food-acceptance skills: She enjoyed eating and managed meals comfortably. Eventually she got the bonus of being "*almost* an adventurous eater." She was able to take pleasure in eating a greater variety of food. Andrea's parents' accepting her eating demonstrated they accepted *her*. That acceptance has supported Andrea in continuing to learn and grow with eating—and likely with life.

It's hard to imagine how exquisitely sensitive Andrea was to the taste and texture and even the *appearance* of food. Had her parents jollied her along or even put pressure on her to eat more foods, Andrea simply would not have been able to do it, and family mealtimes would have disintegrated into a series of fruitless struggles. With less supportive feeding, Andrea could have easily grown up to be an extremely picky eater. Rather than being relaxed and comfortable with what she was able to eat, she could have grown up feeling conflicted and anxious about eating and being ashamed of the short list of foods she enjoyed. Andrea mentioned ARFID: That would be Avoidant Restrictive Food Intake Disorder. In her case, ARFID would be extreme picky eating to the point of nutritional deficiency and weight loss and likely interference with her social functioning: being afraid to eat anywhere besides home. Chapter 12, Feeding Your Preschooler, discusses ARFID, page 445.

Andrea was a particularly late bloomer. The same as with Andrea, with gentle parenting around food, there is hope for your child. Late bloomers continue to add on foods they enjoy, generally in their teens but often even later. Andrea was in her forties when she told her story and was still adding on foods. Jennifer's daughter was 28 when she started eating fresh greens; Anne's son discovered vegetables in college and wondered why he hadn't been given them at home. He had. We talk more about late bloomers below.

Parents preserve food-acceptance skills

Despite her extreme selectivity, Andrea emerged from childhood feeling positive about food, comfortable with what she could and couldn't eat, and enjoying family meals. Andrea's parents preserved those food-acceptance skills by putting their trust in family meals and in Andrea to manage her own eating. For them, pleasant family meals were the primary goal. They set aside any wish they had for Andrea to eat a larger variety of food. They may have even experimented to see if they could make it happen but observed that it spoiled meals. I expect they *were* concerned about her nutritional status, but they kept their concern to themselves, kept their nerve with feeding, and persisted in having family meals. In the process, they gave Andrea *years* of repeated neutral exposure to food.

Andrea's parents were not neglectful in any way because they hung in there with sDOR, and sDOR let them have pleasant family meals.

It seems they even had to let Andrea leave home with her short list of acceptable foods still intact. Even so, she was able to cope with the food world. I hope her parents are still around to share Andrea's enjoyment of a wider variety of food, and I hope they realize what an important part they played.

SUPPORTING YOUR CHILD'S FOOD-ACCEPTANCE SKILLS

Supporting your child in being relaxed and positive about food and inclined to eat it when they can is similar to your supporting your child in learning skills with, say, batting a ball. ESI faculty member Carol Danaher used the example of how parents do their jobs by throwing the ball, again and again. The child swings and misses, again and again. They have fun together and that keeps them both going. The parent doesn't have to persuade the child to swing at the ball, and they certainly don't put pressure on the child to hit the ball because the child already really *really* wants to do that, and applying pressure will get them so flustered that they will miss the ball all the more. The parent remains calm, keeps pitching, and the child keeps swinging. Then, one day, the child hits it! Being able to hit a ball allows the child to play softball and tennis and volleyball and go bowling and feel comfortable in the worlds of people who play ball games. It is a life skill that, once mastered, does not go away.

A child who feels relaxed and positive about eating sneaks up on unfamiliar food. They watch you eat and enjoy it, allow the serving dish to be close to them, put some food on their plate and look, smell, and maybe take a bite and then take it out again (and again and again). Eventually they swallow. Children whose food-acceptance skills have been spoiled by trying to get them to eat get freaked out by unfamiliar food and can't do any of that.

With feeding, you keep pitching and your child keeps learning. One day you can take them to California or Kenya on a family trip without having to worry about whether they can manage the food. They may not be able to *eat* everything that is offered, but they can be relaxed and confident about picking and choosing from what is available.

Understand your child's eating behavior

Is your child relaxed and comfortable at mealtime? Are they pleasant to have at the table? Then your approach to feeding and their food-acceptance skills are working, even when they eat in their usual quirky ways. Children eat a lot one day, little another, enjoy a food one day and ignore it another. One child loves to eat; another is ho-hum about it. All you can do, and it is a *lot,* is hang in there with following sDOR.

Try not to become preoccupied with *what* they eat. The important thing isn't your child's eating certain foods *today*. It is supporting your child in feeling relaxed and positive about food for a *lifetime*. That's more easily said than done. There is something about children's eating that sucks us into worrying. What they eat is so erratic and unpredictable and they are so slow to warm up to new foods that it appears their food acceptance is anything but okay. Like Andrea, some children are particularly slow to experiment with new food and their parents need particularly steady nerves not to interfere with their eating.

Children are extremely sensitive to the taste and texture of food. In contrast to adults, who are likely to eat what is available, they eat only what appeals to them—at that moment. What appeals one day doesn't appeal another day. When you provide a child with repeated neutral exposure, they don't get stuck there. Well, all right, they may *seem* to get stuck because what appeals to them can take quite a while to change. Have courage and hang in there. Eventually, after weeks, months, or even *years*, your child will learn to eat a variety of food.

Some children seem to eat "too much"

Some children particularly enjoy food and look forward to mealtimes: Their parents are less likely to pressure them to eat and, in fact, even swing over into restriction. They may interpret the child's food enjoyment as a sign that the child will get "too fat," assume they will eat too much, and restrict them. Whereupon the child becomes preoccupied with food, eats too much, and their weight accelerates. Allow me to remind you: sDOR works with children of all temperaments and degrees of enthusiasm about eating. Giving children regular and emotionally supportive access to as much as they want of food they enjoy allows enthusiastically eating children as well as those who are more blasé about eating to matter-of-factly satisfy their food needs.

Some children are *really* selective eaters

Really selective eaters are unbelievably slow to warm up to new food. As long as they are reassured that they don't have to eat anything they don't want to eat, even such children can participate comfortably in family meals. They can enjoy eating what they can manage and be matter of fact about ignoring food that they don't want or aren't ready to learn to eat. Children can be really selective eaters when they are unusually sensitive to the taste, texture, smell, and even appearance of food. Pressuring them to eat can activate their strong gag reflex and even make them throw up. Chewing and swallowing problems can make a child appear to be a selective eater, and an occupational therapist or speech and language pathologist can be helpful. They do in-office oral-motor work to help the child get their mouth and throat muscles working properly. At the same time, they do not exert pressure in any way on the child to put anything in their mouth or even touch, lick, or smell any food. Professionals grounded in the trust paradigm support parents in following sDOR at home and do not try to get a child to eat anything they aren't ready to eat.

ESI faculty member Cristen Harris tells of her son Noah who was diagnosed with ADHD in seventh grade. Noah remembers and can clearly describe how unpleasant they found certain textures of food. (Noah prefers the pronoun "they.") Noah learned to ignore or politely refuse what they didn't want to eat. To their parents carefully concealed astonishment, sometime in middle school Noah said, "Please pass the broccoli—I'd like to try it." A decade or more later, Noah enjoys eating broccoli and has turned into an adventurous eater.

Emphasizing *what* destroys food-acceptance skills

Trying to get children to eat certain amounts or types of food takes away their good feelings about eating and is *way* more common than uncommon. Over 90 percent of parents in focus groups said they tried to get their child to eat by preparing special food for them, bribing them with sweets, and persuading their child to eat more when the child said they were full.[4] In 150 families of kindergartners observed at dinner time, 75 percent of parents served their child whether or not the child wanted the food and 85 percent rewarded, praised, and threatened to get their child to eat more than they wanted. Children gave in to their parents' pressure: Over 80 percent of children ate beyond the point where they said they were finished.[5] Parents who do not eat fruits and vegetables put particular pressure on their child to eat them and children do not eat them.[6]

Those parents are crossing the middle line pictured in the Figure 1.3 analogy, "Trust is a two-way street," page 12. In the process, they are making their child's eating worse, not better. Children are so sensitive to pressure that even "nice" pressure takes away their interest in food.

Parents are to be forgiven for their pressure tactics: They have gotten the message that fruits and vegetables are critically important, and they try to get their children to eat them. It doesn't work. A study of almost 300 parents of preschoolers found that passing the message along to children that fruits and vegetables are good for them does not make them eat more—in fact, they eat less. Monitoring, pressure to eat, and restriction of other foods all make children eat fewer fruits and vegetables, not more. What works? Eating dinner together as a family.[7]

GIVE *YOUR* FOOD ACCEPTANCE A BREAK

Before we dive into your role in providing meals, let's get you off the hook with respect to *your* food-acceptance skills. Do you enjoy food? Are you comfortable with what you eat? When you think about what to eat, do you consider what you enjoy, or do you concentrate on what you should avoid? Avoiding food is so much a part of our culture that you may not even be aware you are doing it. Where does your food avoidance come from? Do you attempt to follow the US Dietary Guidelines "healthy eating pattern" recommendations and try to eat lots of vegetables, fruits, and whole grains? Avoid fat in dairy products, meat, poultry, and fish? Try to stay away from high-sugar, high-fat food?[8] Do you have personal standards for "healthy" food, such as clean eating or following a vegetarian, vegan, Paleo, gluten-free, or low-carbohydrate diet? Are you committed to organic, locavore, or low-carbon-footprint food selection?

Whatever your standards, they are working for you if you are comfortable at meals where you don't have control of the menu. You don't have to actually *eat* a variety of food. All you need to do is preserve and protect your own food-acceptance attitudes and behaviors: enjoying food and meals, not being freaked out by unfamiliar food, being able to ignore or politely refuse food you don't want to eat. Trusting your own food-acceptance skills will let you provide for yourself nutritionally at the same time as you show your child what they have to learn. Even if you have a relatively short list of foods you enjoy and provide for meals, your child can learn from other grown-ups to eat a greater variety of food. They can get repeated neutral exposure to other foods at school, at the grandparents', and at the neighbors.

Some parents are picky eaters

You are entitled to eat and enjoy some foods and not others, even if your "enjoy" list is short. If you are positive and matter of fact about simply not eating a food, that's just fine. Foods you don't enjoy are unlikely to show up at family meals. That too, is fine, but it need not necessarily be so. You can still include not-enjoyed foods in meals as long as you don't force yourself to eat them. Who knows? You might even benefit from the repeated neutral exposure and learn to enjoy the food. *But you don't have to eat it if you don't want to*! The same as your child, you can eat and enjoy what you want, ignore what you don't want, and be relaxed and polite about it.

Whatever you do, do not force down foods you do not enjoy. Your child will be onto you in a flash and be as turned off by the food as you are.

Chapter 5, Discover the Joy of Eating, discusses adult food acceptance.

Some parents are epicures

At the other end of the spectrum, some parents take particular pleasure in food and enjoy experimenting with many different foods, and that is fine as well. Children who can politely say yes or no to food learn to eat even the challenging variety of food their parents eat. It just takes longer. If stir-fried tofu shows up only every few months, it will take children a while to accumulate the repeated neutral exposures they need to learn to enjoy it. In the meantime, children can eat rice and gradually get used to the stir-fry.

MEALS SUPPORT FOOD-ACCEPTANCE SKILLS

Your child absolutely depends on enjoyable family meals and sit-down snacks to support their food-acceptance skills and therefore eat what they need. *What you have* at meals is far less important than *having* them. Meals reassure your child that they will be fed. In combination with family meals, your child's erratic eating works for them nutritionally by allowing them to eat a variety of food. Sit-down snacks are also important nutritionally. Children given even nutritious food handouts rather than participating in family meals do not gain food-acceptance skills and do not do as well nutritionally.

Providing your child with the structure of family meals and sit-down snacks relieves you of worry about whether your child is getting the nutrition they need. Think how great it is to go to meals not having to fuss about what and how much your child eats! Such worry doesn't just crop up at mealtime—it follows parents and children around. Parents who establish sDOR and resolve struggles around eating say they and their child feel better all day.

Research backs them up: Children identified as being problematic selective eaters suffer from anxiety and depression, and family functioning is often impaired.[9] Before you freak out at being reminded of still another parenting pitfall, remember: You don't resolve your child's selective eating by getting them to eat a greater variety of food. You resolve it by getting the pressure off what they eat. You relieve pressure by having pleasant sit-down meals and snacks and trusting your child to eat whether and as much as they want. Parents who follow sDOR have better quality of life: They feel better, sleep better, and have lower stress levels.[10] Remember, the outcome you can achieve is your child's positive food-acceptance attitudes and behaviors. The outcome you *can't* achieve is your child's eating a greater variety of food.

Meals correlate with parent well-being

Whatever foods family meals contain, being able to *have* meals correlates with parents' well-being. A key item in sDOR.2-6y, the questionnaire about following sDOR, is "My family has meals about the same times every day." Parents who responded positively to that item said they experienced greater overall enjoyment, concentration, and self-confidence in their lives and less stress and depression.[11]

This is not to say that having meals is the magic bullet for mental health. Rather, it means that having family meals is an accessible task that allows parenting to fall into place. Achieving that task reduces stress and provides a sense of well-being. Keep in mind that parents who filled out sDOR.2-6y also gave their children autonomy with eating. They didn't try to control what they couldn't control. They answered positively to "I let my child eat until s/he stops eating and doesn't want more," and negatively to "If I think my child hasn't had enough, I try to get him or her to eat a few more bites." That, too, likely relieved their stress and increased their sense of well-being. There is nothing so stressful as trying to achieve the impossible: Getting a child to eat.

A meal or not-a-meal?

Now let's consider what *not* to do: Making the bar so high with food selection that you simply can't succeed.

A study of St. Paul, Minnesota, families[12] found that parents consider some foods "meal foods" and some foods not a meal at all. Due to their rigid ideas of what is "healthy," they give little value to perfectly wholesome foods, such as fast, prepackaged, and take-out food. They give such foods so little value, in fact, that they do not sit down together for family meals unless food is "healthy" and "home-cooked." Otherwise, everyone goes off and eats by themselves.

It's not easy to lighten up. Parents in the study gave a glimpse of the ferocious attitudes that underlie food avoidance:

- "You have to buy healthy foods . . . don't buy the prepackaged stuff because it's just a bunch of junk that's not even food."

- "We don't eat healthy food at family meals because the healthy stuff costs so much . . . that is another reason we don't eat together that much."
- "It's cheaper to eat grease and garbage as opposed to buying healthy foods for dinner."

Soothe your food conscience

Your food conscience may not be quite that fierce, but it could still be causing you problems. It may be made up of a hodgepodge of any or all of the above as well as dos and don'ts from every web article you have ever read and every diet you have ever been on. Wherever your food conscience comes from, it can trip you up with respect to providing family meals.

Why not teach your food conscience new ways? Consider expanding your definition of "healthy" to include food you enjoy, irrespective of the label that is applied to it by some outside "authority." Giving yourself permission to eat honors *all* foods allows you to benefit from their nutritional value. The Satter Eating Competence Model (ecSatter) does that and Eating Competent adults do splendidly nutritionally. They get as much as they need of nutrients that make up a healthy diet and even have a higher Healthy Eating Index (HEI) score than the general population.[13] HEI tests people's adherence to the US Dietary Guidelines. Ironically, Eating Competent adults consume diets of high dietary quality without their getting hung up on the "healthy eating pattern's" good-food-bad-food distinctions. That's ironic because I have been telling you that "dietary quality" standards set the bar too high; that going by nutritional adequacy standards is more realistic.

HELP YOUR CHILD BE COMFORTABLE WITH FAMILY MEALS

Your child who feels positive about food and comfortable with family meals will learn to eat the food you eat, if not sooner, then later. In the meantime, keep *yourself* comfortable. Make family meals achievable and let your child attend to their own eating. Understand where your child is coming from. Young children lack experience with food. Moreover, children's survival instinct makes them skeptical of unfamiliar food. A popular theory is that young children are particularly skeptical of green food because green plants in nature are often toxic. We don't really know if this is true, but why not remind yourself of that little factoid while your child takes years and years to learn to eat broccoli or spinach?

We do know that some children—and grown-ups—are particularly sensitive to the bitter undertones in cabbage-family vegetables such as broccoli, cabbage, and cauliflower. Eventually they eat them, but it takes a long time and lots of opportunities to learn. Consider the argument that bitter foods can stimulate the body's defense system, which enhances our antioxidant system to protect against disease. That argument is generally made by folks who go on to talk about what bitter foods you *should* eat, so take it for what it is worth. *Should* is a pressure word.

Relax about nutrition

It's not about the food; it is about the feeding relationship. As long as you follow sDOR, you can ditch good-food/bad-food and restriction and avoidance. Shape what you eat now into family meals and your child will do well nutritionally. Food-seeking—being Eating Competent—*is* the path to nutritional excellence. Eating Competent adults provide themselves with meals, eat as much as they want of food they enjoy, and are healthy nutritionally, medically, and even psychosocially.[14] Eating Competent adults raise Eating Competent children who do the same thing.

You may eat food because it is good for you, but children only eat food that tastes good to them. Your child won't be impressed by being told food is "healthy," and, in fact, saying a food is "healthy" takes away its appeal.[15] You know for yourself that trying to eat more than you want of *any* food renders it unappealing and even repulsive. Ask any weight-loss dieter how much they enjoy the quantities of vegetables they force down to try to fill up on fewer calories.

For some, it seems to be an impossible choice: Do you continue to have dreary food and feel deprived, or do you eat food you enjoy and feel guilty? The families I talked about earlier eat what they consider "junk" and "grease and garbage," but they disrespect it and disrespect themselves for eating it.[12]

The Minnesota researchers concluded with recommendations for making "healthy" meals easier to provide and suggested involving the whole family in food preparation. Certainly, streamlining cooking is a good thing and involving the family is great. However, insisting on "healthy" food is limiting. Family meals have enormous value, no matter the food. As my ESI colleague Jennifer Harris says, "No meal is perfect. Eat together anyway."

Trust your child to eat

It's not easy to trust a child to learn to eat unfamiliar food. Three-year-old Oscar's parents were convinced that his eating the right food would protect him from calamity, although they weren't sure what that calamity was. Oscar ate just a few foods and rejected most others on sight. His parents were experts in positive pressure: rewards, high fives, applause, elaborately enjoying foods he rejected, and occupational-therapist type coaching (looking, smelling, touching food with fingers, touching with the tongue, tasting). As I said earlier, those behaviors are all part of children's food-acceptance skills and how they learn to eat new food. *Making* Oscar look, touch, smell, and taste took those skills away from him and spoiled their effectiveness. They once tried withholding Oscar's favorite foods, but for a week everyone left the table in tears and Oscar still didn't eat anything new. What to do instead?

Be considerate (without catering)

The solution was following sDOR, including Oscar's favorite foods in meals, and trusting him to eat. I am not talking about restricting menus to food the child readily accepts, which is what his parents had been doing. I am talking about being *considerate without catering*: Including with meals one or two *side dishes* that a child generally eats. That doesn't mean baking a pizza when you have stir-fry. It means letting your child eat the rice and ignore the stir-fry and then having pizza another time. Sometimes the child gets lucky and the main dish is something they enjoy; other times, it is somebody else's turn.

Familiar side dishes are important for both your child and you. Your child needs to come to the meal and see some food that they recognize and generally eat; you need to feel successful with feeding your child. Your child might eat one of the starchy foods you have already included or perhaps some other side dish such as fruit. They are examples of what my readers call "safe foods."

Another way of thinking about being considerate without catering is to combine familiar and enjoyed food with unfamiliar and not-yet-enjoyed food. When you plan meals with not-yet-enjoyed food, also provide enough familiar food so everyone can eat as much as they want: You don't want to give the impression that you are preparing that food just for your child. That would be short-order cooking, and *that* puts pressure on your child to eat. Think how you feel when your grandmother says, "I made this especially for you."

Be prepared for your child to eat a lot of the preferred food before they turn their attention to the new food. Parents complain that the considerate without catering strategy isn't working because their child eats slice after slice, meal after meal, of bread and butter. Actually, it *is* working because the child enjoys mealtime. Be patient. Consider yourself successful.

Children tire of even their favorite food—and then they eat a different food, probably meal after meal, day after day.

Stated in another way, providing your child with a "safe food" won't get them stuck on a few familiar foods. In reality, children are more likely to experiment with new food when they can fall back on a familiar food. Remember that the bottom line in your child's doing well nutritionally is having family meals be pleasant for you and your child. For that, both you and your child need to feel successful.

Avoid catering (while being considerate)

As for the *without catering* part of the advice: Catering would be making your child a separate meal. That's you desperately and even resentfully making two or three meals for your family, feeling you have to please every family member with every food, all the time. Catering deprives family members of developing food-acceptance skills. One of those skills is being able to politely refuse food. Another is being comfortable about leaving a meal having eaten nothing at all—after all, a snack is coming soon. When you desperately search for something your child will eat, they learn it is desperately important *to* eat. It isn't. There are lots of opportunities to eat.

Pleasing everybody all the time is the impossible dream, and it has led many family cooks to give up altogether on providing family meals. The exception was the exhausted and exasperated mother who brought her husband and teenagers in to see me. For decades she had been making two or three meals for her demanding and self-satisfied family, each of whom had a short list of foods they would eat.

She was sick of it. The costs to her were obvious: She was sacrificing her time and comfort and reaping a lot of frustration. The costs to her children were less obvious: She was raising a crop of extremely picky eaters who would have trouble providing for themselves after they left home.

I was tempted to advise her to feed them liver and boiled cabbage, but I restrained myself and told them all about being considerate without catering with meal-planning. (I enjoy liver and boiled cabbage, but they are challenging foods and I doubted if they did.) Even having to settle for some foods they enjoyed was a big deal for them. It felt wrong to her to stop catering to them and wrong to them to no longer be catered to! But they all pulled through the bumpy early weeks and eventually they all settled down to their new mealtime routine. The husband and sons also developed some food-acceptance skills: Instead of being freaked out by food that was not exactly to their liking, they learned to ignore food they didn't want to eat and to be polite about it.

The moral of the story is that making your child a special meal is catering, and catering will not turn out well. Keeping peanut butter or cereal on the table is also catering. Remember, I said a *side dish*. Peanut butter and cereal are alternate *entrees*—main courses—and that is short-order cooking.

Figure 11.6, "Be considerate without catering with meal-planning," page 363, discusses the strategy in more detail. It is in Chapter 11, Feeding Your Toddler, where you will *really* need it!

Relax about "forbidden" food

You have likely gotten the message that you aren't supposed to let your child have what I call "forbidden" food, known elsewhere as "junk" food: sweets, salty and fatty snacks. It doesn't work. Restricted children eat more, not less of those foods.[16] A nurse who approached me at a conference was upset about her 11-year-old daughter's passion for candy and potato chips: "I didn't raise her this way, but she stops at the store on the way home from school and buys junk with her own money and eats it on the way home, and then she won't eat her dinner. Or she hides it. I find candy wrappers and potato chip bags in her room."

I had just finished my presentation about sDOR and children's learning to be comfortable with all kinds of food, but parents need to ask their own question in their own words to be sure I really mean what I say. "I am afraid you have some making-up to do," I told her, "but it's not too late. Your job is to take the 'special' and 'forbidden' out of those foods by including them regularly."

Then I went into my standard forbidden-food schtick: Restricting access to "forbidden" foods has made them "special" for your daughter. Turn them into ordinary food by including them regularly. Put one serving of dessert at each person's place when you set the table. Let children and other people eat it before, during, or after the meal. No seconds. When you have chips or fries, include them at mealtime and offer enough so everyone can eat their fill.

To make up for limiting sweets at mealtime, periodically offer unlimited sweets at snack time, such as a plate of cookies or snack cakes. If your child is preoccupied with sweets, have sweets more often. Offer milk and you have a nutritious snack. Let your child (and yourself) eat as many cookies as they want. As I warned the mother of the 11-year-old, at first your child will likely eat a lot. But the newness will wear off, and they won't eat so many.

Consider more "forbidden" food exposure

I often hear about 11- or 12-year-olds whose eating is "out of control," because it generally takes children until they enter late school age to start getting "forbidden food" on their own. Restricted younger children do the same eating-to-excess at birthday parties and potlucks, but their embarrassed parents feel they can keep a lid on things. With older kids, it is obvious that the lid is off. It's better to lighten up on "forbidden food" when your child is younger.

From the perspective of the "healthy eating pattern," high-fat, high-sugar, high-salt is to be avoided on the grounds that it is inconsistent with good nutrition. From the perspective of the trust paradigm, because such appetite-enhancing, soul-satisfying foods contribute to the enjoyment of family meals, they contribute to the nutritional welfare of family members. People who regularly include those foods in their meals and snacks get enough of them and don't overeat them. People who try to avoid them altogether periodically cut loose and eat a lot to the exclusion of other food.

ESI faculty member Cristen Harris, whom you may remember as the mother of Noah-with-the-broccoli, tells a potato chip story that she says helps her eating-disordered clients. During a televised football game at a friend's house, her toddler, preschooler, and school-age child stood over the potato chip bowl eating constantly. They couldn't go play; they couldn't watch TV. Cristen realized that she had inadvertently been depriving her children of potato chips: Since she didn't particularly enjoy them, she rarely bought them. She changed her shopping ways, and soon her children were relaxed about potato chips—they still enjoyed them, but they weren't the big deal they had been at the friend's home.

For more about the how and why of sweets, see Figure 11.7, "Regularly offer 'forbidden' foods," page 366.

Don't hide the vegetables

I was surprised when a reporter asked to interview me about the topic of parents hiding vegetables in other foods in order to get their child to eat them. I thought it was old news, but apparently the idea is alive and well today.

I don't like the idea. Not only would it take a *lot* of beet-laced brownies to get a serving of beets, it is trickery, and trickery undermines trust. Sooner or later, children catch on, and instead of being interested in food, they become wary. My friend Lisa, then employed as a preschool teacher, talked about the rabbit food buffet that capped off their week-long series of lessons on all things rabbit. As the children eagerly lined up for the meal, a little girl heard her teacher talking about her carrot cake. "What?" she screeched. "Carrot cake? Everybody, don't eat that! It has carrots in it!"

I think we can guess the tactics her parents used to get her to eat carrots! *Books* have been written about sneaking vegetables into children's food and social media is full of strategies. Parents share their ingenuity in concealing grated carrots in the meatloaf, chopped zucchini in the spaghetti sauce, and pumpkin in the muffins. Nutritionally it is fine, but it is controlling and controlling tactics spoil feeding.

Again, the point of following sDOR is not to get your child to eat vegetables *today*. It is to raise them to feel positive about vegetables and possibly even eat them *for a lifetime*. It would be far better to invite your child to help wash and chop vegetables and even grow them, always reassuring both of you that the point isn't getting them to *eat* vegetables but rather allowing them to *feel good* about vegetables. It is certainly okay and even lovely to prepare vegetables in appealing ways by cooking them well and using sauces, dips, and seasonings. Enjoy them yourself and depend on repeated neutral exposure to bring your child along with respect to eating vegetables.

I do enjoy zucchini and carrots in spaghetti sauce and love baked goods that contain pumpkin, but I told my children they were there. The rule of thumb is that if you are working harder than your child to get food into them, you are crossing the lines of sDOR. If you are dishonest with children about their food, they become suspicious, cautious, and reluctant to try new food.

CHILDREN WHOSE "WHAT" IS LIMITED

It's not easy to keep providing meals when eaters have only a short list of foods they enjoy. It's especially difficult to keep having meals you enjoy when you are a single parent and it is just you and your child. We all hope for a child like my youngest, Curtis, who would see a new food, try it, and in most cases eat it enthusiastically. My other two children were not like that. Lucas, my middle child, was skeptical. "What's that?" he would say. I would tell him. "I don't like it," he would announce. "You don't have to eat it if you don't want to, but you might like it if you try it," I would respond. (That maneuver made Curtis mad the one time I used it with him.) Lucas would try it and generally enjoy it enough to eat more. Lucas knew I was fully prepared to take no for an answer, and that freed him up to experiment. Kjerstin, my oldest, was extremely picky. She ate few foods and vegetables did not cross her lips. When she approached her teens, she began eating a wider array of food and now she eats a great variety and enjoys experimenting with unfamiliar food.

It's just the way children are, and you can't change them. My three children demonstrated the observations of Clara Davis, the doctor I told you about in Chapter 1, who did the feeding experiments with transitional infants. In another article, Davis described three patterns of children's learning to eat unfamiliar food: what I call the early adopter, the skeptical experimenter, and the late bloomer.[17]

With all three patterns, you have to hang in there with sDOR. As I discovered with my grandchildren, hanging in there is really difficult with late bloomers. With my own children, I was too busy to worry about what they ate and I assumed if they didn't eat certain foods, there was nothing I could do about it. I was correct about that, although it was years before I came up with sDOR.

Late bloomers are challenging

With my grandchildren, I had time to be challenged. Kjerstin's daughter Marii enjoyed family meals, but she was a late bloomer with respect to eating a variety of food. I visited her family only so often and then as a guest, so I was interested but not bothered by her eating patterns. My grandson Zakkary was another matter, and his frequent visits at mealtime tested my convictions. For years and *years*, Zakkary ate from only a short list of food. He enjoyed family meals but ate few of the foods there. I had to settle for including one of his acceptable foods at each meal. It was not easy, but his parents, his other grandmother, and I did not make an issue of it. Somewhere in his early teens, Zakkary began eating a wider variety of food. Now when he visits, we experiment with Pad Thai and have regular chili instead of the smooth and soft version that we learned to make by copying the chili-like-food from his favorite restaurant.

I don't comment on Zakkary's newfound interest in a greater variety of food, and he seems unaware of it. Marii is well past her teens, so I asked her what she remembered from her selective-eating days. She said it was the texture of the food that was challenging for her, more than the flavor. I am waiting to have that conversation with Zakkary.

It seems to me that the moral of the story is obvious, but you know me: I will tell you anyway. With late bloomers, difficult as it is, you have to hang in there with sDOR. You must not make an issue of what your child eats even when their selective eating goes on and on. Provided you have been able to stay in your lane with feeding, when your child approaches their teens, they are likely to begin eating more foods. Who knows why? Probably something to do with maturation, but there it is. Children *mature*. They are *driven* to mature. They are driven to master their parents' world, and part of that world is food.

You can't force a child to bloom

You may have heard enough on this topic for now, but I have one more story from my clinical years that I really want to tell you. Parents, and siblings as well, came into my office wanting me to get 12-year-old Carter to eat more "healthy" food. The family confirmed my suspicions about what was going on with feeding: Parents pressuring Carter to eat; siblings getting no recognition for choking down food they didn't enjoy, to please their parents and make up for Carter's pickiness; everyone suffering through years of conflict at family meals.

Most parents would have given up on family meals altogether, but to their credit, Carter's parents hung in there. To their further credit, they remained concerned enough about Carter's nutrition to ask for help. Parents and siblings chimed in on the family story of Carter's eating. They all regarded the now-robust Carter as sickly. He had been an especially small child who grew slowly. Almost from the first, his parents were urged by well-meaning professionals and extended family to get him to eat more. The feeding struggles that started with nipple-feeding and solids introduction persisted as Carter made the transition to family food and through all the ages and stages from then to now.

"It's clear you all care about Carter and want the best for him," I told them. "His list of foods *is* pretty short, but I am more concerned about the negative way he *feels* about food. Would you be terribly upset if I told you that your trying to get him to eat has been creating the very problem you were attempting to address?"

I went on to tell them how trying to get Carter to eat was spoiling family meals and making him reluctant to try new food. I introduced sDOR and we discussed how that would play out: Parents could take a break at family mealtimes from trying to get Carter to eat, Carter could stop being so defiant and simply attend to his eating, siblings could stop gagging down food they didn't enjoy. Eventually Carter might get to the point where he enjoyed eating a greater variety of food, but that was up to him. In fact, Carter's eating more foods wasn't the important outcome. That was letting Carter and the rest of the family be comfortable and relaxed at enjoyable family meals.

The family came back for a handful of sessions until we got everything ironed out, and for that I admired them. Another family would have told me I was out of my mind and gone off to find someone who would tell them how to get Carter to eat. My family therapy colleagues reminded me that the family's issues went deeper than feeding, and that could be so. I have also found that families who successfully address feeding struggles discover new possibilities for addressing other parenting issues.

Lighten up on "healthy" food

Annie's desperate parents complained that the only time Annie ate much was at the neighbors'. To their credit, they wanted to know why. After all, their food was so excellent compared with the neighbors' food. They were careful to use very little fat, avoided sugar, provided lots of fruits and vegetables, and offered lean meat and skim milk. Most people who try to live by such dietary rules are inconsistent: They adhere and feel deprived sometimes, fall off and feel guilty other times. But Annie's parents did not deviate. They were absolutely convinced of the rightness of their ways, and they adhered to those ways without exception.

Thanks to the neighbors, Annie still had food-acceptance skills—she was interested in food and enjoyed eating. However, her skills depended on her being offered enjoyable food, and she wasn't getting that at home. The concept that food is supposed to be enjoyable was novel to Annie's parents. To them, food was fuel.

I didn't want to hurt their feelings, but they wanted Annie home at dinner time, so I told them: "I am afraid your food doesn't interest Annie. Children don't eat what is good for them. They eat what *tastes* good." I advised them to use more fat in cooking, to butter the vegetables, to offer unlimited amounts of butter and regular salad dressing at mealtime, to deliberately include forbidden food, to be considerate without catering, and let Annie eat whether and as much as she wanted from what they provided.

It was difficult for them to allow more fat into the house, but they bought whole milk, made sauces for meats, showed Annie how to put butter on her vegetables, and made a dip for raw vegetables. I reassured them they didn't have to eat the higher-fat food if they didn't want to. Alarming as these strategies were for them, they were reassured by Annie's joining them for dinner. It didn't happen right away: Annie took a few weeks to trust that her parents really were having better-tasting food and that they weren't going to try to get her to eat. I have this fantasy that after a while the parents even lightened up and started eating some of the flavor-enhancers they offered to Annie.

You can make up for past feeding mistakes

You may have made some of these same mistakes with feeding. Nobody's perfect. My ESI colleague Jennifer Harris worked with parents who confessed that they routinely forced their school-age child to eat and that he routinely threw up on his plate. Because the parents had been so rigid about feeding, Jennifer was surprised when they were willing and able to start following sDOR. Family meals immediately became enjoyable, but it took a long time for the child to voluntarily eat the foods he had been forced before to eat. Children in the laboratory who had been pressured, praised, or rewarded at home for eating did not increase their short-term food acceptance with neutral exposure.[18] However, we find clinically that over the longer term they do come to accept a greater variety of foods. If you change your ways with feeding, your child will change too—but it will take time.

Have a "we are going to change this" conversation with your child, then establish sDOR. When you let up on pressuring your child to eat, your meals will soon become more enjoyable. After that, it could take a while to get the routine of family meals and sit-down snacks in place. Then you will need some time to catch on to the ways you put pressure on your child's eating—and stop doing it.

Your child needs time to change, as well. Their eating will become more extreme at first: They will eat even fewer foods. They need time to trust that you really mean what you say about not pressuring them to eat. After a while, they will settle down to eating the same as any other child: a variety sometimes, only one or two foods another, a lot sometimes, hardly anything other times. Don't pin your feelings of success on what your child eats—vegetables or anything else. Given your previous struggles with feeding, it could take months or even years.

Remember, *the key outcome indicator is pleasant family meals.* The hoped-for-but-can't-force-it bonus is your child's eating a greater variety of food. Pleasant family meals support your child's food-acceptance skills. Eventually, to the best of their ability, your child will learn to eat a variety of food. Conversely, if you let sDOR slip, meals will go back to being unpleasant, your child's food-acceptance skills will disappear, and they won't have a prayer of learning to eat new food.

Allow me to harp on this: You absolutely *must* settle for pleasant family meals in order to be successful with feeding and your child successful with eating. You absolutely must *not* hold out for your child's eating the food somebody else wants them to eat. Your child *will* learn to eat a greater variety of food, but that could be *years* in coming.

MASTER FAMILY MEALS

Let's be realistic: Family meals are about getting home late and nothing sounds good and everyone is tired and cranky and the kids whine about the food. Forget about the perfect home-cooked meal and pleasing everyone with all the food. Hang on to sDOR, prepare one meal for everyone, and be considerate without catering. Your job is done when the food goes on the table. After that, other family members have a job to do: Eat or not eat. You don't whine about doing your job; they don't whine about doing theirs.

Adjust your expectations—for yourself as well as for your child. It will make all the difference with respect to your being able to follow sDOR. Researchers in Atlanta, Georgia, examined hundreds of parents and found them, to a greater or lesser degree, to suffer from "resource depletion": They were overwhelmed. Those overwhelmed parents were more likely to get controlling with their children's eating: They resorted to food restriction and pressure to eat.[19]

Do what you can to keep yourself from being overwhelmed. Have enjoyable family meals that relieve your stress rather than contributing to it:

- Develop a meal and snack routine that works for *you and your family.*
- Include foods you truly enjoy. Don't be ruled by lists of food-to-eat and food-to-avoid.
- Make eating times pleasant. Relax. Pay attention. Take your time.

Start successful and let yourself grow

To get started with family meals, eat what you eat now even if you aren't being "good." Keep control of the schedule: Have meals and sit-down snacks at more or less set times that you determine, don't just have meals when you feel hungry or someone else asks for something to eat. Everyone's hunger rhythms soon adjust to family mealtimes. Instead of leaving a pizza, macaroni and cheese, or some chicken nuggets and chips on the counter for family members to help themselves and wander off to eat on their own, turn it into a meal. You don't even need a table, sitting around a blanket on the floor will do. Put out the food, add a beverage, and call everyone together to sit down to eat.

Have what you have when you get home late, and everyone is tired and cranky, and you couldn't care less. Whatever you have, dignify the food. Treat it with respect. It is, after all, *food*, and it sustains life. Have a mealtime ritual. Wait to start eating until everyone is present, greet each other with *bon appétit*, and pass the food.

Don't panic if the food you enjoy is on someone's "bad" list. A web search for *Most popular American dishes* reveals a lot of fried food; food that conventional nutrition advice condemns as unhealthy. Sadly, most feel guilty about eating the high-fat food that we love based on the unproven assertion that it makes people fat and prone to early heart attack and cancer. Nutritional-doom-saying hasn't changed our food preferences that much, but it has made us feel bad about what we eat! It isn't nice to disrespect other people's food. The kids say it best: Don't yuck my yum.

But wait, you may say, you can't possibly know how bad it gets! I doubt if you would give me any surprises. Well, all right, if your meal is soda and Pop-Tarts and that's it, I might try to interest you in whole milk instead of soda. Or I might suggest a peanut butter sandwich and some chips and enlighten you on their nutritional value. But really, from the sDOR perspective, meals are about *ritual*. It's a meal when you sit down together and share the same food. It's the ritual that is so important for your child's well-being and nutritional status, not the good-food/bad-food commotion. To reassure you that you can eat what you enjoy, see the Chapter 11 section, "Celebrate food," page 395.

You will find yourself offering sit-down snacks

To help you establish and maintain the family-meal routine, consider offering yourself and your child sit-down snacks between meals. Small children—and perhaps big children and adults—can't comfortably last from one meal to the next. Trying to get by on in between food-and-beverage-munching spoils meals—it fills up family members so they aren't interested in eating at mealtime. Planned, sit-down snacks midway between meals allow eaters to come to meals hungry but not starved and interested in the food there.

You will find yourself planning

Planning grows out of the family-meal routine. Do it when you are ready, and make it your servant, not your master. Start with a *little* planning, say knowing in the morning what you will have for dinner, maybe even figuring out meals a day or two ahead. Only do as much planning as you can tolerate.

You will find yourself adding on food

Once you get the ball rolling with family meals, you will naturally learn and grow. When you sit down and pay attention to eating, you may find that you are tiring of eating the usual fare and look for a bit of variety. You might add canned peaches to your pizza meal or peas to your macaroni and cheese meal.

You will find yourself needing sDOR

Children and other adults may tire of the usual food, as well, but it is familiar to them, and they enjoy eating it. When you add on food, reassure them that you are not taking away their usual food. Not only that, but they don't have to eat any of the add-ons if they don't want to. Remember sDOR and remind them that they don't have to eat anything they don't want to. Along with adding variety, you are applying the sDOR-consistent strategy of being considerate without catering.

The Minnesota parents, the ones who consider their usual food to be "grease and garbage," say "the biggest challenge to having family meals is coming up with ideas that everyone likes." One said, "all three of my kids are picky eaters so most of the time we don't eat together to avoid the fighting and complaining about food." Following sDOR and being considerate without catering addresses the dilemma and lets you make one meal for everyone. Making food "that everyone likes" is the impossible dream. Catering to children puts pressure on them to eat and is likely to precipitate fighting and complaining about food. Both are a drag.

You will find yourself cooking

It will help if you can do a bit of cooking. "How to cook" in *Secrets of Feeding a Healthy Family* helps the beginning cook succeed. It gives simple, delicious recipes, includes method summaries and recipe notes, suggests menus, and gives tips for including kids in the kitchen. You can do just fine with frozen, order-in, take-out, or canned meals. Jumpstart your cooking by using pre-prepared ingredients. Check out the table in *Secrets* Chapter 11, "Grocery list of convenient foods and ingredients." Consider chicken, beef, pork tenders, fillets, or stir-fry, prewashed salad ingredients, and frozen or canned vegetables and fruit.

Give yourself permission to cobble together a meal from whatever you have on hand in your pantry and freezer. Get some ideas from the Secrets Chapter 9 section on grab-and-dump meals. Consider meals you can get done in a hurry, such as canned hearty soups with crackers, boxed rice and bean dishes, or tuna-noodle casserole. Searching dump dinners on the web could be helpful, although those meals are generally a bit more complicated than what I have in mind for those can't-think-of-dinner occasions.

You will find yourself considering food groups

You may have already been at this stage when we started this discussion, and now we have caught up with you. The time-honored meal-planning strategy is including something in a meal from each of the food groups. Meal-planning just works that way and needn't get in the way of eating foods you enjoy. The four food groups are a protein, one or two starches, fruit or vegetables or both, and milk. Include fat in food preparation and at the table—butter for bread, gravy for potatoes, regular salad dressing, dip for raw vegetables. Fat makes food taste good and lets the littlest and/or hungriest eaters get filled up. Four food groups may seem like a *lot*, but think about it: Consider pizza (starch, protein, vegetable), hamburger and fries (starch, protein, vegetable), chicken nuggets and fries (ditto—consider the breaded coating), tacos (ditto). Add milk as the beverage and you have four.

If your food budget is tight, let family members get filled up for less money by choosing higher-calorie versions of your usual foods: whole milk, fruits canned in heavy syrup, fried meats, butter or margarine for bread. Ration the expensive food—say have one pork chop or only so many strawberries for each person—but have enough potatoes, rice, and/or bread so everyone can fill up. For more about coping with a tight food budget, see the Chapter 5 section, "Address food insecurity," page 142.

Forcing down food doesn't work

If you are eating a food so your child will eat it, spare yourself. You can't fake it. Your child will know and in their child's way think, "That must not be so good so I'm not going to eat it." If you want to, you can learn to enjoy a wider variety of food, but you don't have to. See the Chapter 5 section, "Picky eating," page 149. Your following sDOR lets your child retain the food-acceptance skills that they need to learn to eat unfamiliar food at someone else's meals.

Along those same lines, about the time you get family meals well in hand, you are likely to find yourself tripping on your personal guidelines for "healthy" food. *Don't go there!* Getting caught in the dos and don'ts of food selection can be an unfortunate and destructive spin-off from getting organized with food. It will spoil your eating and get in the way of you having family meals. Not to worry—being Eating Competent means you eat nutritious food because you *enjoy* it, not if you don't. In contrast, with control-based, eat-this-don't-eat-that thinking, enjoyment is an afterthought.

MAINSTREAM ADVICE IS CONTROLLING

The mainstream way of talking, thinking, practicing, and doing research with respect to what your child eats is based on *control*. If feeding dynamics are taken into account at all, it is from the perspective of using feeding to manipulate the child's eating certain amounts or types of food. That controlling don't-eat-so-much, eat-this-don't-eat-that, and weigh-the-right-amount thinking is everywhere, and it has been around for so long that it can seem to be the only way. Because of that and in their defense, controlling health professionals are doing what they think is right and may even think they are following the division of responsibility.

In contrast, sDOR is based on trust: Trust in your child, once you have done your jobs with feeding, to eat what they need to have a nutritionally adequate diet and be healthy. Embracing the trust paradigm requires ignoring oh-so-readily-available controlling advice. Little wonder that in the face of children's erratic eating, many parents and health professionals lose their nerve and interfere. That interference undermines the child's interest in food and enjoyment of eating and creates the very problem they are trying to address, that of children's eating only a limited variety of food.

What clues can help you tell the difference between information and advice that is trusting and recommendations that are controlling?

Consider the intent

Is the intent of the advice to support you in trusting your child to enjoy food, learn to eat what you eat, and grow and be well in their own special way? Or is the intent controlling: getting you to get your child to eat certain foods and grow in certain ways? Trusting makes family meals possible; controlling complicates family meals and makes it difficult to continue having them.

Consider vegetables

With respect to vegetables, it's not easy to go with trust. Vegetables have taken on a sort of magic bullet status: A child's eating enough vegetables seemingly ensures their nutritional welfare and health. Trusting your child to eat their vegetables means letting them have the weeks, months, or even years they need to learn to enjoy eating vegetables on their own. Controlling your child's vegetable-eating is satisfying your own need to get vegetables into them *today* or even *soon*. Hiding vegetables in the brownies is controlling because it tricks the child into eating them rather than trusting that they will, sooner or later, eat vegetables on their own.

Control-based research explores ways to get children to eat their vegetables, and funding agencies are guided by nutrition policy: They readily fund such research. That research investigates tactics such as mixing fruits and vegetables with food the child enjoys,[20] serving vegetables first,[21] increasing vegetable portion sizes,[22] and making fruits and vegetables available for the child to snack on throughout the day.[23]

Let's have a little test: Which of the strategies I just listed is trusting and therefore consistent with sDOR?

If you answered "none of the above," you are correct. The available-for-snacking strategy is inconsistent with sDOR because even fruit and vegetable handouts spoil children's appetite for meals.

The control-oriented research I just cited showed that children *do* eat more fruits and vegetables when they are rewarded, but compared with what? What happens when you simply follow sDOR and give children repeated neutral exposure to vegetables as they show up on the family menu? A group at University College in London found that the latter children were more likely to continue to eat the vegetables than children who were rewarded for eating them.[18, 24]

Consider scare tactics

The control stance is that your child is doing poorly—or potentially so—and something must be done about it. Control is reflected in research insisting that "dietary intakes of US toddlers are nutritionally inadequate."[25] The trusting stance is that you and your child are doing well, and you will benefit from encouragement and support. Trust is reflected in research indicating that, for the most part, children do well nutritionally.[26] Control uses the *nutritional quality* defined by the "healthy eating pattern," which mandates children eat over *two cups* a day of fruits and vegetables, two ounces of lean protein foods, three adult servings of breads and cereals, and two cups of low-fat milk or other dairy foods. The difference is in the yardstick. Trust uses the *nutritional adequacy* standard. According to that, young children need five *child-size* servings of fruits and vegetables a day. A serving is a tablespoon per year of the child's age, or five tablespoons total—just over a fourth cup of fruits and vegetables.

You will hear more from the control perspective. Conventional nutrition advice is to insist you have to get children to eat their vegetables and stay away from chips and sweets. Some warn that you can't raise healthy children in today's food world.[27] The media loves fearmongering because it captures an audience. The well-publicized slogan, "Count every bite to make every bite count,"[8] strikes fear into parents' hearts. There is simply no evidence to support such a warning; children and the rest of us have considerable nutritional margin for error. We can satisfy our nutritional needs and have calories left over to spend on sugar and fat. Moreover, we don't have to count calories to do it. Hunger and appetite do the work.

Fearmongering feeds on control and I would like to get rid of it: It freaks parents out and makes them put pressure on children's eating. In reality, you don't expose your child to the food world. You expose them to meals and sit-down snacks made up of foods *you* choose from the grocery store and your kitchen. You include those foods again and again, meal after meal, day after day. In the process, your child learns to eat the variety of food that you eat, so they, in turn, can grow up to manage their food world.

Here's a little test: What happens to your following sDOR when you try to "make every bite count?"

Did you answer that you swerve into your child's lane with sDOR and your child eats less well, not better? You got it! Not to mention what it does to the peace and comfort of family meals.

Be alert to mixed-up tactics

Mixed-up approaches to feeding draw on both trust and control. It doesn't work. Trust is saying, *without reservation*, that when parents follow sDOR, children will eat what and as much as they need to grow well and be healthy. Control is keeping your fingers crossed, even when the controllers *say* they are following a division of responsibility or doing "responsive feeding."

Consider the University at Buffalo review of "positive parenting approaches" that recommend "goal-directed feeding practices to shape the types and amounts of food children consume."[28] Consider the Pennsylvania State College infant obesity-preventing INSIGHT "responsive feeding" intervention that used repeated neutral exposure "to increase food acceptance."[29] With both, note the contradictions in terms: You can't *both* do positive parenting *and* be goal-directed; you can't both be neutral *and* get children to eat certain foods. The alert reader will note that goal-directed advice drives on both sides of the sDOR road (Figure 1.3, page 12). In the research literature, such mixed-up approaches to feeding are often labeled "responsive feeding." The problem is that "responsive feeding" isn't well defined so it might or might not be goal-directed and therefore inconsistent with sDOR.

A review by Texas nutrition professionals of fruit and vegetable parenting practices includes getting children to eat "healthy" food by experimenting with *positive pressure*: praise, encouragement to take a bite, cutting food into cute shapes, enthusing about how great the food is, telling the child the food is healthy, makes them strong, or that their favorite cartoon characters eat it.[30]

A group of researchers from Britain propose the concept of *covert control*—a concept that is frequently cited by conventional nutrition professionals. Covert control is pressure that "can't be detected by the child" and includes tactics such as telling a child that a food tastes bad or is bad for them. Covert control transforms the structure that is essential to sDOR into a means for controlling children's eating: not buying sweets and crisps; only eating those foods when children are not around; avoiding cafes and restaurants that sell high-fat, high-sugar foods; stripping children's environment of all sweets and fatty food.[31] Covert pressure can be giving an approving look, saying "That food is good for you," putting the food closer to your child, or elaborately praising food you want your child to eat. I don't think I need to point out to you that covert pressure or restriction are still pressure or restriction, and that sooner or later children catch on.

Answer me this: Which of these covertly controlling strategies is consistent with sDOR? If you have trouble making the distinction, consider your intent: Which strategies have the intent of supporting your child's positive eating attitudes and behaviors? Which have the intent of getting your child to eat or not eat certain foods?

If you answered "none of the above" is consistent with sDOR, you get a gold star. If you said the strategies and intent are controlling, you get another. Imagine sneaking out to eat food you won't allow your child to eat! How long do you think you could get away with that? Children catch on to what you are doing, know that other children eat those foods, want them too, and eat them all the more when they get the opportunity. What is accomplished by "covert" restriction, and it is seriously negative, is that children feel bad about eating food they know their parents don't want them to eat. Longitudinal studies find that such restricted girls get fatter over time.[32]

In their defense, nutrition and health professionals who use goal-directed covert strategies have been trained in control, and the professional world in which they function is controlling. They care deeply about children's nutrition and wellness. It is not easy for them to trust parents to do their jobs, then let go of trying to influence what and how much children eat. Like parents, health professionals feel pressure to get children to eat well.

Consider the backstory

Trust depends on repeated neutral exposure to allow children to learn to eat a variety of foods. Control tries—generally unsuccessfully—to get children to eat certain foods. Consider the media release, "Tasting game increases children's vegetable consumption," praising the work of a London research group. Children increased their vegetable-liking more over two weeks when parents offered them, every day, a single very small piece of a target vegetable and rewarded them for eating it.[33]

More? More than whom? The context—the backstory—was that the comparison children never *saw* the vegetables. How can children learn to eat *anything* if they are never *exposed* to it?

Trust is knowing that parents and children who are Eating Competent can eat as much fat and other high-calorie food as they enjoy and their weights will be what their genetics indicate they will be. Control is a press release from a Pennsylvania State University child-obesity laboratory saying, "Eating fat makes children fat."[34] The backstory of the Penn State study is that many of the parents were dieters. They restricted their own and their daughters' fat intake, which made fatty foods "forbidden" and therefore highly desirable. When parents fell off their diets, both parents and children ate more fatty foods and gained weight. It wasn't the fatty food per se that disrupted children's weight, but the restriction and disinhibition.

WILL YOU BE TRUSTING OR CONTROLLING?

You choose. Raising your child with eating is about the long haul. Will you be more likely to hang in there with feeding if you try to get your child to eat their vegetables, worry about whether they drink too much or too little milk, or try to get them to weigh within certain limits? Or are you more likely to stay the course with feeding if you relax, have enjoyable family meals, trust your child, and assume their nutrition will be all right?

Is it realistic for you and your family to single your child out and play a two-week "tasting game," which may or may not be effective? To consistently hide vegetables in other food? To play games or make vegetables cute in order to get your child to eat them? Or is it more realistic for you to include vegetables in meals, enjoy vegetables yourself, and thereby give your child repeated neutral exposure to vegetables?

Of course, I advocate repeated neutral exposure, but as I have said before, my point of view is in the minority. To stick to sDOR, you have to ignore almost everyone around you who tells you which foods your child *should* eat and how to get them to eat those foods. It's not easy to ignore all the racket. As I said in Chapter 1, even if you know better than to go along with destructive advice, it is difficult to ignore what you are told. It happens. You may even give in and go along with the prevailing ideas, but paying attention to your child lets you self-correct. You observe that feeding is going poorly, you go back to following sDOR, and your child goes back to doing well with eating. Kids are resilient and change rapidly when we do.

You can't have it both ways. You can't both follow sDOR and try to get your child to eat "healthy" food. For you, the same as for health professionals, researchers, and policy makers, it comes down to *trust.* Will you follow sDOR, then trust your child to take it the rest of the way with whether and how much they eat and how they grow? Or will you doubt your child's natural inclinations and try to control their eating?

Consider your feelings

Let's consider your *feelings* about your choice: Will you be comfortable if you steer clear of playing the tasting game, being a cheerleader for vegetables, or hiding beets in the brownies? Will you feel you have done enough if you simply have pleasant family meals with your child, meals that include vegetables? You will be doing a *lot* when you consider the day-in-day-out, year-in-year-out of keeping family meals going. Even so, given the degree to which we have been steeped in controlling attitudes about food and eating, at first the repeated neutral exposure route is likely to feel *wrong*, even if your head knows otherwise. Hang in there: As with behavior change in any other area, your head changes first and your feelings catch up. It doesn't help that while you wait for your feelings to catch up, your child's short list of foods may get even shorter. Courage. Your child's food list will get longer as they come to trust that you really will let them eat what they want and not try to get them to eat anything they don't want.

Consider your preconceptions

If your conscience insists that you do something to *get* your child to eat "right," consider your preconceptions: Parents get caught in the shoulds and oughts, as well. More than one parent has told me that sDOR doesn't work because their child only eats vegetables when they—the parents—insist. Sure enough, when parents stop insisting, the child stops eating vegetables—for a while. That is to be expected. Their child needs time to recover from feeding pressure before they begin to trust they don't have to eat vegetables. After that, they can begin to take an interest in them. Their taking an interest might not happen for months or even years, and it is difficult to wait that long. In the meantime, pay attention to how much more pleasant family meals are for everyone without the hassles with children about eating.

I might add that only the compliant child can be forced to eat. Parents of more determined children discover to their chagrin that their child will sit *for hours* in front of a congealing plate of food without taking a bite. Remember that the goal is not to get children to eat vegetables *today* but to support them in learning to *enjoy* vegetables for a *lifetime*. If they are forced to eat vegetables when they are growing up, children will avoid them in later life—or the same as their parents, force them down because they feel obligated.

REFERENCES

1. Nas Z. Nature and nurture in fussy eating from toddlerhood to early adolescence: findings from the Gemini twin cohort. *Journal of Child Psychology and Psychiatry*. 2024. doi:10.1111/jcpp.14053
2. Cardona Cano S. Trajectories of picky eating during childhood: A general population study. *Int J Eat Disord*. 2015;48:570–579.
3. Davis CM. Self-selection of food by children. *The American Journal of Nursing*. 1935;35:403–410.
4. Sherry B. Attitudes, practices, and concerns about child feeding and child weight status among socioeconomically diverse white, Hispanic, and African-American mothers. *J Am Diet Assoc*. 2004;104:215–221.
5. Orrell-Valente JK. "Just three more bites": an observational analysis of parents' socialization of children's eating at mealtime. *Appetite*. 2007;48:37–45.
6. Fisher JO. Parental influences on young girls' fruit and vegetable, micronutrient, and fat intakes. *J Am Diet Assoc*. 2002;102:58–64.
7. Peters J. Associations between parenting styles and nutrition knowledge and 2-5-year-old children's fruit, vegetable and non-core food consumption. *Public Health Nutr*. 2013;16:1979–1987.
8. U.S. Department of Health and Human Services. *Dietary Guidelines for Americans. 8th Edition*. 2020.
9. Zucker N. Psychological and psychosocial impairment in preschoolers with selective eating. *Pediatrics*. 2015;136. doi:10.1542/peds.2014-2386
10. Lohse B. Valid and reliable measure of adherence to Satter Division of Responsibility in Feeding. *J Nutr Educ Behav*. 2021;53:211–222.
11. Lohse B. Use of an observational comparative strategy demonstrated construct validity of a measure to assess adherence to the Satter Division of Responsibility in Feeding. *Journal of the Academy of Nutrition and Dietetics*. 2021;121:1143–1156.e6.
12. Berge JM. Perspectives about family meals from single-headed and dual-headed households: a qualitative analysis. *Journal of the Academy of Nutrition and Dietetics*. 2013;113:1632–1639.
13. Lohse B. Diet quality is related to Eating Competence in cross-sectional sample of low-income females surveyed in Pennsylvania. *Appetite*. 2012;58:645–650.
14. Satter Eating Competence Model (ecSatter): Evidence-based research. *https://www.needscenter.org/resources/satter-eating-competence-model-ecsatter/*
15. Wardle J. An experimental investigation of the influence of health information on children's taste preferences. *Health Educ Res*. 2000;15:39–44.
16. Entin A. Parental feeding practices in relation to low diet quality and obesity among LSES children. *J Am Coll Nutr*. 2014;33:306–314.
17. Davis CM. Feeding after the first year. In: McQuarrie I, ed. *Brennaman's Practice of Pediatrics*. W.F Prior; 1957.
18. Anez E. The impact of instrumental feeding on children's responses to taste exposure. *J Hum Nutr Diet*. 2013;26:415–420.

19. Tate AD. Association between parental resource depletion and parent use of specific food parenting practices: An ecological momentary assessment study. *Appetite*. 2024. doi:10.1016/j.appet.2024.107368
20. Spill MK. Hiding vegetables to reduce energy density: An effective strategy to increase children's vegetable intake and reduce energy intake. *Am J Clin Nutr*. 2011;94:735–741.
21. Spill MK. Eating vegetables first: The use of portion size to increase vegetable intake in preschool children. *Am J Clin Nutr*. 2010;91:1237–1243.
22. Mathias KC. Serving larger portions of fruits and vegetables together at dinner promotes intake of both foods among young children. *Journal of the Academy of Nutrition and Dietetics*. 2012;112:266–270.
23. O'Connor TM. Parenting practices are associated with fruit and vegetable consumption in pre-school children. *Public Health Nutr*. 2010;13:91–101.
24. Wardle J. Modifying children's food preferences: the effects of exposure and reward on acceptance of an unfamiliar vegetable. *European Journal of Clinical Nutrition*. 2003;57:341–348.
25. Dwyer JT. The Feeding Infants and Toddlers Study (FITS) 2016: Moving forward. *The Journal of Nutrition*. 2018;148(suppl_3):1575S–1580S.
26. Welker EB. Room for improvement remains in food consumption patterns of young children aged 2-4 years. *J Nutr*. 2018. doi:10.1093/jn/nxx053
27. Savage JS. Parental influence on eating behavior: conception to adolescence. *J Law Med Ethics*. 2007;35:22–34.
28. Balantekin KN. Positive parenting approaches and their association with child eating and weight: A narrative review from infancy to adolescence. *Pediatr Obes*. 2020;15. doi:10.1111/ijpo.12722
29. Paul IM. Preventing obesity during infancy: a pilot study. *Obesity (Silver Spring)*. 2011;19:353–361.
30. O'Connor T. Health professionals' and dietetics practitioners' perceived effectiveness of fruit and vegetable parenting practices across six countries. *J Am Diet Assoc*. 2010;110:1065–1071.
31. Ogden J. Expanding the concept of parental control: a role for overt and covert control in children's snacking behaviour? *Appetite*. 2006;47:100–106.
32. Birch LL. Learning to overeat: maternal use of restrictive feeding practices promotes girls' eating in the absence of hunger. *Am J Clin Nutr*. 2003;78:215–220.
33. Fildes A. Parent-administered exposure to increase children's vegetable acceptance: A randomized controlled trial. *Journal of the Academy of Nutrition and Dietetics*. 2014;114:881–888.
34. Fisher JO. Fat preferences and fat consumption of 3 to 5-year-old children are related to parental adiposity. *Journal of the American Dietetic Association*. 1995;95:759–764.

CHAPTER 3

Your Child Knows How Much to Eat

Every child is entitled to eat as much as they are hungry for. Let me up the ante on that one: Even the fat child is entitled to eat as much as they want; even the thin child is entitled to eat as little as they want. For a child, being allowed to eat as much or as little as they want is the same as being given warmth, love, and acceptance. Being allowed too little food feels cold and rejecting. Being expected to eat too much food feels disrespectful.

You don't have to go there. You are entitled to relax and trust your child to know how much to eat. You can enjoy your child, hang on to your curiosity, and let yourself watch them grow up. "It ain't over," said baseball great and home-spun philosopher Yogi Berra, "'til it's over."

DEPEND ON EATING COMPETENCE

Your baby was born Eating Competent—they know how much to eat. You choose whether to breast- or bottle-feed or use some combination (Chapter 6). Then you preserve your baby's Eating Competence—their knowing how much to eat—by guiding feeding based on information coming from them about how much, how often, how fast—the list goes on. In the process, you also preserve your child's positive feelings about themselves and about you.

As your child gets older, they still have that instinctive knowing about how much to eat, and they still depend on your leadership and acceptance with feeding to continue to do well with food regulation. Food selection becomes more complex but following the Satter Division of Responsibility in Feeding (sDOR) with respect to food regulation remains the same: You do your jobs and let them do theirs. You go by your child's developmental readiness to choose what to offer—food that supports their making the transition to family food—and you continue to trust their ability to regulate their food intake. You defer to them to determine whether and how much they will eat from what you make available. It's a circular process: You trust your child from birth to know how much to eat, and they, in turn, are trustworthy. You continue to be willing to go by information coming from them—from birth—and they trust you to meet their needs. That mutual trust gives both of you a firm basis for the challenges and rewards to come.

This box demonstrates how Eating Competence works.

EATING COMPETENCE AND *HOW MUCH* YOUR CHILD EATS

Structure + food regulation capabilities =
energy balance and therefore constitutionally appropriate growth

Be wary of interference

The problem, as I have said before, is *interference*. That interference comes from the prevailing conviction that your child "should" eat the "right" amount to grow within "certain" limits. That interference characterizes control-paradigm thinking and doing with children's nutrition and growth. Folks laboring under the constraints of the control paradigm may warn you that your relatively high BMI or enthusiastically eating infant or child will get "too fat." The same control-paradigm thinking is behind warnings that your relatively low BMI or indifferently eating infant or child is growing poorly. Acting on those warnings—trying to get your child to eat less or more—makes them feel bad and takes away their ability to regulate their food intake. The restricted child reacts by trying to eat more; the pressured child by trying to eat less—exactly what the warning tells you to prevent. It takes courage to resist such interference. Following the *trust* paradigm—preserving your child's Eating Competence rather than trying to get them to eat and grow in a certain way—lets you act on behalf of your child. It's all about following sDOR and trusting your child.

As I emphasized in Chapter 1, following sDOR is trusting; interference is controlling. Trust supports your child's ability with internal regulation. Control undermines it. Figure 3.1 describes what helps as opposed to what hinders children's ability to eat the amount they need to grow in the way that is right for them.

FIGURE 3.1: SUPPORTING CHILDREN'S ABILITY WITH INTERNAL REGULATION

Children can be trusted. They have a strong and resilient ability to eat as much as they need.	
WHAT HELPS: TRUSTING YOUR CHILD'S EATING	**WHAT HINDERS: CONTROLLING YOUR CHILD'S EATING**
Letting your child pick and choose from the available food. Letting your child eat a lot. Letting your child not eat much. Letting your child eat more or less than other children eat. Letting your relatively fat child eat a lot. Letting your relatively thin child not eat much. Trusting how much your child eats meal after meal, day after day.	Trying to get your child to eat certain foods. Trying to get your child to avoid certain foods. Trying to get your child to eat less, more, or certain portion sizes. Pressuring or rewarding your child to eat. Having skimpy, uninteresting, unpleasant, or unappealing meals and snacks. Trying to get your child to grow in a certain way.

I will explain growth charts and percentiles in Chapter 4, Your Child Knows How to Grow. For now, know that each child tends to grow along a particular trajectory on the growth chart maintained for them by their health professional. That trajectory may be a high, low, or in-between percentile curve on their growth chart. Your child's growth is appropriate when it generally follows a particular percentile, even when that percentile is above the 85th or below the 15th. On the other hand, your child's growth may be concerning if it accelerates or falters: if it suddenly and considerably shifts up or down. Even such growth-shifting has to do with the feeding relationship. Children's accelerating or faltering growth doesn't happen for no reason. Something causes it, and that cause is highly likely to include a distortion in the feeding relationship.

IN THIS CHAPTER

This chapter addresses how your child's knowing how much to eat, from birth, depends on your trusting them and acting on that trust by following sDOR. sDOR continues to be important as your child gets older and depends on your respecting and trusting their natural ways with activity as well as eating. Throughout, the evidence supports following sDOR and trusting your child's natural ability to eat the amount they need to grow in the way that is right for them. The section at the end of the chapter, "Suspect prevailing 'evidence' and practice," reviews and critiques research and information in the media that can lead you astray. Your being able to identify the flaws in research allows you to ignore it.

FOLLOW THE SATTER DIVISION OF RESPONSIBILITY IN FEEDING

Your child will be Eating Competent—they will eat as much as they need to grow in the way that is right for them, provided you follow sDOR. Here is sDOR for your toddler-through-adolescent child:

> You are responsible for the *what, when,* and *where* of *feeding*.
>
> Your child is responsible for the *how much* and *whether* of *eating*.

Rather than trying to get your child to eat the "right" amount to grow within certain limits, sDOR raises your child to be Eating Competent: to eat and grow in the way that is right for them. When your child has good food regulation skills, they will:

- Eat as much as they are hungry for.
- Be relaxed about getting enough to eat.
- Enjoy their body and be relaxed about size and shape.
- Grow in the way nature intended for them.

sDOR works for all children

Because it is so important and because you may need reassurance, let me repeat what I said in the first two chapters: sDOR works with children of all sizes and temperaments, degrees of enthusiasm about eating, and eccentric ways with eating. It works with children who are neurodiverse, those with autism, those who have medical conditions such as diabetes and cystic fibrosis, and children who have syndromes such as Down syndrome and Russell-Silver syndrome. It works with relatively large and relatively small children and with children of all sizes in between.

sDOR supports "how much" for all developmental stages

Following sDOR and respecting your child's messages about *how much* are critical for their emotional and social development. Following sDOR with your newborn's sleeping and eating supports their achieving homeostasis—being calm and understandable—and, a few months later, supports their attachment—falling in love. Following sDOR as you respond to your child's readiness to make the transition to family meals supports their beginning separation/individuation—being their own person. Following sDOR with your toddler and preschooler allows you to do authoritative parenting, accept your toddler's continuing separation/individuation, and support your preschooler's initiative—confidently exploring the world. The stage-related chapters—7, 10, 11, and 12—discuss child development in more detail.

Following sDOR at every stage lets you establish feeding patterns that support your child's eating the amount that is right for them, both during the early years and beyond. Young adults who were raised with family meals tend to provide meals for themselves. Your child's positive and relaxed eating attitudes and behaviors growing out of your following sDOR support their eating as much as they need to grow in the way that is right for them. Conversely, their relaxed and positive eating attitudes and behaviors reassure you that feeding is going well.

The school-age child gradually begins to take on some of the *what*, *when*, and *where* for themself as they choose food at school, at the local store, and at friends' homes. With your guidance, school-age children who are Eating Competent can manage their own after-school snacks and contribute ideas for and even help prepare family meals. The adolescent is even more on their own with eating, but family meals remain important. The adolescent can be expected to show up for dinner on time and hungry and provide themself with meals and snacks when they are away from home. The adolescent needs to learn to manage food so they can learn to provide for themself after they leave home. The two booklets, *Feeding with Love and Good Sense: 6 through 13 Years* and *Feeding with Love and Good Sense: 12 through 18 Years* offer guidance in brief for feeding your older child. They are available from the Ellyn Satter Institute.

Crossing sDOR lines creates crashes

With respect to how much your child eats, it is particularly important to stay in your own lane with feeding. I told you in Chapter 1 that trust is a two-way street and have told many stories describing the crashes that result when parents cross the double yellow line between their jobs and their child's jobs. Staying in your lane means providing regular and enjoyable meals and snacks; supporting your child's being in their lane means, within that context, letting them determine whether and how much to eat from what you provide.

When parents cross the lines of sDOR, some children eat too much, and their growth accelerates; other children eat too little and their growth falters. Some children are such good regulators that they manage to eat the amount they need and grow consistently despite lack of support with *what*, *when*, and *where* and interference with *whether* and *how much*, although their eating attitudes and behaviors suffer. Remember, your long-term goal is to raise a child who is relaxed and confident about their eating. Crossing the lines of sDOR creates conflict, makes children anxious about eating, and impairs their Eating Competence.

TRUST YOUR CHILD TO KNOW HOW MUCH TO EAT

When family meals are in place, you can trust your child to eat as much as they need. By *family meals* I mean the package: Sit-down meals + sit-down snacks. I also mean sitting together and sharing the same food: not "perfect" food—just food.

Structure frees you from micro-managing

What is your knee-jerk response when your child who eats a lot of food asks for second or third helpings? Is it to provide the food, or do you cross over into their lane? Do you try to interest them in the salad? Do you say, "Here you are," or do you say, "Are you sure?" or "You already ate a lot!" or do you give them the "look?" What if your child is exceptionally large? Can you still say, "Here you are?" What if someone you value is calling your child's growth into question? Can you still say, "Here you are?"

At the other extreme, how do you react when your child asks to leave the meal having eaten very little? Do you say, "Okay, but that's it until snack time." Or do you say, "You hardly ate anything!" or "Eat your cheese and then you can go." What if your child is exceptionally small? Can you still say, "Okay, but that's it until snack time?" What if you just came from an appointment where your child's growth was called into question? Can you still say, "Okay, but that's it until snack time?"

These are tricky questions, so if you answered no to some of them, be gentle with yourself. Micro-managing what and how much children—and we ourselves—eat is so common it seems automatic. But your child knows they are being managed and is likely to react. Be a pressure detective. What upset your child? What made you cross into your child's lane and/or doubt their abilities?

Keep in mind that children are resilient. When you stop micro-managing, your child will stop reacting—after a while. They need time and reassurance to know they won't have to eat any more, less, or different food than they want to.

Structure lets you trust your child

Following sDOR is feeding with love and trust, and it isn't necessarily easy. When you faithfully and accurately follow sDOR, you stifle your misgivings and give your child those helpings and you let your having-barely-eaten child leave the table. At first their eating will become more extreme, but then it will moderate. You will come to trust your child to know what they are doing, and they will come to trust you to let them eat what and as much as they want—from what you provide.

You are not throwing open the refrigerator door and letting your child eat anything they want: You are providing the structure of regular, sit-down meals and snacks with food that you choose. That gives you a great deal of influence over your child's eating without having to interfere with what and how much they eat. Getting rid of interference, in turn, lets your child enjoy family meals, learn to eat the food you eat, and eat as much or as little as they need. They have such firm conviction that they will get to eat that they don't even think about it. Having that conviction lets them tolerate being a bit hungry before the next time to eat, be matter of fact about exploring new foods, and be relaxed about "forbidden" food.

Parents who follow sDOR provide leadership that is open, accepting, and supportive of their child's independence. That leadership supports children's natural tendencies to eat as much as they need to grow in the way that is right for them, tendencies that they retain as they grow up. "Well, all right" detractors say, "Babies know how much to eat but children lose that ability by the time they are toddlers—or preschoolers—or in grade school—or in high school." Nonsense! Children continue to know how much they need to eat as long as parents follow sDOR. But when parents try to control whether and how much they eat, children can lose track of eating as much as they need. That loss can start in infancy. I say, "*can* lose track," because as I just told you, some children are such good regulators that no amount of interference disrupts their growth. Most lose track.

Your child may be bigger or smaller than average

If you are relaxed and curious about your child's growth, more power to you. You can skip this section! If not, this section is intended to help you.

Parents can have a natural and often unconscious tendency to try to moderate their child's growth extremes. I have told you before that policy makers define "normal" growth as being between the 15th and 85th BMI percentiles, and health professionals are expected to go by those guidelines. In my view, children outside those cutoff points are growth *diverse*, not abnormal. Labeling relatively large or small children as "abnormal," whatever euphemisms are used, leads to pressure or restriction with feeding and exacerbates the very issues it is intended to address. Such judgments are destructive because they take away trust in children's ability to grow in the way that is right for them.

To protect yourself from interference, remember that upward and consistent growth is normal at any level; accelerating or faltering growth is concerning at any level. Stated in another way, from the trust perspective, children's growth is normal when it follows along at a particular percentile level, even if that percentile is very high or very low. Children's growth becomes concerning only when it accelerates or falters from its usual growth trajectory.

Even when children's growth is concerning, it is critical not to restrict their food intake to get their growth to slow or pressure them to eat more to get their growth to go faster. Instead, check yourself to make sure sDOR is in place. Be particularly alert to whether you are pressuring your child to eat or doing something that makes them afraid of going hungry. If you are at a loss for what is going on, get outside help. I typically found that I had to be a detective to uncover the source of distortion and source of support over several sessions to help parents take leadership with feeding and give their child autonomy with eating.

Your child may eat a little or a lot

Structure works to support internal regulation with children who eat unusually large or small amounts. All three of my children looked average in size and shape but plotted relatively tall and heavy on their growth charts. All three ate relatively small amounts of food. All three instinctively ate as much as they needed. As adults, they have kept those instincts, have continued to eat moderately, are about average in size and shape, and are relatively heavy. I was astonished the first time my daughter Kjerstin stopped eating in the middle of a bowl of ice cream. I am sure the boys did the same, but I was no longer astonished—I assumed that was normal child eating behavior. None of my children felt deprived because they couldn't eat as much as their big-eating friends. Even sturdy Curtis, who had a relatively small appetite, was unaware that his slender friend Jason ate at least twice as much as he did.

It's okay to *love* to eat

Loving to eat is about *feelings*, and your child needs you to accept those feelings about eating as much as they need you to accept any of their other feelings. Some children particularly enjoy eating, others are ho-hum about it. For them all, sDOR works to support internal regulation. The problem arises when parents can't *accept* and don't *trust* their child's normal inclinations for eating and react by trying to get their child who loves to eat to eat less, or the one who is blasé about eating to eat more. Parents react out of love and concern, but from the child's point of view, their parents' reaction means there is something wrong with them—with the child. Parents cross into their child's lane with feeding, hurt their child's feelings, and run the risk of creating problems with the child's eating and growing.

Being alarmed by a child's eating enthusiasm is so common that even your well-meaning health professionals could encourage you to put on the brakes with how much your child eats. Judging by the number of journal articles on the topic, researchers are attracted to the idea that variations in children's eating attitudes and behaviors can make them "too fat." Consider a review from Britain of over 1,000 studies demonstrating that children have a greater tendency to "obesity" when their parents rate them as being eager and enthusiastic about eating, preoccupied with food, having a poorly defined stopping place, and eating for emotional reasons.[1] Consider an article from Pennsylvania State University Nutritional Sciences saying one-year-olds who particularly enjoy eating become eight-year-olds who are fatter: They eat more when given large portion sizes and free access to high-calorie snacks.[2]

These studies leave the impression that there was something wrong with children that made them get fat. Think of that! What does it do to children to blame them for their fatness? There is so much stigma about being fat, and then to pile self-blame on top of that—it boggles the mind! But I digress. Those hundreds of studies all had a missing piece, and it was an enormous one: they failed to observe the parent-child feeding relationship. You simply cannot understand a child's eating unless you observe and understand what goes on between them and their parents with feeding. Had the researchers examined the parent-child feeding relationship, they likely would have found that there was something wrong with *feeding*. Enthusiastically eating children become preoccupied with food and eat seemingly without stopping only when they can't trust that they will get enough to eat. Children eat for emotional reasons when parents give food handouts for any and all upsets.

On the other hand, enthusiastically eating children eat as much as they need and grow consistently when parents follow sDOR. They have a stopping place. Children whose parents follow sDOR do not learn to eat for emotional reasons because they don't get food handouts when they are upset.

For a discussion of parent BMI and child weight, see the Chapter 4 section, "People of size do not eat poorly," page 117. The control assumption is that "obese/overweight" people eat too much of the wrong food (and get their child to do the same). A few might, but most make the mistake of restricting their children's food intake, hoping that doing so will keep children from being fat. Parents of all sizes and shapes do well with respect to feeding their children when they follow sDOR.

A large child who loved to eat

The word *avid* is used to describe some children's eating. It is defined as a child who particularly enjoys food and responds to the food in their environment. They also eat for emotional reasons and seemingly eat more than they are hungry for.[3] Enjoying and responding to food are inborn characteristics. Eating for emotional reasons and eating more than they are hungry for grow out of distortions in feeding dynamics.

The subjective meaning of *avid* is "desirous to the point of greed." In today's austere food world, normal food enjoyment may be viewed as avid. Sarah, a chubby baby, *loved* to eat. She loved eating so much that her eyes would light up and she would sit bolt upright in her high chair, eyes fixed on the food, eagerly anticipating each bite. When food was in her mouth, Sarah would *moan* with pleasure. Sarah loved feeding herself with her hands, folding her fingers over to capture the food and pressing it into her mouth.

Sarah's mother was humiliated. She thought Sarah's passion for food was greedy and therefore indecent, and she feared Sarah's passion would make her fat. She was particularly embarrassed that their friends and family so enjoyed Sarah's eager eating that they gathered around to watch, laughing and exclaiming.

Sarah's weight did accelerate, but the real problem was not Sarah's eating enthusiasm; it was *food restriction*. Her mother tried to get her to eat less, whereupon Sarah ate more and appeared even more enthusiastic about eating. Sarah's audience contributed their own interference by goading Sarah to eat. Sarah couldn't win. On the one hand, she was being restricted; on the other, she was being cheered on to eat a lot. Once she felt on firmer ground with feeding, Sarah's mother told Sarah's audience to cease and desist. It took a while for Sarah to recover from the contradiction of being both restricted and encouraged to eat. However, after a while she went back to enjoying eating and having a stopping place. She ate a lot sometimes, not so much other times.

Sarah was learning that there was something wrong with her that needed to be changed in order for her mother to truly love her. It was the last thing her mother intended, but there it is. Freeing Sarah's mother to trust her daughter with eating freed her to accept Sarah for the fine little person that she truly was.

GET COMFORTABLE WITH NOT KNOWING

You can know what's on the menu for meals and sit-down snacks. You can know that your family meals are enjoyable and that your child enjoys being there. You can know there is enough food so that everyone gets enough. But you can't know how much your child *should* eat. I know this is quite different from what you have been led to believe. The diet culture predicts how much we need and says that we should control it. But the truth is, we can't predict how much we need to eat, and we certainly can't predict that for our children. But, hey, we still want to *know*, and some generalities might even be helpful.

We can't predict how much

Even though you can't predict, considering how much children eat *is* interesting and *can* help you remain calm when your child eats extreme amounts. Duke University Health Sciences professor Asheley Skinner, PhD, analyzed the food intake of almost 13,000 children, ages 1 to 17 years. Average intakes for the two days surveyed for 1- to 3-year-olds was 1,350 calories. There was nothing surprising about that number but consider this: The range was 180 to 3,700 calories! That is, the least-eating toddlers ate 180 calories per day, the most-eating toddlers 3,700 calories. For 3- to 5-year-olds, the average intake was 1,600 calories, the range 400 to 4,500 calories. For 6- to 8-year-olds, the average was 1,850 calories, the range 600 to 4,500 calories.[4]

Not only is there huge variation child to child, but there are also many metabolic moving parts within each child. The first paragraphs in Chapter 4 introduce the concept of children's physical homeostasis: how they instinctively balance energy in and energy out and grow in the way that is right for them. Even exceptionally large and exceptionally small children maintain homeostasis. Small-eating children seemingly eat astonishingly little but still do well. Big-eating children eat more than their parents but still grow consistently. Children designated "overweight" or "obese" by policy makers often eat less than their "healthy" weight peers.[4]

Children vary day-to-day

I suppose it is possible that some of Skinner's children consistently got along on a few hundred calories every day and that others required thousands. It's more likely that surveyors happened to catch the children on days that their food intake was extreme. Allow my granddaughter Marii to illustrate. When she was a toddler and preschooler, Marii ate very inconsistently. Some days—many days in a row, in fact—Marii ate very little—bites, fingerfuls, sips. Other days, she ate more than you could imagine such a small and slender girl could even get *inside* her. She grew consistently at the 25th weight percentile.

DO NOT TRY TO CONTROL HOW MUCH

The folks who define a child as "overweight" when their BMI is at or above the 85th percentile offer the solution of eating the "right" foods and avoiding the "wrong" foods. Do a web search for *diet for childhood obesity*. You will come across the "healthy eating pattern," which encourages eating lots of fruits and vegetables, whole grains, low-fat dairy and meat, and few if any sweets and chips. Those recommendations come from the US Dietary Guidelines.[5] Although the advice to follow this "healthy eating pattern" is repeated so often by so many that it seems true, there is *no evidence* that it "allows children to achieve lower BMI percentiles."

In defining a "healthy eating pattern," the Dietary Guidelines is addressing an entire population and attempting to promote variety, but they are doing it in a prescriptive fashion. As is typical of food-management prescriptions, very few people actually follow the guidelines; more are left feeling bad about what and how much they and their children eat, still others ignore the guidelines altogether. There is no way to say from far away and about everybody what and how much they should eat. There are just too many intricacies in food availability and economic reality, not to mention individual metabolic variation.

You don't need a prescription, nor does your child. Being Eating Competent and following sDOR allow you and your child to function on a far more sophisticated level. You can trust hunger, appetite, and satiety to address nutritional needs as well as accommodate the continually shifting homeostasis of growth, body weight regulation, and illness and health. You can trust your child to grow in the way that is right for them. You do not need to try to force your consistently growing child's weight down to the 85th BMI percentile or below. Growing according to outside standards is a *control* concept. The trust concept is letting your child grow in the way that is *right for them*.

Being controlling with feeding does harm

Consider five-year-old Penelope. Penelope was big and had always been big—her weight and height were both consistently at the 95th percentile.

Because her weight and height were the same, her BMI was at the 50th percentile. To her very great credit, Penelope's doctor reassured her parents that she was just fine. But the parents had learned their societal lessons about risks for childhood "obesity," and they did what they thought was right to try to slim Penelope down. They were concerned about nutrition, ate organic, and their diet was a model of the "healthy eating pattern." They struggled with Penelope to get her to eat her fruits and vegetables. Penelope was only mildly interested in the food at family meals. She was likely not the only one, as her mother threw out a lot of food.

Penelope was, however, highly interested in the food at birthday parties and at the Friday-night neighborhood buffets. She hung around the food and ate as much as her parents would let her. Penelope would rather eat than play with the other children, and her mother's friends laughed at the how enthusiastically Penelope ate. Despite all the interference with her eating, Penelope was an excellent regulator. Her weight consistently followed the 95th weight percentile.

The problem was that any and all dealings with food were miserable. To their equally very great credit, Penelope's parents picked up on Penelope's distress—and their own—and sought help from a professional well-versed in sDOR. They shifted from withholding and restricting to providing enjoyable food at mealtimes and giving Penelope permission to eat. It was scary for them at first because Penelope ate a lot of their newly more-appealing food and particularly ate a lot of the sweets they let her have for sit-down snacks. However, the parents hung in there and Penelope's eating settled down to the point where on Friday evenings and at birthday parties she became more interested in playing than eating.

Mary's parents kept the restriction going

I generally spare you stories of feeding intentions gone *very* wrong, but this issue is so important it needs to be emphasized. Let me begin with a word in defense of parents: Our diet culture can leave them terrified of their child's being fat. Particularly if they have struggled with their own weight, they can assume the way to keep their child happy and safe is to keep them thin. Sadly, such efforts do a lot of harm: They spoil feeding, and they teach the child there is something seriously wrong with them. Feeling bad about themself makes a child a target for bullying. Ironically, restricting children's eating is likely to make them grow up to be fatter than nature intended them to be.

This story is extreme because the parents persisted in their attempts to restrict the child's eating and weight despite the fact that it was causing her a great deal of distress. Therein lies the saving grace for you and provides, up front, the moral of this story. You know when your child is unhappy, and you seek solutions. Mary's parents were so committed to keeping her from being fat that they could not let themselves be aware of how deeply unhappy she was.

Nineteen-year-old Mary was bulimic. She threw up every time she ate because she felt miserable about herself and was trying to address that misery by losing weight. Mary's earliest memory of eating was of being dished up small portions of very carefully chosen food. And she cried, because to her, not getting enough food seemed very much like not getting enough love. Mary felt profoundly hurt by her parents' actions, singled out, and deeply ashamed of her longings for food and her actually quite lovely body. She was notorious in her family for "stealing" food from the cupboards and refrigerator, and she was ashamed of herself for wanting to eat so much more than her parents wanted to feed her.

Unlike Penelope's parents, Mary's parents couldn't, or wouldn't, tune in to Mary's misery. They were determined to make Mary thin, and they persisted in withholding food from her year after year, even though it wasn't working. Mary's weight remained higher than her parents wanted despite all their efforts. When Mary got out on her own, she sought help and had to work for a long time to become positive and self-trusting about her eating and feel better about her body. It took even longer for her to feel better about herself.

It is all such a waste. Despite the almost universal handwringing, children of size do not become "too fat" and, in fact, tend to become taller and learner as they get older.[6] Restricting children's eating is likely to cancel this natural growth process and convert it into gaining excessive fat. Let me say that in different words, because it is *so* important: Large children's weight tends to gradually shift toward average as they get older. It does, that is, unless parents restrict them. Then, they tend to gain more weight than nature intends them to.

Let your child grow at their own pace

Now let's consider parents who struggled to get their child to eat more and be bigger. Timothy comes to mind, a prematurely born baby whose weight perked along at a consistent and gradually increasing low percentile level on his growth chart as his parents devoted themselves to getting on his wavelength with feeding. Feeding and growth went well, that is, until at an appointment his doctor said, "He should be growing faster." This was their wonderful doctor, who had taken care of Timothy during his early months in the NICU. Of course, they trusted his advice to get Timothy to eat more, and overnight feedings changed from lovely times of being on the same wavelength to unpleasant struggles. Timothy's parents woke him up to feed him, tried to get him to finish bottles, and constantly worried that the amount of formula he ate was less than the amount he was *supposed* to eat. Despite their best efforts, Timothy's weight fell off the growth curve and they started to feel like failures with feeding. Soon after, they got a feeding consultation. It was an easy fix: Go back to trusting him as they had done before. Feeling comfortable with trusting him was the hard part.

To their credit, they talked with Timothy's doctor and told him what he had missed: Before they started pressuring him to eat, Timothy had actually been slowly gaining weight. To his equal credit, the doctor took a closer look at Timothy's growth chart, agreed with the parents, and acknowledged that their original approach to feeding was the right one.

It is all too common for parents of preemies and other very small children to be advised to get their child to eat more and grow faster. They get into the same struggles with feeding that Timothy's parents did. It is especially sad because those parents have already been through so much! Feeding struggles that start early can go on month after month, year after year, and often produce a picky eater whose growth falters.

It is not unusual to get contradictory patterns. Children whose parents struggled to get to eat as infants and toddlers gain too much weight as older children: their weights accelerate upward from their seemingly normal curves. Rather than resisting early feeding pressure, those children gave into it and lost track of their sensations of hunger and fullness. They learned to chronically eat more than their body told them to, and that made them gain weight later on.

Right-food/wrong-food doesn't control how much

Provided parents follow sDOR, low-calorie food doesn't fool children into eating less and high-calorie food doesn't fool them into eating more. Their bodies know, and children are instinctively aware of the hunger and fullness sensations that give them that information. Adults, not so much. We have learned to ignore and override those sensations, to our detriment. Studies show that children offered a high- or low-calorie snack before a meal ate less at mealtime when they were given a high-calorie snack and more when they were given a low-calorie snack. They ended up eating the same number of calories overall. They did, that is, provided they weren't restricted at home. If they were restricted, they ate the same at the meal, no matter whether their snack had been high- or low-calorie, and they were fatter. Adults, the same as the restricted children, ate the same at the meal no matter what.[7]

The alert reader will note that this study is over 20 years old. I continue to use it because it is so complete: it observed children's actual food consumption and measured their and their mother's eating attitudes and behaviors. Children's biopsychosocial drives and their eating attitudes and behaviors do not change. They depend on positive feeding to do well with eating and they do less well when parents or other adults cross the lines of sDOR. A more-recent Australian study that used questionnaires and no observation found that same thing. Parent feeding restriction correlated with children's food preoccupation and tendency to eat as much as they could whenever they could.[8] It is typical of many other current studies using the same experimental strategies.

Your child will eat more or less of the food available to get as many calories as they need. As I emphasized in Chapter 2, they will learn to enjoy a variety of food provided they are given repeated neutral exposure to those foods. Children's fatness or thinness is not related to their food preference. Relatively fat children are no more partial to fatty or sugary foods and no less partial to fruit and vegetables than relatively thin children.[9] Children eat what they like, they don't eat food they find unappealing (even if it is good for them), and, when they get it regularly, they do not overeat on food they find particularly appealing. In fact, telling them a food is good for them makes them less inclined to eat it, not more.[7]

Sweets and chips don't make children fat

Children overeat on sweets and chips when sweets and chips are being restricted. When high-fat, high-sugar foods are treated as dietary no-nos, children want them and eat a lot of them when they can.

A series of *Eating in the Absence of Hunger* feeding experiments at the Pennsylvania State University Child Obesity laboratory found that children whose parents didn't let them eat as much as they wanted, particularly of "forbidden" foods, ate a lot of those foods when they could. Children who had not been restricted at home ate "forbidden" foods in moderation, irrespective of their weight. That's important, so allow me to restate it: The difference in children's food consumption came from whether they had been restricted at home, not from their relative size. Nonetheless, researchers targeted the children. They recommended that children should be taught to like "healthy" food and consume "appropriate" portion sizes. In other words, children should be taught to restrict themselves.[10] These were the same researchers who, two years earlier, interpreted their findings to mean that children know how much to eat and that you can't fool them.[7]

A later group from the same laboratory repeated the experiment and found that "normal" weight girls who ate a lot of "forbidden" foods in the laboratory had somewhat higher levels of body fat a year later. The feeding relationship was ignored, leading to the inevitable conclusion that the children who eat in the absence of hunger are *just that way*: They eat a lot for no apparent reason. Building on that conclusion, authors recommended keeping sweet and savory foods out of the home and teaching children to resist their food cravings.[11] That is, of course, a control-paradigm approach, in contrast to the trusting sDOR approach of moderating children's tendency to eat in the absence of hunger by regularly letting them have sweet and savory foods at meals and snacks.

In short, studies that examine feeding dynamics conclude that in order to be able to eat "forbidden" food in moderation, children need regular access. That is certainly the experience of ESI faculty members and other sDOR-informed clinical practitioners. These findings form the basis for the advice in the Chapter 2 section, "Relax about 'forbidden' food," page 50.

Let your child determine their own portion size

Parents want to know *how much* to give their child to eat. Whether they are going by portion sizes or some notion of how much their child "should" eat, almost all parents try to get their child to eat more when they say they are full.[12] Children who give in to the pressure and clean their plates lose track of their internal regulators: their sensations of hunger, appetite, and satiety. They eat in accordance with how much food is *there*, not how hungry or full they are. That leads to errors in food regulation: Children eat too much or too little and grow too rapidly or too slowly.

As the Skinner studies illustrated, you can't know or predict *how much* a child *should* eat (there's that pressure word again). Rather than leaving you totally up in the air, it may help to have an idea of a realistic serving size for a child: a tablespoon per year of age and offer more if your child wants it. That guideline is to keep you from overloading your child's plate, overwhelming them, and having a lot of food waste. It isn't to control how much they eat. It is even better to let your child serve themself—even toddlers can learn to be surprisingly good at it.

Although it is well established that children know how much to eat and that portion-sizing undermines that knowing,[7] portion-size research is popular in the nutrition world. Research highlights the importance of "right-sizing" children's portions with findings that children eat more calories when they are offered larger portions, particularly larger high-calorie portions. The results seem plausible until you take a look at the back story, which shows that children whose parents did not try to control how much they ate at home were unaffected by portion size, even of highly appealing food. This held true even for children whose parents rated them as particularly enjoying food.[13]

A spin-off of portion-sizing research is a study exploring serving dessert with the meal as a way to get children to eat less and, presumably, weigh less.[14] That advice misuses my long-standing sDOR-based advice on the dessert topic, offered with the intent of avoiding using dessert for leverage to get children to eat their vegetables. As I observed in Chapter 2, controlling tactics make children eat more dessert and fewer vegetables.

RESPECT YOUR CHILD'S NATURAL ACTIVITY

Manipulating activity can be a last-ditch effort to manipulate weight. Don't do it. Activity just *is*, and your child is entitled to enjoy it for its own sake. Children are born loving their bodies, curious about them, and inclined to be active. By moving, they learn about their body and hold on to their good feelings about it. Don't make today's common mistake of using activity to burn off calories, slim down, bulk up, or be generally "healthy." That will take all the fun out of it and is, in fact, demoralizing. Joyful activity is sustainable—it has a chance of developing into a lifelong habit of movement. Good parenting with activity involves following a division of responsibility:

You provide *structure, safety,* and *opportunities.*

Your child determines *how much* and *whether* to move and the *manner* of moving.

Figure 3.2 gives more detail about the division of responsibility in activity.

Let your child be naturally active

What you can do, and it is a *lot,* is to set up the environment so your child can do what comes naturally for them: move. Get your baby out of the infant seat onto a blanket on the floor so they can wiggle and kick. Develop your tolerance for noise and commotion. Inform yourself about reasonable levels of physical risk, find your child a safe place to play, and let them move. Keep a time limit on the TV. Free yourself from electronic babysitters by making your child responsible for dealing with their own boredom. Don't try to persuade or pressure your child to be active or you will experience the same kind of whiplash that you get from trying to control how much they eat.

FIGURE 3.2: THE SATTER DIVISION OF RESPONSIBILITY IN ACTIVITY

Children are born loving their bodies, curious about them, and inclined to be active. Good parenting with activity preserves those qualities. The division of responsibility with activity changes as the child grows.

The Satter Division of Responsibility in Activity for infants:

- Parents are responsible for *safe opportunities.*
- The child is responsible for *moving.*

The parent provides the infant with a variety of positions, clothing, sights, and sounds. Then the parent remains present and lets the infant enjoy moving.

The Satter Division of Responsibility in Activity for toddlers through adolescents:

- The parent is responsible for *structure, safety,* and *opportunities.*
- The child is responsible for *how, how much,* and *whether* they move and the *manner* of moving.

Parents' jobs:

- Develop judgment about normal commotion.
- Provide safe places for activity the child enjoys.
- Find fun and rewarding family activities.
- Provide opportunities to experiment with group activities such as sports.
- Set limits on screens but not on reading, writing, artwork, other creative sedentary activities.
- Remove the screens from the child's room.
- Make children responsible for dealing with their own boredom.

Parents trust children to do their jobs:

- Children will be active.
- Each child is more or less active depending on their constitutional endowment.
- Each child is more or less skilled, graceful, energetic, or aggressive depending on their constitutional endowment.
- Children's physical capabilities grow and develop.
- Children experiment with activities that are in concert with their growth and development.
- Children explore and find activities that are right for them.

Some children are more active than others

Children are naturally active, but each child is more or less active, skilled, graceful, energetic, or aggressive. As children grow and develop, their physical capabilities grow as well, and they experiment to find activities that are right for them.

Researchers who had children wear activity monitors found that about a fifth of children had high activity, both with physical and sedentary pursuits and another fifth were at the opposite extreme: low for both. The rest of the children showed combinations of the two: They had high or low physical activity paired with the opposite tendency in sedentary pursuits.[11]

Research doesn't identify or distinguish between low-activity and high-activity sedentary pursuits or make correlations with health.[15] It seems to me that you can find that out yourself by observing your child. Is their screen-viewing sedentary? My grandson Henry does not sit still when he watches TV! What about when they pursue other screen-time activities (e.g. writing, texting, emailing, video games)? Then there is studying, drawing, crafting, and/or doing puzzles. Jennifer's daughter was relatively inactive, but her sedentary pursuits were active: She preferred arts and crafts and reading, hunting for salamanders, and walking the beach looking for agates. My daughter Kjerstin showed similar patterns until she joined crew as a high school senior. My boys were relentlessly and exhaustingly active at all times. I didn't try to change any of them, although I did dream of ways to slow the boys down and I looked forward to their daily television allotment.

Activity fine-tunes *how much*

Research done with adults shows that being moderately active makes the food-regulation sensations of hunger, appetite, and satiety (feeling full and satisfied) more accurate and easier to detect and trust. That, in turn, supports homeostasis—automatically keeping energy systems in balance. That would be balancing calories in with calories out and maintaining stable weight or, for a child, growing predictably. On the other hand, being especially *inactive* appears to disrupt homeostasis by fooling the appetite into wanting more rather than less food, and weight goes up.

I think the research is fascinating, so bear with me, or skip it if it bores you. My favorite study is another of my oldies-but-goodies, done over 60 years ago by Harvard nutritionists with men in a jute factory in Bengal, India. That setting was chosen because there was such a range of activities, from men who sat all day to those who spent their days hauling huge and heavy bales. Men in the sedentary range—the ones who sat all day—ate more than they needed, and their weight accelerated. Once the men got into the active range their food consumption and weights became proportional and remained proportional at increasing activity levels.[16] The researchers called the weights across the activity range "J-shaped," meaning weights were balanced in upper activity ranges but excessive in the lower ranges.

More recent research from the Sport and Physical Activity Academy in the UK found the same J-shaped relationship between energy intake and activity. Inside the sedentary ranges, subjects gained weight. Outside the sedentary ranges the more active the research subjects were, the more they ate—and their weights were stable.[17]

The question, of course, is how much activity your child needs to get out of the sedentary range. I don't know, but it may be less than you think. For yourself, you can probably tell that when you are more regularly active it is easier to know when you are hungry and when you are full.

Limit your child's screen watching

As I noted earlier, only television watching is correlated with children's weight.[15] A nationwide analysis of almost 5,000 US children ages 8 through 16 in the 1988 to 1994 National Health and Nutrition Examination Survey found good news: 80 percent of parents reported three or more bouts of vigorous activity per week, and 40 percent of children watched one hour or less of television per day. On the other hand, one-quarter of US children watched four or more hours of television each day. Those children were heavier than those who watched fewer than two hours per day.[18]

Extrapolating from the J-shaped relationship between activity and body weight provides a logic for the relationship between high TV-watching and excess weight gain. Children who watched enough TV to put them in the sedentary range were heavier. Studies in a Memphis metabolic laboratory explain why: 8- to 12-year-olds watching television burned calories at a 15 percent lower rate than children doing other sedentary activities.[19] It would be fun to see how children's TV-watching has changed since the 1990s when these studies were done, but I could not find more recent studies. Today's children watch cell phones and tablets more than TV sets, and research doesn't distinguish among the type of electronic usage.

Children deprived of TV appeared to increase their activity level and energy expenditure even when they did other sedentary activities.[20] And that is good news: Reading, coloring, and doing puzzles use more energy than watching TV. Video games? I don't know. There is little research on the topic, and it is contradictory. Cell phone and tablet usage? Now, there's a question for you and certainly applies as your child gets older and chooses being on their portable electronic device over other activities!

While we don't have research evidence, we *can* consider good parenting. The American Academy of Pediatrics advises avoiding media for children under two years old and limiting it to one hour or less a day of "high-quality programming" for preschoolers. For grade-schoolers through teens: "Don't let media displace other important activities such as quality sleep, regular exercise, family meals, or 'unplugged' downtime." I might add socializing face-to-face rather than electronically.

Don't be your child's entertainment committee

Shutting down screens need not—in fact, must not—mean that you will become your child's entertainment committee. Certainly, you will take an interest, be companionable, and set aside a regular 15 or 20 minutes to play; it doesn't have to go on forever for you and your child to connect. With playing, as with eating, children benefit from taking the lead while you are a supportive presence. Your child may want you to lose at Candyland for the hundredth time, and they will find it as fresh and exciting as the first time.

However, once you have done that, it is up to your child to take it the rest of the way. Your child benefits from being bored. Rather than wearing yourself out trying to entertain your child, let them figure out what to do with themself. Let them discover they enjoy their own company by doing something creative and wonderful.

FOLLOW sDOR IN FEEDING *YOURSELF*

Whatever your weight or attitudes and beliefs about food and eating, for the sake of your child if not for yourself, consider lightening up. Support your eating in the way you support your child's by applying the sDOR routine-plus-trust principles to feeding yourself:

- Provide yourself with regular and reliable meals and snacks made up of food you enjoy.
- Let yourself eat what and as much as you want and then stop, knowing another meal or snack is coming soon and you can do it again.

Chapter 5, Discover the Joy of Eating, talks more about your Eating Competence. It introduces you to The Joy of Eating: Becoming Eating

Competent (sBEC). My wish is for you to free yourself from the misery of struggling with your eating and weight.

Accept your own eating and weight

sBEC, the same as sDOR, requires routine plus trust, supports your dietary excellence, and makes it possible for you to know how much to eat. sBEC is feeding yourself faithfully and giving yourself permission to eat. It means making time to eat, paying attention while you do it, and eating as much as you want of food you enjoy.

Following sBEC allows you to trust your body to know how much to eat and how much to weigh. Trusting yourself allows you to trust your child. Conversely, worrying about your weight and trying to control your eating interferes with your ability to trust your child's eating. Despite your best intentions, struggling with your own weight can make you a restrained feeder: You are likely to try to get your child to eat less and less appealing food in hopes of keeping them slim. It doesn't work and, instead, creates the very problem it is intended to prevent.

Resist stereotypes

The conviction that fat people eat too much and pass that tendency on to their children is so strong that it distorts the way research is interpreted. "Obese" mothers are said to eat too much fat, feed it to their daughters, and the daughters are heavier.[10] Let's reexamine that interpretation of the Penn State Child Obesity Laboratory study, taking feeding dynamics into account. Daughters who ate relatively large amounts of fat had mothers who chronically restrained and disinhibited—who dieted and fell off diets. When mothers restrained, they ate little fat and when they disinhibited, they ate a lot of fat. Their daughters experienced the same famine-and-feast cycle and ate more fatty food when it was available. Unlike people who regularly have fat-containing food and eat moderate amounts of it, those self-restricted mothers and their children overate on fat when it was available.

SUSPECT PREVAILING "EVIDENCE" AND PRACTICE

I have said before and will undoubtedly say again: Following sDOR requires steady nerves and a leap of faith. Prevailing thought can get on your nerves and undermine your faith. The prevailing control-paradigm thinking is that unless they are controlled or coerced, children will eat too much and get "too fat," and they won't eat their vegetables. Not only that, but most controlling thinkers fail to consider the child in the context of the feeding relationship. They warn that an eagerly eating child could gain too much weight or develop an eating disorder. Such thinking neglects the reality that eager eaters grow up to have eating and weight distortion only if parents are so spooked by their child's eating enthusiasm that they attempt to restrict and control what and/or how much their child eats.

As in previous chapters, this evidence section is meant to help you avoid interference. A lot of the interference comes in the form of spin—interpreting research so that it conforms to prevailing thought. That conviction is that children have to be managed or coerced in order to eat and grow well. I touched on spin in my Chapter 2 criticism of studies claiming children eat vegetables better when parents play a tasting game. There was spin in the study I just discussed—the one that concluded that eating fat will make children fat. The trusting stance is that, in the context of sDOR, children will get around to eating their vegetables. Not only that, but they will eat as much or as little fat as they need to make their food taste good and satisfy their energy needs.

Ignore insistence that your large child needs to lose weight

Child "overweight/obesity" hysteria is hard to ignore, and the pressure on you to do something about your exceptional child's weight is considerable—even enormous. Those who preoccupy themselves with slimming down "overweight/obese" children by getting them to eat less and move more keep trying and, when it doesn't work, try harder. The 2023 American Academy of Pediatrics Clinical Practice Guidelines for Child Obesity recommends diagnosis and treatment starting at age two years with children whose BMI exceeds the 85th percentile. This treatment includes intensive health behavior and lifestyle treatment and, in extreme cases, use of weight-loss drugs and bariatric surgery in children as young as 13 years old. Intensive health behavior and lifestyle treatment is up to and even over one year-long intervention with doctors, nutritionists, exercise physiologists, and mental health professionals.[21]

Aside from the fact that very few busy pediatricians in clinical offices come anywhere near to being able to offer such intervention, it doesn't work! Multidisciplinary weight interventions of 52 to 114 contact hours show reductions of less than one BMI point: say, from the 95th to the 94th percentile. Nonetheless, this is the path recommended by AAP for all parents of large children, even though authors of the recommendations realize full well that such treatment is characterized by relapse and must be applied again and again.[21]

Following sDOR and letting children grow in the way that is right for them lasts a lifetime.

Food restriction can make children gain weight

Clinically, we often see children whose growth abruptly accelerates after they are diagnosed as being "overweight" or "obese" and parents begin trying to restrict their food intake. Typically, parents attempt to follow standard weight-management guidelines (lots of low-calorie food, hardly any high-calorie food) reinforced by restrained feeding: controlling the child's portion sizes, saying, "Are you sure you really want that?" and giving them "the look."

The research supports our clinical observations. Particularly convincing are the large-scale studies I review in the Chapter 4 section, "Protect your child against diagnosis," page 121. Children perceived by their parents as being "overweight" or "obese" tended to get heavier over time than children perceived by parents as being about the right weight.

As I just said, even intensive and highly organized weight-reduction efforts do not work any better for children than they do for adults,[22] if by "working" you mean forcing children to lose weight. Part of the challenge of such interventions and long-term weight maintenance is neutralizing the obesogenic influence of food restriction: Children and adults fed restrictively tend to overeat periodically and get fatter over time! Nonetheless, child "obesity" thought-leaders ignore the data, insist that parents accept child "obesity" diagnoses,[23] and come up with ever more forceful interventions.[21] Such thought-leaders definitely do *not* consider addressing the issue in a way that it can be solved—following sDOR and letting children grow in the way that is right for them.

TRUST YOUR CHILD AND ENJOY FEEDING

Following sDOR means trusting your child and resisting interference; it does not mean doing nothing at all. In fact, it means doing a *lot*. It means providing regular meals at predictable times and sit-down snacks between times throughout your child's growing-up years. It means being so reliable with feeding that your child doesn't even have to *think* about whether they will get to eat. It means—and perhaps the most difficult part—managing your anxiety, ignoring your well-meaning but interfering advisors, and trusting your child to eat as much as they need so they can grow up to get the body that is right for them. With such an enormous job, why would you ask for more by trying to manage what or how much your child eats?

Following sDOR is the gift that keeps on giving. Every day, every *meal*, feeding your child will give you joy. At the same time, your child will develop positive attitudes and behaviors about eating and about themself that will serve them throughout life.

REFERENCES

1. Kininmonth AR. The relationship between the home environment and child adiposity: a systematic review. *Int J Behav Nutr Phys Act*. 2021;18. doi:10.1186/s12966-020-01073-9
2. Keller KL. PACE: a novel eating behavior phenotype to assess risk for obesity in middle childhood. *J Nutr*. 2024. doi:10.1016/j.tjnut.2024.05.019
3. Edwards KL. Examining parents' experiences and challenges of feeding preschool children with avid eating behaviour. *Appetite*. 2024/07/01/2024;198:107372.
4. Skinner AC. Self-reported energy intake by age in overweight and healthy-weight children in NHANES, 2001–2008. *Pediatrics*. 2012. doi:10.1542/peds.2012-0605
5. U.S. Department of Health and Human Services. *Dietary Guidelines for Americans*. 8th *Edition*. 2020.
6. Wright CM. Breast-feeding in a UK urban context: who breast-feeds, for how long and does it matter? *Public Health Nutr*. 2006:686–891.
7. Birch LL. Family environmental factors influencing the developing behavioral controls of food intake and childhood overweight. *Pediatr Clin North Am*. 2001;48:893–907.
8. Say A. The correlation between different operationalisations of parental restrictive feeding practices and children's eating behaviours: systematic review and meta-analyses. *Appetite*. 2023;180. doi:10.1016/j.appet.2022.106320
9. Hill C. Adiposity is not associated with children's reported liking for selected foods. *Appetite*. 2009;52:603–638.
10. Birch LL. Learning to overeat: maternal use of restrictive feeding practices promotes girls' eating in the absence of hunger. *Am J Clin Nutr*. 2003;78:215–220.
11. Bhat YR. Eating in the absence of hunger is a stable predictor of adiposity gains in middle childhood. *The Journal of Nutrition*. 2024;154:3726–3739.
12. Sherry B. Attitudes, practices, and concerns about child feeding and child weight status among socioeconomically diverse white, Hispanic, and African-American mothers. *J Am Diet Assoc*. 2004;104:215–221.
13. Kling SM. Double trouble: portion size and energy density combine to increase preschool children's lunch intake. *Physiol Behav*. 2016. doi:10.1016/j.physbeh.2016.02.019
14. Huss LR. Timing of serving dessert but not portion size affects young children's intake at lunchtime. *Appetite*. 2013;68:158–163.
15. Chaput J-P. 2020 WHO guidelines on physical activity and sedentary behaviour for children and adolescents aged 5–17 years: summary of the evidence. *International Journal of Behavioral Nutrition and Physical Activity*. 2020;17. doi:10.1186/s12966-020-01037-z
16. Mayer J. Relation between caloric intake, body weight and physical work. *American Journal of Clinical Nutrition*. 1956;4:169–175.
17. Beaulieu K. Does habitual physical activity increase the sensitivity of the appetite control system? a systematic review. *Sports Med*. 2016;46:1897–1919.
18. Andersen RE. Relationship of physical activity and television watching with body weight and level of fatness among children: results from the Third National Health and Nutrition Examination Survey. *JAMA*. 1998;279:938–942.

19. Klesges RC. Effects of television on metabolic rate: potential implications for childhood obesity. *Pediatrics*. 1993;91:281–286.
20. Epstein L. Effects of manipulating sedentary behavior on physical activity and food intake. *Journal of Pediatrics*. 2002;140:334–339.
21. Hample SE. Executive Summary: clinical practice guideline for the evaluation and treatment of children and adolescents with obesity. *Pediatrics*. 2023. doi:e2022060641
22. O'Connor EA. Screening for obesity and intervention for weight management in children and adolescents: evidence report and systematic review for the US Preventive Services Task Force. *JAMA*. 2017;317:2427–2444.
23. Gerards SM. Parental perception of child's weight status and subsequent BMIz change: the KOALA birth cohort study. *BMC public health*. 2014. doi:10.1186/1471-2458-14-291

CHAPTER 4

Your Child Knows How to Grow

In your child's mind, trusting their growth is about trusting and accepting *them*. Trying to control and modify their growth is about controlling and rejecting *them*. Even when they get older, no child should have to worry about their eating, moving, or weight. Such worries amount to lack of self-acceptance and are deeply wounding. I realize I am being blunt, and that is exactly how I mean it. My intent is to protect you and your child. Today's concern about "overweight/obesity" prevention has reached epidemic proportions. Acting on that concern by becoming controlling with feeding can harm your feeding relationship and therefore your child. It can also create the very problem you are trying to prevent.

sDOR LETS YOU TRUST YOUR CHILD'S GROWTH

Follow the Satter Division of Responsibility in Feeding (sDOR) and let your child grow in the way that is right for them. Your child was born knowing how much to eat to support their distinctive size and shape. It is the same with activity: They were born with a tendency to be more or less active, and their level of activity supports their distinctive size and shape—and their eating. When they are the *Competent Eater* that we have been discussing, they don't have to work at it: They just *live* it. This is trust-paradigm thinking and doing, based on accepting and depending on children's capabilities with eating, moving, and growing *in the way that is right for them*. This is in contrast to control-paradigm thinking and doing, which attempts to manage children's eating and activity and thereby get children to eat and grow *in certain ways*.

Your child will be a Competent Eater when you follow sDOR. If you recall, a Competent Eater enjoys family meals, picks and chooses from the food you provide, and eats as much or as little as they want. Those positive eating attitudes and behaviors let them instinctively eat in the way that keeps all their systems in balance and allows them to grow in the way that is right for them: They maintain *homeostasis*. Chapter 3 defined newborn *emotional and social* homeostasis as being calm and understandable. In this context, we are talking about *physical* homeostasis: maintaining a state of balance within the body. Both have to do with being able to adapt to external and internal conditions and remain stable.

Growth, *what*, and *how much* are so tied together that I debated whether to make growth a separate chapter. Discussing growth issues often demands straying into *what* and *how much*, with particular emphasis on *how much*. I tried putting growth in the *how much* chapter, where you will also find *activity*, but that gave the chapter too much to do. So, let's bash on and put up with the overlapping areas while we consider growth.

IN THIS CHAPTER

This chapter continues the discussion from previous chapters by addressing what you can do to let your child eat, move, and grow in the way that is right for them—even when that growth is at the extremes. Because control-paradigm thinking and practice is such a part of addressing children's weight, this chapter reviews research as we go along rather than saving it for a separate section toward the end. You can still skip the parts that are particularly heavy going, such as "Children's growth adjusts," and "What about weight and health?"

The research supports the trust-paradigm perspective of trusting infants and children to know how to grow. In the first six months to a year, growth can be unpredictable, but after the first year children's growth generally settles down to follow a particular growth curve, with minor zigs and zags. Consistent growth at any percentile is likely to be appropriate. Abrupt, rapid, and prolonged acceleration or faltering after the first year may not be appropriate and calls for detecting and addressing any disruptions and following sDOR. The task is not, *ever*, to try to get a child to eat more or less.

sDOR SUPPORTS HOMEOSTASIS

Your child will keep their eating and activity in balance and grow in the way that is right for them when you follow sDOR. Here is sDOR for your toddler-through-adolescent child. For other feeding stages, see Figure 1.2, page 8, Satter Division of Responsibility in Feeding.

You are responsible for the *what, when,* and *where* of *feeding*

Your child is responsible for the *whether* and *how much* of *eating.*

Here we arrive at one of those places where *growth* and *how much* are tied together. Children's knowing how much to eat depends on the food regulation capabilities we discussed in the last chapter. A child does well with food regulation and therefore growth when they:

- Eat as much as they are hungry for.
- Are relaxed about getting enough to eat.
- Enjoy their body and are relaxed about size and shape.
- Grow in the way nature intended for them.

Your job is to support your child's eating: It is to drive in your lane, as we discussed in Chapter 1, and stay out of your child's lane. That is a saying a *lot,* but you don't have to be perfect. Your driving won't always be the greatest and you may even stray into your child's lane. You will know when you are because feeding will become a hassle and your child's positive eating attitudes and behaviors will erode. Take heart: Your child is resilient and so are you. You can go back to sDOR, and feeding will go back to being relaxed and rewarding.

sDOR works for all children

sDOR supports children in growing in the way that is right for them. sDOR works with children of all sizes and temperaments, degrees of enthusiasm about eating, and strange ways with eating. It works with children who are neurodiverse, have medical conditions such as diabetes and cystic fibrosis, and those who have syndromes such as Down syndrome and Russell-Silver syndrome.

Trusting your child's growth is a celebration

It is lovely to be able to trust your child's growth, even when it is extreme or unusual. My daughter Kjerstin's weight followed the 75th percentile throughout her growing-up years. Lucas had catch-up growth in his first few months and plotted at the 95th percentile by one year. Curtis plotted at the 95th percentile from the first. Both boys weighed above the 95th percentile as older infants and toddlers and tracked at lower percentiles later on. I am not sure why I didn't track Lucas, but you can see Curtis's growth curves from birth until age 12 years in Figures 4.2 and 4.3, pages 105 and 106. I followed sDOR with all of them, was entertained by tracking their growth, and celebrated not having to interfere. It was before these days of obesity hysteria, so none of my health advisors questioned my boys' exceptionally large size. I will talk more later about understanding growth curves.

The loveliness gets spoiled when a child's size and growth are deemed inappropriate, as they too often are. Health professionals may, however reluctantly, apply health policy guidelines saying "normal" growth is only between the 15th and 85th BMI percentile (see below). Such control-paradigm thinking even judges natural infant catch-up growth to be a risk factor for "obesity" and encourages taking steps to prevent it.[1] Interviews with mothers of children deemed "overweight" or "obese" based on those cutoffs, whether or not they really are, show those mothers suffer from weight stigma. They say they feel ashamed, guilty, sad, and responsible for their child's weight. They say that family members, children's physicians, and others blame them for letting their child get fat.[2] Children suffer as well. Children who get the idea they are "too fat," whether or not their BMI is relatively high, feel flawed—not smart, not physically capable, and not worthy.[3] While social attitudes are not as virulent about low-weight children, parents still feel self-conscious and cringe at even well-meaning comments about their child's small size.

It's easier said than done but be aware of the cluelessness inherent in shame-laden comments and advice and protect yourself and your child against them.

Owen's parents resisted interference

Owen's parents did the right thing but raising him would have been a lot easier had they had support with respect to trusting his growth. Here is their story—in his mother's exact words (I do not edit what parents say).

> *Owen's well-child checks were all the same. "He needs to weigh less." "Don't let him eat so much." "What are you feeding him?" What can I say? I lied. Owen ate a lot. He had a lot of bottles when he was a baby, was passionate about solid food, and was eating table food by age eight months. He got a bit picky as a toddler, but his appetite definitely did not fall off. He ate a lot at mealtime and had to have snacks or he fell apart.*
>
> *It was hard. My sister is morbidly obese, and I was so afraid Owen would have her problems. Looking back, I suspect food restriction made my sister so fat. In spite of my worries, I am happy to say that I did not restrict Owen, but I did watch him carefully to make sure he didn't sneak and hoard food like my sister did. Now at age 23, Owen is a lean 6'3" tall, still has a big appetite, and gets crabby when he is hungry. It seems that what I worried about—his big size, big appetite, and the*

way he loved to eat—were just natural for him. Withstanding all that pressure to get Owen to eat and weigh less was hard on me, but I am so happy that I did the right thing!

Trust your child to grow in the right way

Owen's parents trusted him and accepted his natural size and shape despite the interference from his pediatrician. Contrast Owen's story with Mary's story in Chapter 3. From the way feeding was conducted, Mary learned that there was something seriously wrong with her. Owen learned that he was just fine and that getting hangry—crabby when hungry—was just the way he was. Explaining to a child that they are being fed restrictively to get their weight down doesn't prevent the damage. In fact, it highlights the child's understanding that there is something wrong with them. To prevent doing such damage, the same as Owen's parents, you must keep your nerve, trust your child, and accept their natural size and shape.

Guard against your inclinations and those of others to react and try to compensate for any extremes in growth. Owen's advisors, the same as most of the health world, practiced based on the control paradigm. Exacerbated by today's preoccupation with prevention and treatment of "overweight/obesity," your health advisors may give interfering advice about eating and activity to get your exceptionally large or small child's growth to be more toward average—between the 15th and 85th BMI percentiles. Your advisors are mandated by their standards of practice to intervene with your exceptionally large or small child. Perhaps you can help free them from those standards by showing them the evidence in this chapter and introducing them to the possibilities of trust-based practice.

Here is an example of that evidence. Despite the almost universal hand-wringing, children of size do not become "too fat" and, in fact, tend to become taller and leaner as they get older.[4] Infants and children who are restricted become frightened of going without, eat more than they are hungry for, and are at risk of having their weight accelerate. Infants and children who are encouraged to eat more than they want get turned off to food and are at risk of having their weight falter.[5] On the other hand, they may acclimate to eating more than they want and their weight will accelerate.

Rather than trying to change your child's natural body, take care of your child's spirit by feeling good about them and helping them be all they can be. Help them develop good character, common sense, ways of coping with emotions, problem-solving skills, self-confidence, and the ability to get along with others. All children are unique. Any child can be teased for the strangest reasons. Lucas's friends called him "Lucas the pukas." I hesitate to say how Curtis's friends misused his name. Both Lucas and Curtis just smiled and ignored them.

Be wary of interference

It is certainly all right to take an interest in your child's growth and follow it over time on their growth chart. Chances are that at health checkups your child is weighed and measured, and those measurements are plotted on standard percentile growth graphs. In the US, standardized growth charts are provided by the Centers for Disease Control (CDC). The rest of the world depends on the World Health Organization. The CDC website gives growth charts for weight-for-age (W/A), height-for-age (H/A), weight-for-height (W/H), and body mass index (BMI). Do a web search for *CDC growth charts* to see what they look like.

Consider the trust paradigm with growth

Figure 4.1 summarizes the trust-paradigm approach to assessing children's growth.

FIGURE 4.1: NORMAL GROWTH FROM THE TRUST PERSPECTIVE

Compare each child with themself and evaluate their growth consistency over time. Avoid diagnosing children whose growth is above the 85th percentile or below the 15th percentile.

Understand the basics

- A child's growth generally plots along a particular growth percentile: high, low, or in-between.
- Normal growth can be high and fast or low and slow.
- A single measurement tells little about growth, even when it is plotted on a growth chart.
- Children's growth can slowly diverge toward average—unless we spoil it by being controlling.
- Compare children with themselves; avoid cutoffs for "overweight" or "failure-to-thrive."

Distinguish normal growth adjustment from a potential growth problem

- Normal growth adjustment generally starts slowly and proceeds gradually.
- Growth faltering—abrupt, rapid downward adjustment—can indicate a problem.
- Normal growth can be high and fast.
- Growth acceleration—abrupt, rapid upward adjustment—can indicate a problem.

The trusting approach with determining whether a child is growing well is comparing them with themself: assessing their growth based on their previous and ongoing growth pattern. That is, does the child's growth follow consistently (with a bit of zigging and zagging) along a particular growth percentile, even if it is relatively high or low? It is still trusting to be concerned about a child's *sudden and considerable* divergence up or down on their growth chart—say crossing two to four percentile curves over several months or longer. It is trusting because rather than trying to get the child to eat or move less or more to correct that divergence, we consider the issue from the child's point of view. We say essentially, "It is normal for this child to grow consistently. What happened to disrupt that consistent growth pattern?" The section, "Address growth issues," page 113, answers that question.

Monitor for consistent growth

Your child's consistent growth over time is one of the best overall indicators of how things are going with them medically, nutritionally, emotionally, and in terms of the feeding relationship. The same applies to a pattern of slow divergence over considerable time. The same holds true for relatively small children: It is not unusual for their growth to ever-so-gradually diverge upward. However, sudden divergences up or down indicate that something could be the matter medically, nutritionally, emotionally, and/or in terms of the feeding relationship. Why emotionally? As I have said before, in order to eat and therefore grow well, children need their emotional needs met. Feeding based on sDOR meets those emotional needs; trying to get a child to eat more or less does not. In fact, such efforts are likely to accomplish the opposite of what is intended. Putting a child on a weight-reduction diet can make their weight accelerate; trying to get a small child to eat more can make their weight falter. Some illnesses can make both weight and height suddenly diverge downward, such as thyroid dysfunction or kidney disease.

AVOID APPLYING BMI CUTOFFS

In contrast to the trust approach of comparing children with themselves with respect to growth, health policy sets up standards and cutoffs for "normal" growth: It states that your child's BMI is "normal" if it is between the 15th and 85th BMI percentiles and recommends diagnoses and intervention if it is above or below those percentiles. Children whose BMIs are at or above the 85th percentile are defined as "overweight;" those whose BMIs are at or above the 95th percentile are defined as "obese."

Health policy is less prescriptive at the lower percentiles, but common clinical practice is to define children whose BMI is below the 15th percentile as being "underweight," and those whose BMI is at or below the 5th percentile as "failure to thrive." Using those statistical cutoffs makes two mistakes: Diagnosing children whose growth is at the extremes but is consistent, and failure to track for divergence children whose growth plots within "normal" limits. A child whose growth suddenly increases from the 25th to the 80th percentile could escape notice and so could a child whose growth falters from the 80th to the 25th percentile.

Remember: The trust perspective is that *tracking* is important; the control perspective emphasizes cutoffs. I leave the control folks to argue their case; here, we think in terms of trust. From that perspective, what you need to focus on when you walk into your child's doctor's office is the *consistency* of your child's growth. Are they following along at or near a particular percentile, even if that percentile is above the 85th or below the 15th percentile? If so, they are growing just fine.

WEIGHT FOR AGE CHARTS

Let's get a feeling for reading growth charts by taking a look at Figures 4.2 and 4.3 showing my son Curtis's early growth. As you can see, Curtis started out growing at or above the 95th percentile, slimmed down to around the 85th percentile by age seven years and to the 50thth percentile at age 10 or 12 years. I show you Curtis's W/A growth charts rather than his BMI charts because, clinically, I have found that W/A gives the most immediate information about a child's nutritional status. H/A is also useful but less immediate: It tells you about your child's nutritional status long term. Stated another way, height takes longer than weight to respond to changes in a child's eating, activity, and overall environment, and therefore gives evidence of the child's longer-term nutritional status. When a child's weight accelerates or falters significantly because of nutritional issues, height does the same a few months later.

Weight-for-length (W/L), W/H, and BMI combine weight and height measurements and indicate how dense your child is: the heaviness of their bones and muscles. While considering body density is interesting, I tend not to use W/L, W/H, or BMI clinically to track children's growth. Conflating weight and height measurements makes it hard to know what is going on nutritionally. If both weight and height go up or go down the same amount at the same time, *even a lot*—as the plottings would if a child has thyroid or kidney problems—W/L or BMI would not change.

W/L is generally used for children under age two years, BMI over two years. I don't show you this, but Curtis's W/L and BMI were relatively high; Timothy, the small and slender boy we talked about in Chapter 3, had relatively low W/L. Children's hands offer a clue to children's body density. My high-BMI children had such sturdy little hands that I was startled by the neighbor girl's slender, flexible hands. My neighbor girl's BMI was low.

Health policy uses BMI as an indicator of child "obesity" and equates BMI with health. Those assumptions carry stigmas and are riddled with flaws, as we discuss in the section, "More about BMI cutoffs," page 120.

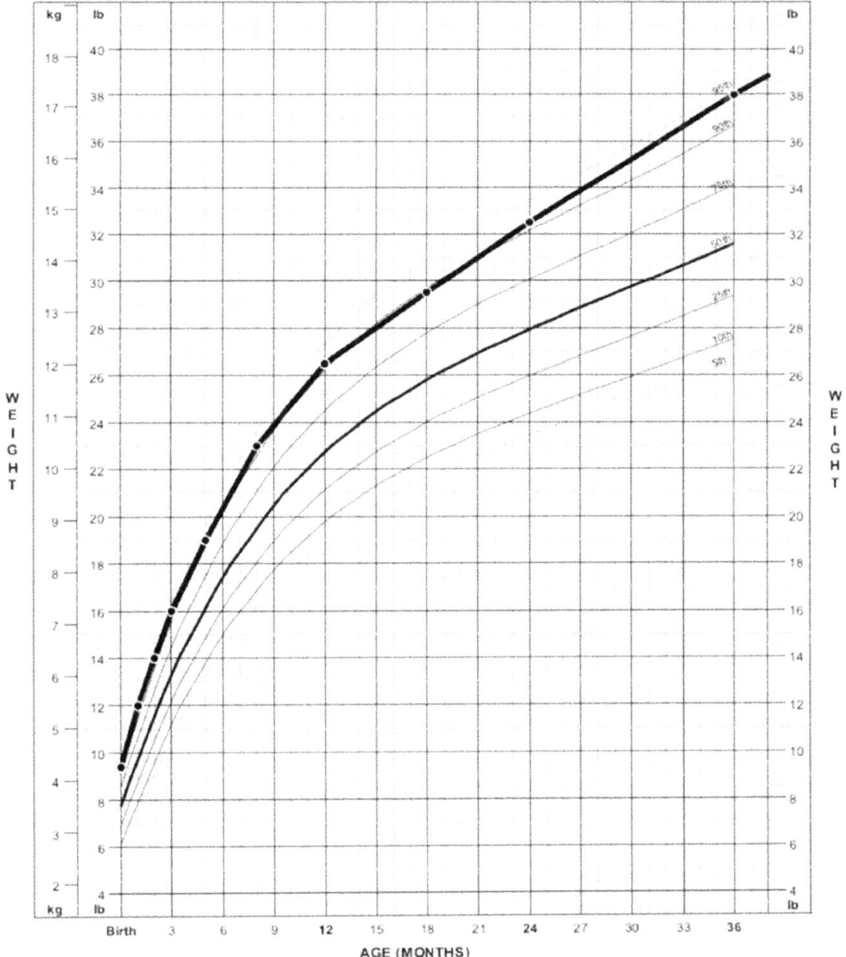

FIGURE 4.2: CURTIS'S WEIGHT-FOR-AGE 0 TO 36 MONTHS

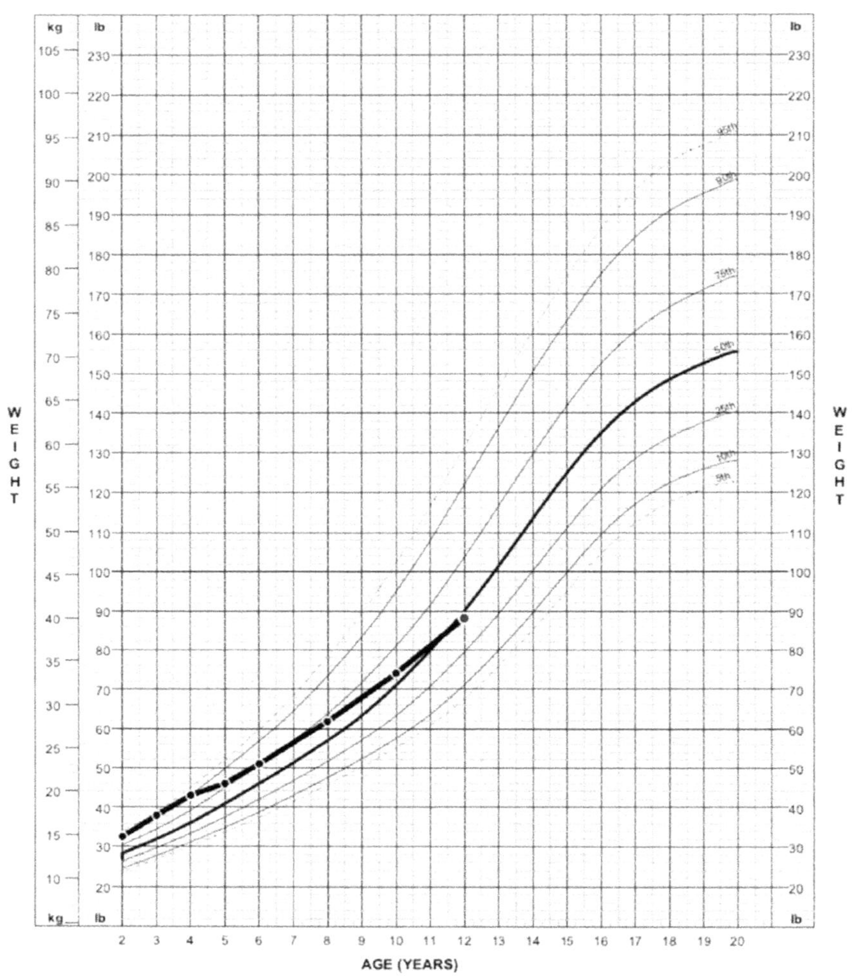

FIGURE 4.3: CURTIS'S WEIGHT-FOR-AGE 2 TO 12 YEARS

Not the least of those erroneous assumptions is that BMI "works" as a measure of body fat. It doesn't. It could just as well be a measure of muscle mass, bone density, and/or overall body composition. It is an even more erroneous assumption to equate BMI with health.

CHILDREN'S GROWTH ADJUSTS

The same as Curtis's did, the weight of relatively large children tends to diverge downward slowly as they get older. Unlike Curtis, that divergence tends to start in infancy, where babies who are larger at birth tend to grow less rapidly; those who are smaller at birth tend to grow more rapidly.[6] That means children in the "diagnosable" range according to health policy tend to grow out of that range. They do, that is, unless their homeostasis has been interfered with by trying to get their growth to change—by trying to get the big child to eat less and move more, the small child to eat more. Happily, small children's activity generally isn't a target for intervention—yet.

Between birth and age seven years, it is typical for children's height to gradually adjust toward the average when their two parents' height varies a lot. That is, children tend to become taller than the shorter parent, shorter than the taller parent, and their eventual height ends up somewhere in between.[7]

Growth blips

While a child's growth tends to follow a certain percentile, it is not absolutely consistent. It tends to zig and zag and once in a while you see a blip that disappears the next time the child is weighed and measured. While it is likely that the blip is normal, it is worth doing some investigation to be sure all is going well. A few simple questions work just fine: Has anything changed in your family or the child's life? How is feeding going? Is there anything about your child's eating that concerns you?

Newborn growth adjusts

It takes a while for newborn growth to settle down to a consistent percentile. Newborn growth adjustments can look like upward or downward divergence, so keep your nerve, feed well, and trust your child's growth pattern as it emerges. Feeding well is following sDOR. Following sDOR for your infant is respecting their sleep rhythms, helping them to be calm and awake during feeding, and depending on their hunger and fullness signs to determine how much to feed them.

A study of over 45,000 eastern Massachusetts children followed from age 1 month to almost 11 years provides fascinating insights on growth adjustments. Sixty-one percent of 1- to 6-month-olds crossed upwards one percentile and 18 percent crossed upwards two or more percentiles. Twenty-one percent crossed downwards. Children's growth continued to adjust in the second year. By 18 to 24 months, 28 percent of children crossed upwards one to two or more percentiles and 43 percent crossed downwards. Children whose growth crossed upwards tended to be larger at ages 5 and 10 years old.[8]

From the trust perspective, infants who show rapid weight gain and get big are are just fine as long as they follow their consistent growth trajectory, even if it is above the $85^{th}/95^{th}$ percentile. From the control perspective, infants who show rapid weight gain are "at risk" of growing above the $85^{th}/95^{th}$ BMI percentile and are "overweight/obese."

The eastern Massachusetts data *supported* the trust perspective but was *interpreted* from the control perspective.[8] It is one of a number of studies of rapid infant weight gain done in the past 15 years. Ironically, the studies give insights on normal growth but define growth at the rapid end of the spectrum as a risk factor for "obesity" later in life. Do a web search for *Satter rapid infant weight gain*.[9]

This discussion with all its contradictions may be as challenging for you to read as it was for me to write! Let me conclude by saying that if hundreds of thousands of children do it, they must be on the right track.

Applying labels does harm

Without observing the feeding dynamics of infants who are doing catch-up or catch-down growth, it is difficult to know whether those growth patterns are normal or distorted. Unusually small and prematurely born infants tend to attract pressure to eat more, but parents and practitioners who are tuned in to rapid weight gain research may try to restrict them to prevent normal catch-up growth. Unusually large babies who grow rapidly may attract restriction. Pressured or restricted infants lose track of their internal regulators and either eat as much as their grown-ups want them to eat or resist so strongly that they eat and grow poorly. Children's weight may accelerate or decelerate, which signals a feeding problem even when growth is between the 15th and 85th percentiles. Parents and professionals become concerned about the child's "excessive" or "deficient" weight and apply even more pressure. Whereupon the child's ability to regulate their food intake is further impaired and they are set up for even more weight dysregulation.

In the best of all worlds, this cascade of errors can be prevented by following sDOR from the first and trusting the child to grow in the way that is right for them.

Rapid gainers become dense, not fat

Contrast the Massachusetts control-based conclusions that rapidly gaining infants get "too fat" with trust-based conclusions that rapidly gaining infants become relatively heavy but *not* "too fat." A study of over 1000 Glascow Scotland infants showed rapid weight gainers were heavier because they were taller and leaner at seven to eight years of age, not fatter. Researchers observed that parents were more likely to discontinue breast-feeding infants and start solid food early in response to this rapid early weight gain, not that ceasing breastfeeding and starting solids *caused* the rapid weight gain. Those rapidly gaining babies enjoyed eating and were demanding with food, and their mothers had difficulty keeping up with their hearty appetites![10]

Larger than average children tend to become larger than average grown-ups and, from the trust perspective, that is fine. Four hundred children studied at age nine years and again after 50 years were found to have correlations between early and later heavy build (leanness and heaviness independent of fatness). No surprises there, but here is the surprise, at least to those of the control-paradigm persuasion: The heaviest were the healthiest. Adults with heavy builds had significantly lower blood lipids and glucose and women had lower blood pressures. Being thin in childhood offered no protection against adult fatness and the thinnest children tended to have the highest adult degenerative disease risk at every level of adult obesity.[11]

ACCEPT GROWTH EXTREMES

What can we conclude from this somewhat convoluted discussion of growth adjustment? It is that we need to keep our nerve, trust our children's growth, and wait to see how it turns out. Accepting your child's consistent growth at any percentile supports your feeding relationship. Applying BMI cutoffs and growth standards undermines it. It takes courage to resist advice to interfere with your child's growth, but it is *so* important. Otherwise, as these parents did, you and your child will pay a considerable price.

Lauren's parents tried to get her to eat less

Lauren's parents brought her into treatment when she was six years old, complaining she was a compulsive eater. Lauren's parents saw her as eating *a lot*, and she regularly embarrassed them at family gatherings by hanging around the food and eating as much as she could hold. The parents were looking for help being more "successful" with restricting her. When we considered her backstory, it became apparent that more restriction was the *worst* thing to do.

"Obesity" cutoffs are not supposed to apply to infants, but Lauren's weight-conscious parents still cringed when their friends hefted her and exclaimed, "What a *big* baby!" To her parents, Lauren's being a big baby meant she would be big for life, and they set out to prevent that. They didn't let her eat quite as much formula as she wanted and it made her fussy and wakeful, although they didn't connect her fussiness with her being constantly hungry. They continued to restrict how much she ate until she became a relentlessly food-begging toddler whose constant refrain was "I'm hungry, I'm hungry." Her busy and preoccupied parents simply weren't able to withstand her relentless raids on the food supply and constant demands for food, and her weight abruptly and rapidly accelerated to far above the 95th percentile. By the time she was six years old, Lauren weighed 95 pounds. The absolute number wasn't the problem: That she got there via weight acceleration was the problem.

Even though Lauren's parents were afraid that she would gain even more weight when they stopped restricting her, their misery around feeding Lauren made them desperate enough to go ahead with treatment. They started following sDOR, and, at first, Lauren confirmed their worst fears: She ate like there was no tomorrow. But they hung in there despite their anxiety and after two or three weeks, Lauren's eating began to settle down. Instead of begging for food, she asked for reassurance: "I can have as much as I want, right?" After another two or three weeks she began eating like any other child her age—a lot sometimes and hardly anything the next. Sometimes she forgot all about her snack, which pleased her parents, but I advised them to offer it anyway because Lauren needed to trust that they would remember to feed her.

None of us can take our children where we haven't gone ourselves, so Lauren's parents had to learn to trust their own food-regulation processes as well. I worked with both parents to increase their Eating Competence, with particular attention to discovering their own ability to detect their hunger and satiety cues and use those cues to guide how much they ate.

The treatment succeeded. Within six to eight weeks, Lauren's "compulsive eating" had gone away, and she became relaxed and casual about meals and snacks. She had fun with the other kids at family gatherings and would go off to play without finishing the second helpings she still asked for. She was reassuring herself she would get enough to eat.

Most touching of all, Lauren's mother discovered what her preoccupation with Lauren's weight had been doing to their relationship:

> *I finally realized what you mean by positive feeding relationship. I can now look at her and appreciate her and not have food be the end-all. Allowing her to be her own little person has freed me up to just enjoy her, and I appreciate her in a whole different way. Even if it is her fate to be heavier, have her be happy and not feel that you have to be thin to be happy, which is what my life has been about.*

Erica was a *very* large baby

Erica's story reflects Lauren's. Since we had a glimpse of Erica's long-term outcome, I am telling you about her to remind you that following sDOR is about the long haul. Erica weighed over nine pounds at birth and for the first few months her weight increased rapidly to well above the growth chart and climbing. In retrospect, I don't think that early gain was weight acceleration but simply catch-up growth. It is unusual for such a big baby to do catch-up growth, but she did it nonetheless. Erica, the same as other infants who do catch-up growth, appeared to need more room to grow than she had had in the uterus. My twin granddaughters did catch-up growth. They were each born at just under six pounds—at around the 15th percentile. By age one year, the weight of one increased to the 50th percentile, the other to the 85th. It was easier for us to be relaxed about our average-sized girls' rapid growth than it had to be for Erica's parents because Erica started out exceptionally big and got even bigger.

Not only was she big, Erica *loved* to eat. At first her parents reluctantly let her eat as much as she wanted—or thought they did—but by age six months they began restricting her in earnest—or they tried. She put a lot of pressure on eating, including looking absolutely bereft when she wasn't allowed to eat as much as she wanted, and her parents were too soft-hearted to hold out against her longing for food. They held out and then gave in, over and over. Erica learned to eat all she could whenever she could get it, and her weight truly accelerated.

When Erica was about a year old, a dietitian friend introduced her parents to sDOR. It made sense to them, and they were relieved not to have to make Erica so unhappy. It wasn't easy for them to change their ways with feeding. Both parents were weight-conscious, Erica had an older brother whose weight was relatively low, and they had been trying to get him to eat more. They resolved to follow sDOR with both children.

At first it took a lot of nerve for the parents to follow sDOR because Erica ate even more than before and her brother ate even less. But family meals immediately became more positive and rewarding and both children were happier. That kept the parents going. Eventually both children settled down to eating the same as other children their ages. I don't know about the brother, but by the time she was six years old, Erica had slimmed down from way above the 95th weight percentile to the 75th percentile. Erica was lost to follow up once the feeding problem was resolved, but the dietitian friend saw her when she was a teenager and she had an average, relatively sturdy body.

Samantha wasn't *really* teeny tiny—at first

Given Samantha's history of food allergies and her parents' seeing her as "teeny-tiny," it was little wonder that her parents got pushy with feeding.

Samantha grew consistently at the 50th percentile, but at age three months her weight began to falter. That faltering continued until at age 15 months her weight had dropped to below the 5th percentile and her parents brought her into treatment complaining that she wouldn't eat.

A video of a typical 45-minute mealtime showed Samantha's exhausted and despondent mother enticing Samantha to eat every single bite. Well, not *every* bite. When her mother was distracted, Samantha readily ate with her fingers. Once her mother went back to trying to get her to eat, Samantha cheerfully clamped shut her mouth, twisted her head away, and pushed food back out on her chin. Samantha wasn't allowed to be her own little person, and she was settling for second best: attention! But she was paying a price because her weight was faltering. Samantha's parents were able to institute sDOR although it was hard for them to let go of their efforts to get food into her and trust that she would eat enough. Samantha's eating recovered and at last report she ever-so-gradually had begun to gain back some of her lost weight.

Interference hurts children

Children do not compartmentalize. If parents do not feel good about a child's hair or freckles—or weight—and try to change those features, children feel that everything about them is bad. Of course, the issues are not quite the same because parents generally don't feel they caused their child's hair or freckles except to pass on their genes. When it comes to a child's weight, parents often feel they caused it. I hope our discussions will help get you off that particular hook.

Not being allowed to have enough to eat made Lauren and Erica feel bad all over. We can get a glimpse of what it must have been like for them by watching eight-month-old Andrew on the downloadable video *Feeding with Love and Good Sense I by Ellyn Satter*. Andrew is so excited to eat that he can't sit still in his highchair. But his excitement is tinged with anxiety, and it isn't long before we know why. Andrew's child care provider has been instructed by the parents not to let Andrew eat as much as he is hungry for. His parents are convinced that Andrew "has no stopping place." Being forced to stop eating when he is still hungry has happened often enough that even at eight months of age, Andrew anticipates going hungry.

Andrew's parents were wrong: Andrew had a stopping place—at least he did until they started restricting him and he became food preoccupied. Andrew's child care provider could have broken through his parents' misguided certainty if she had said, "No way am I going to make him go hungry." A good child care provider is more valuable than rubies, and those parents might have listened to her. However, the provider bought into the idea that Andrew didn't have a stopping place. After she saw the video with my comments, she felt bad: Getting some distance from what she was doing let her tune in on Andrew's misery. She was so loving with the children she cared for that I am sure she learned from that mistake and didn't try to make other children go hungry. My fantasy about Andrew is that when he got to be a toddler, he turned into a relentless little cupboard-raider like Lauren and Erica and made himself such a nuisance that his parents were forced to get help straightening out their approach to feeding. Often, situations have to get worse before parents can see there is a problem.

Andrew is chubby, but that's all right because many children are naturally chubby by the end of the first year. The chubby infant has no greater risk of growing up fat than the thin infant.[4] However, Andrew's chances of slimming down as he gets older are decreasing before our very eyes, because he is learning there won't be enough food and he had better eat as much as he can whenever he can, whether he wants it or not. To understand what it is like for Andrew, imagine you are on an international airline trip without food or beverage service or a whitewater rafting trip where the provisions have fallen over the side. Hunger becomes harsh if there is no way to make it go away.

Perhaps worst of all, Andrew was learning there was something wrong with *him* for wanting to eat more than his grown-ups wanted him to eat. Children feel bad all over when you try to get them to settle for less than they want, and it is just as negative for them to be expected to eat *more* than they want. Consider having to force down food when you aren't hungry, or remember your nauseated, too-full feeling when you have overdone it. A mother who sought my advice about getting her "too-small" two-year-old to eat more said it best: "When you don't want the food," she observed, "it feels like it grows in your mouth." Despite her sensitivity to his feelings, the mother was so desperate about her son's very *survival* that she put food in his mouth and held his lips shut until he swallowed. That mother was only able to follow sDOR when I analyzed the boy's growth from birth and was able to demonstrate that his weight fell off at the same time she started force-feeding him.

ADDRESS GROWTH ISSUES

Are you caught in a struggle with your child's eating and weight? I am sorry for your misery. You can dig your way out, and your child's eating attitudes and behaviors will recover. You may or may not be able to do it on your own. Erica's parents were dealing with a lot, and they were still successful in following sDOR just from reading my book. Samantha's and Lauren's parents needed help to detect and trust their children's capabilities with growth, and they needed help keeping their nerve with following sDOR.

Why did you lose trust with feeding?

Earlier I posed the problem solving question, "It is normal for this child to grow consistently. What happened to disrupt that consistent growth pattern?" Then answer is that something happened that took away trust in the child to do their part with feeding. As Lauren and Erica illustrated, it could have been their size. With Samantha, it wasn't her *actual* size but the way her parents *viewed* her size: they were concerned that she was too small. Your child may have been or continue to be medically vulnerable. That vulnerability can be made to seem even more frightening by being urged to get them to eat. The problem may have even come from you: If you don't trust your own ability to regulate your food intake, you have no basis for trusting that your child can eat what and as much as they need.

Solving the problem requires following sDOR, but being advised to do so could come across to you as just one more of the piecemeal bits of advice you have gotten in the past. You may have even been told to follow the division of responsibility by people who don't understand how to apply it properly. Often, uninformed advisors will say "division of responsibility" then go on to tell you what and/or how much your child should eat or suggest ways to get them to eat it. You may need an sDOR-trained professional to sit down with you, fully understand what you have been through with feeding your child, and take all your child's and family's complications into account as they work with you in finding your way out of your dilemma. As part of the assessment, such professionals observe videos of family meals or typical feeding interactions. Concerned parents often pressure or restrict with feeding without realizing it.

My colleagues and I at the Ellyn Satter Institute have trained many professionals to work with parents to solve such established feeding problems. Get in touch with the Ellyn Satter Institute to get help finding an informed and experienced person to work with you.

Identify growth acceleration or faltering

At the same time as you accept your child's consistent growth, be alert to growth *divergence*—when your child's growth suddenly crosses several growth percentiles. Growth divergence does not call for you to restrict your child or try to get them to eat more, but rather to detect whether there is a problem and correct that problem.

It takes a *lot* to cause the rapid crossing of growth percentiles that I described with Lauren, Erica, and Samantha: Lauren's and Erica's weights went up; Samantha's went down. Their stories illustrated distortions in feeding that can disrupt growth. Their rapid and pronounced weight shifts were quite different from Curtis's growth *adjustment,* where his relative decrease in weight started gradually and proceeded slowly.

Poor food selection or a child's occasional over- or under-eating will not derail a child's growth, but a feeding problem can. Abrupt and extended weight shifts indicate that feeding may not be going well and that other factors in the child's life may be disrupting feeding and the child's homeostasis. Getting to the bottom of why a child's growth accelerates or falters requires doing well-informed detective work to tease apart what is going on in the child's life medically, developmentally, nutritionally, and with respect to feeding dynamics.

Wherever the problem starts, feeding dynamics are always distorted. Often feeding problems start with a child's size or medical condition. Parents consciously or unconsciously compensate for their child's perceived vulnerability, feeding becomes disrupted, and each stage of feeding becomes a struggle of trying to address current issues while at the same time compensating for earlier errors. Parents get a lot of advice, much of it conflicting, which further distorts feeding.

It is difficult, but I have seen parents work their way out of these struggles on their own: They are able to accurately establish sDOR, then trust their child to do the *whether* and *how much* of eating. Others start and stop, alternatively letting the child do *whether* and *how much* and then taking it away when the child's at-first-extreme eating scares them off. Professional help supports them in holding steady with sDOR until their child's eating stabilizes and becomes more apparently trustworthy.

YOUR CHILD MIGHT INHERIT YOUR SIZE AND SHAPE

Provided your relative weight has been fairly consistent during your adult years, your child's body will tend to resemble yours. If your weight has gone up or down a lot, it is difficult to know what is natural for you and natural for your child. To accept what is natural for your body, you need to understand your own transition to having an adult body. Women tend to achieve their adult height about the time they graduate from high school and their adult weight somewhere in their early twenties. Women develop a mature woman's body by putting on fatty tissue. Men tend to grow in height and weight until they are in their mid-twenties by gaining muscle and developing longer and heavier bones. Trust-paradigm thinking is that this late-teen, early-twenties weight gain is normal and desirable; control-paradigm thinking is that it is abnormal and undesirable.

What if your weight has been inconsistent?

If your weight has been inconsistent, it is hard to predict your child's body inheritance. If you had already started dieting and trying to lose weight—or force-feeding yourself and trying to gain weight—by the time you got into your twenties, your natural weight may have been distorted. If you have continued to have a lose/regain pattern over the years, your weight is likely higher than is natural for you. Many of my adult patients and those of my ESI colleagues were put on weight-reduction diets when they were young, and by their twenties they had already started the regrettable pattern of losing weight and then regaining to a higher level. Wrestlers show the same stair-step pattern of weight regain when they diet to make weight, then gain it back and more besides in the off season.

I am reminded of Nora and Charlie, who are raising four wonderful children. Both parents are markedly fat; all their children are of average weight or less. Nora and Charlie have learned to accept and respect their bodies and take a steady course with following sDOR. Health professionals who don't know them look them over, consider their children, and congratulate them for their children's slenderness. It never fails to irritate them. Health professionals who know Nora and Charlie remember their instructions: **"Don't—say—anything—about—weight."** When they are wise, those professionals learn from Nora and Charlie about following sDOR and supporting children's natural growth.

Nora and Charlie know from their own experience how destructive it is to interfere with children's growth: It was that very interference that made them fatter than was right for them. From the time they were small, they had been subjected to food restriction and showed rebound weight acceleration. By the time they were in their twenties, their weights were already much higher than if they had been allowed to grow in the way that was right for them.

Nora and Charlie are well aware of the weight bias and misguided thinking behind the congratulations. Control-paradigm thinking is that parent "obesity" is without question a major risk factor for child "obesity." It is assumed that parents who are fat eat too much of the wrong food and exercise too little and raise children who do the same. That couldn't be less true of the two of them: They eat well, are active, and do a good job with feeding their family. For the most part, they ignore weight-biased comments and devote themselves to following sDOR. Nora says, "following sDOR is not for the faint of heart." Following sDOR can be a challenge. For them, it was a particular challenge because they had to learn to accept their own eating and weight. They know they can trust their children to eat as much as they need because they have learned to trust themselves.

People of size do not eat poorly

The common assumption that people of size eat too much of the wrong food is simply not true and is nothing but prejudice. It is far more common for people who see their weight as too high to engage in a chronic struggle to do something about it: To eat less than they want of food they enjoy. There is no way they can succeed. It is simply not possible to spend a lifetime eating less than you want and avoiding food you enjoy. It is typical for people of all sizes, not just those whose weight is high, to periodically give in to their hunger and appetite, eat a lot, and regain any weight they have lost before. Then they diet again, fall off again, and again regain their lost weight and more besides. The biological pressure to regain lost weight is enormous: It is the product of that homeostasis that I talked about earlier.

That off-again, on-again, yo-yo-dieting pattern interferes with family meals and causes problems with children's eating and weight. Based on a questionnaire, obese (not my word) mothers were less likely than normal-weight (not my word either) mothers to manage the *what*, *when*, and *where* of children's eating. However, obese mothers were no more likely than normal-weight mothers to offer food to deal with emotional distress, to use food as a form of reward, or to encourage the child to eat more than they wanted to.[12]

NATURE OR NURTURE?

Is body size and shape the result of nurture or nature? Is it caused by the way children are raised or is it inherited? Control-paradigm thinking is that children of size overeat and underexercise. Trust-paradigm thinking is that there is a strong genetic predisposition to body size and shape *and* the predisposition can be supported or undermined by the feeding relationship.

Genetics contributes 40 to 50 percent of the variability in body weight.[13] Genetic factors predispose some people but not others to weight acceleration when environmental factors overwhelm their food-regulation abilities.[14] Remember the earlier observation that some children's ability to maintain homeostasis is more resilient than others? That is, some children's weights accelerate or falter when feeding goes poorly and others' weights remain stable no matter what. We were talking about genetic differences among children. To repeat: Since you can't know about your child's genetic predisposition to maintain homeostasis, it is best not to take chances. Support your child's food regulation abilities by following sDOR and trust them to grow in the way that is right for them.

Despite the strong research support, the idea of genetic predisposition to weight acceleration remains a hard sell. For that reason, and for the sheer enjoyment of considering some fascinating research, I give you the—well—research. Skip this if you don't share my enthusiasm.

Inherited fatness

Pediatricians Garn and Clark analyzed the fat-fold thicknesses of almost 21,000 parent–child pairs and divided the children into groups depending on whether parents were both "lean," "medium," or "obese"—all arbitrary designations—or had some other combination. Garn and Clark's data clearly illustrates that relative leanness or fatness are normal conditions for some people and that children tend to inherit their parents' relative leanness or fatness.[15] The researchers didn't share my interpretation: Their control-based and data-resistant conclusion was that something should be done about it. Their explanation was breathtaking in its genetics-negating tunnel vision and weight bigotry: Like marries like and couples share their bad habits.[15]

This study was done decades ago, but it applies today: Genetics change over *centuries*, not over years or even decades.

Inherited thinness

A group from the Health Behavior Research Center in London did a more recent study of British children's thinness and found essentially the same body-build relationships between children and their parents. In surveying almost 8,000 children ages 2 through 15 years, the group found that starting at age 2 years, children's BMI was lowest when their two parents' BMI was relatively low. The relationship between parent and child thinness persisted as children got older and was most pronounced after children were 10 years old.[16] In contrast to Garn and Clark, the London group accepted their findings and concluded that "many cases of thinness are likely to represent the low end of the healthy distribution of weight and, as such, are likely to have a primarily genetic origin."

Redo that sentence in your head, substitute *fatness* for *thinness* and *high* for *low*, and you have an accurate conclusion for the Garn and Clark study. In fact, I will do it myself because it captures so well what you need to remember in the midst of all this control-based weight craziness: *Many cases of fatness are likely to represent the high end of the healthy distribution of weight and, as such, are likely to have a primarily genetic origin.* Having written that, I realize I would substitute the word "most" for "many" in both studies: *Most* cases of thinness . . . *Most* cases of fatness . . .

Inherited height and weight

There have been a lot of twin studies: Scientists do them to tease apart nature versus nurture with respect to many characteristics, height and weight included. Consistently, studies have found that genetics is by far more influential than environment. Identical twins who have been reared apart resemble each other a great deal in height and weight—only slightly less than those who have been reared together and far more than non-identical twins or other siblings. In other words, weight, to the same extent as height, is mostly determined by genetics; environment has far less influence. A recent study was conducted as a collaboration by researchers from Canada, Sweden, Denmark, and Australia based on data from 23 twin groups—over 24,000 boys and girls—from those countries. Researchers found that genetics explained 80 to 90 percent of the variability in both height and weight. Those genetic tendencies for height and weight showed up as early as age five months and became increasingly apparent through late adolescence. At the same time, environmental influences became less apparent.[14] What does this mean? The same as indicated by the other studies in this section, nurture is a factor, but nature is more powerful.

Consider body diversity

Body diversity is simply variation in size and shape and does not have to be categorized as "normal" or "abnormal." Why not think of body diversity in the way we think of neurodiversity, as part of a wide range of the way we can be? It makes no statistical sense to apply cutoffs to children's growth, and it makes even less sense (can one make less than *no* sense?) to apply the same standards to children of all ethnic groups. Consider studies of Navajo children: their average BMI was at the 85th percentile.[17] By health-policy standards, they were "overweight" by nature. Consider Mexican and other Hispanic children: their average BMI was also at the 85th percentile.[18] Consider Turkish and Albanian immigrant children living in the Netherlands: again, their average BMI was at the 85th percentile and above. In contrast, Asian immigrant children living in the Netherlands tended to have lower BMIs.[19] These are old studies—there isn't a lot of current interest in finding out what is normal for children. You can still trust the information. Genetics doesn't change much in a few decades, although children's growth patterns will be diluted as parents intermarry.

Definitions of body types tend to be lost in the mists of time, but they are still useful in helping us accept variations in fatness and thinness. Some people are *ectomorphs*: they are slender, likely to be tall, and have relatively light muscles and bones. Some are *mesomorphs*: they naturally have more muscles, heavier bones, and less fat. Some are *endomorphs*: they have softer and perhaps broader and more pear-shaped bodies, with relatively more fat and less muscle.

Now for the quiz: Which body type is preferred in today's world? Which body type makes a child most vulnerable to interference?

You know the answer, but I will give it anyway: Mesomorphs and ectomorphs are preferred, and endomorphs are most vulnerable to interference. Unless that ectomorph is relatively small, then they are vulnerable to interference from people who worry they are too small. It's all quite unreasonable.

MORE ABOUT BMI CUTOFFS

I have been telling you that health policy makers' control-paradigm orientation leads them to consider only BMIs between the 15th and 85th percentile to be "normal." Ignore those BMI cutoffs. Statistically, they make little sense. The BMIs of 15 percent of children *naturally* track at or above the 85th percentile cutoff; BMIs of 5 percent of children track at or above the 95th percentile. At the other extreme, BMIs of 15 percent of children track normally at or below the 15th percentile; those of 5 percent of children track at or below the 5th percentile.

The 85th/95th "overweight/obese" BMI percentile cutoffs come from the CDC and other federal agencies. They are passed on to pediatricians and other health professionals by the American Pediatric Association (APA) as standards of practice, accompanied by food-restriction recommendations. Those standards of practice mean that your health professional is expected to give your child the recommended diagnosis and you the intervention. Those recommendations are all about pressure: Get your child to weigh the "right" amount by eating the "right" food and avoiding the "wrong" food—and "not too much," whatever that is. If all goes well, your advisor will resist those standards on your behalf and support your consistently growing but above-the-85th/95th-percentile child.

Small children also attract interference. According to the World Health Organization control-paradigm advice, a child is "underweight" if their weight/height or BMI is at the 15th percentile or below, and "severely underweight" if their weight/height or BMI is below the 3rd percentile. Such relatively small children are often labeled "failure to thrive," a terrifying diagnosis if there ever was one. Such a diagnosis is often accompanied by recommendations to get the child to eat more, particularly of high-calorie foods. The same as for large children, resist the cutoff-based judgments of your child and concentrate on whether they are growing consistently.

If you impose either set of controlling recommendations on your child, you are being caught up in the hot-potato game: Pressure, the same as a hot potato, gets tossed down the line from policy makers to health professionals to you until it ends up in the lap of the person least able to cope with it: your child. Health policy is unlikely to be changed any time soon, but if all goes well, your health professional will be able to hang on to that hot potato on your and your child's behalf.

Protect your child against diagnosis

Resisting creates anxiety, and your health professional does a great service to you and your child by hanging on to that anxiety and not passing it onto you. If you are not so lucky, you will have to ignore your health professional's assessment that something is wrong with the weight of your consistently growing, relatively small or relatively large child—and deal with your own anxiety. Perhaps you can provide each other with mutual support in following the trust paradigm view of growth.

Weight-based diagnosis harms because it takes away your trust in your child to do their part with sDOR. Often children's growth abruptly accelerates after they are diagnosed as "overweight/obese" based on those cutoff points. Parents feed restrictively, children become afraid of going hungry and react by eating as much as they can, whenever they can, and the child's weight goes up even more.

Similarly, growth often falters when children are diagnosed as being "underweight" and/or "failure to thrive." Parents try to get the child to eat more than they want, the child is overwhelmed and revolted, they eat less than they need, and their weight goes down. My ESI colleague Peggy Crum observes that parents often react to such diagnoses by abandoning structure and pressing food on their child anywhere, any time. For the child, being made to eat when they don't want to, pressure becomes a constant threat and they eat less, not more.

Parents are reluctant to accept diagnosis

Considering a child as being "too fat," worrying they will *get* "too fat," and trying to keep them from gaining "too much" weight is miserable for them and miserable for parents. On some level, most parents realize this up front and resist accepting an "overweight/obesity" diagnosis for their child. They have a good idea about what comes next: Continually trying to get their child to eat less, imposing low-calorie restrictions on family food (or trying to stop the "overweight" child from eating the regular food), giving up Friday night pizza in front of the TV. It is all that Lauren's and Erica's parents endured, and more—and what Owen's parents avoided.

Although parents' reluctance to accept an "overweight/obese" diagnosis is understandable, it causes great consternation among weight-focused clinicians, researchers, and policy makers. Those folks maintain that accepting the diagnosis is essential in order for parents to do something about the child's weight.[20] That insistence is amazingly misguided and data resistant. Not only does the "doing something" not work,[21] study after study shows that such a diagnosis is likely to make children fatter rather than thinner. Consider these two.

A joint United Kingdom-U.S. study followed the BMI of 3,500 Australian children from age 4 to 13 years. They found that children whose parents saw them as "overweight" were fatter after nine years than children whose parents saw them as being "about the right weight." The findings were independent of children's *actual* weight.[22]

Almost 1,500 Dutch parents of children between the ages of 2 and 9 years filled out annual questionnaires. According to study authors, around 80 percent of parents either "underestimated" or "overestimated" their child's weight, meaning parents perceived both "overweight/obese" and "underweight" children as being of normal weight.[20] Good for them—and for you too, if that is what you have to do to resist diagnosing your child's growth as being abnormal! But to go on, at every age, rhe Dutch study found that children whose parents "underestimated" their presumed "overweight/obesity" had a markedly lower BMI than children of parents who "accurately perceived" their weight. That is, when parents resisted seeing their children as being "too fat," their children remained slimmer. When parents saw their children as being "too fat," their children became fatter.[20] The study didn't examine growth on the other end, that is, what happened with the growth of relatively small children when parents did or didn't accept the diagnosis that they were "underweight." There isn't much research interest in "underweight" children.

Just as the children from Australia, the children from the Netherlands had an increased likelihood of showing weight acceleration when their parents saw them as being "overweight." The Dutch study authors' conclusion? "Accurate weight status perception may be an important prerequisite for involving parents in childhood obesity interventions."[20] Words fail me. Why would parents accept a misery-making diagnosis and pursue a "cure" that doesn't work, a "cure" that makes children fatter rather than thinner?

Sigh. So it goes in the control-focused child nutrition and health care world. Keep in mind that the purpose of eating is to *sustain life,* and that the child's most critical nutritional need is to *eat enough* to be healthy and grow well. In spite of those realities, the health care world preoccupies itself with interfering with the food intake and growth of children whose BMI are at the extremes of normal.

WHAT ABOUT WEIGHT AND HEALTH?

During my speaking days, after I made one of my trust-paradigm, child-weight-neutral presentations and opened the floor for questions, someone almost always insisted, "Well that's all very interesting but obesity is still unhealthy." My questioners were thinking about "extremely obese" children, who are generally assumed to be very unhealthy, and applying that assumption to all children of size. Moreover, they were having trouble wrapping their brains around the difference between children who grow consistently at high percentile levels and children whose growth reaches extremely high percentile levels via weight acceleration.

Are extremely obese children unhealthy?

Children are classified as "extremely obese" or "morbidly obese" when their weights are way above the 99th percentile. Are those "extremely obese" children unhealthy? A West Virginia study of over 23,000 children showed that 3 percent of "extremely obese" children had a higher incidence of five cardiovascular risk factors: high blood pressure, high total cholesterol, high HDL, low LDL, and high triglycerides. Those are *risk factors,* not the cardiovascular disease itself: heart disease and strokes. That compares with a 0.5 percent incidence of the same five cardiovascular risk factors among the entire population. Fourteen percent of the "extremely obese" children had no risk factors, compared with 51 percent in the total population.[23]

Studies that follow adults' weights from childhood find health problems only in those whose weights have accelerated. People classified as "overweight" in childhood and who remained at that weight level as adults had no greater risk of heart disease. However, those who became overweight as adults did have greater risk.[24] A summary of 37 studies found that adult "obesity-related" illnesses could not be predicted from childhood "obesity," and that most adult "obesity-related" health problems occurred in "obese" adults who were of average weight or below in childhood.[25]

Which brings us to the consideration of weight instability. There is considerable evidence *in all weight groups* that it is the weight *cycling*—the yo-yo effect—and that even one time weight regain after weight loss contributes to a higher incidence of cardiovascular risk factors among people of size, not the weight, per se.[26] Research concluding that weight cycling (yo-yo effect) is not harmful examined only its impact on subsequent ability to lose weight.[27] In our culture, an "overweight" or "obesity" diagnosis and efforts at weight loss go hand in hand. Weight instability goes along with weight-loss efforts; regain after weight loss, often repeated. Stated in another way, yo-yo dieting—weight cycling as the result of weight-reduction dieting—is part of the history of almost every person of size.

Consider the backstory of "extreme obesity"

If there is an association between elevated weight and health, weight acceleration is likely to be the culprit. It takes *a lot* to make a child's weight accelerate, and an *extraordinary lot* has to go wrong in a child's life for their BMI to get into the "extremely obese" range. "Extremely obese" children were not always in that weight category: They got there as a result of extreme weight acceleration, often in reaction to food restriction or food insecurity. The BMIs of 600 "severely obese" children in the Louisiana-based Bogalusa Heart Study had accelerated from average ranges to extreme weight categories sometime in their early childhood years and stabilized in their teens and twenties.[28] Once a child's weight is extreme, imposing food restriction and forced activity will only compound their misery. However, much can be done to enhance the child's wellness and quality of life.

Consider an "extremely obese" child

Clear as mud? Let's see if an example helps.

In *Your Child's Weight* Chapter 10, Understand Your Child's Growth, I talk about Marcus, whose troubles began early. Marcus grew consistently at the 60th weight percentile for his first 12 months. At his two-year-old checkup, he was diagnosed with "extreme obesity:" his weight had jumped to uncharted territory on his growth chart *way* above the 99th weight percentile—to over 45 pounds. By age 6, Marcus weighed 153 pounds; by age 10, 367 pounds; and by age 13, 447 pounds.

To understand why Marcus gained so much weight, we have to understand his backstory. Marcus's mother saw him from the time he was a newborn as being an avid eater who had no "off button." She said he was always hungry as an infant and as a toddler, he put a lot of pressure on food. He ate as much as he could whenever food was available, and he hoarded food.

Marcus's eating reflected his circumstances. Rather than lacking an "off button," Marcus suffered from extreme food insecurity. His overwhelmed mother was incapable of regularly providing him with food. He had to eat as much as he could whenever he could because he never knew when he would get to eat again. Once Marcus's weight became high, the food insecurity at home was repeated by imposed food insecurity at school—administrators, nurses, social workers, teachers, and school-lunch personnel all devoted themselves to depriving Marcus of food. Little wonder that his food preoccupation and tendency to eat as much as he could, whenever he could, persisted.

Because of troubles of her own, Marcus's mother was neglectful, and Marcus's home life was chaotic. So chaotic, in fact, that Marcus was put into foster care when he was 13 years old. It could have been a perfect setup for treating Marcus's issues—the least of which was his weight. His foster parents could follow sDOR in feeding him: have regular meals and sit-down snacks and let him eat what and as much as he wanted. They could do the same authoritative parenting overall by being tuned in, warm and nurturing, maintaining structure, and accepting and supporting Marcus's autonomy by ensuring his safety and well-being at the same time as they let him make his own decisions and learn from his experience. Such parenting would support his development as an emotionally healthy teenager.

However, the perfect setup didn't happen. Marcus was placed in foster care because of his weight, not because of extreme neglect, and his foster parents were required to restrict his food intake to get him to lose weight. You can't do positive parenting when you are not letting a child have enough to eat.

Understand and address the backstory

Every "extremely obese" child has a backstory explaining why their weight accelerated to such a high level. For "extremely obese" children, intervention is only ethical and responsible when it takes that backstory into account and addresses underlying causes. In today's obesity-crazed world, that is unlikely to happen. Once a child's weight becomes an issue, it is difficult for those working within the control paradigm to see beyond it. Most fail to ask the question, "What caused this child's weight to be so high in the first place, and how can we address those causes?"

Neglect made Marcus weigh 447 pounds, but his weight was the least of his problems. He needed nurturing. With good nurturing, including being fed following sDOR, his weight had a very good chance of going down a bit and, more importantly, as his Eating Competence and activity improved, his wellness had every chance of increasing.[29] Instead, current American Academy of Pediatrics recommendations would have Marcus be put into a multi-year, multidisciplinary weight intervention. If that doesn't make him lose weight, and outcomes even from such ambitious treatment show slight weight loss,[21] the next AAP-recommended treatment step is for him to have bariatric surgery.[30] The AAP recommendations were written before the extreme weight loss drugs came on the market. Given her life challenges, it is difficult to imagine Marcus's mother being able to support him in making use of any extreme measures.

WHAT DO YOU CHOOSE FOR YOU AND YOUR CHILD?

Why should you trust what I tell you when it is so different from mainstream thought and practice? I give you the evidence I showed you in this and other chapters but, more importantly, I give you the evidence of your child. Consider your parent wisdom and your need to nurture. Owen's, Lauren's, Erica's, and Samantha's parents simply could not tolerate making their children miserable with feeding. I couldn't tolerate it either, and I regularly celebrated not having to try to slim my boys down. Weight struggles spoil everything. Letting go of weight struggles and depending on sDOR makes life better for everyone.

It isn't easy to go against prevailing thought, but acting as an advocate for your child is what parenting is all about.

REFERENCES

1. Shin YL. The timing of rapid infant weight gain in relation to childhood obesity. *J Obes Metab Syndr*. 2019;28:213–215.
2. Gorlick JC. "I feel like less of a mom:" experiences of weight stigma by association among mothers of children with overweight and obesity. *Childhood Obesity*. 2020;17:68–75.

3. Davison KK. Weight status, parent reaction, and self-concept in five-year-old girls. *Pediatrics*. 2001;107:46–53.
4. Wright CM. Breast-feeding in a UK urban context: who breastfeeds, for how long and does it matter? *Public Health Nutr*. 2006:686–891.
5. Spill MK. Caregiver feeding practices and child weight outcomes: a systematic review. *The American Journal of Clinical Nutrition*. 2019;109:990S–1002S.
6. Flores-Barrantes P. Rapid weight gain, infant feeding practices, and subsequent body mass index trajectories: the CALINA Study. *Nutrients*. 2020. doi:10.3390/nu12103178
7. Tanner JM. Standards for children's height at ages 2 to 9 years allowing for height of parents. *Archives of Disease in Childhood*. 1970;45:755–762.
8. Taveras EM. Crossing growth percentiles in infancy and risk of obesity in childhood. *Arch Pediatr Adolesc Med*. 2011;165:993–998.
9. Satter E. Internal regulation and the evolution of normal growth as the basis for prevention of obesity in childhood. *J Am Diet Assoc*. 1996;96:860–864.
10. Wright CM. How does infant behaviour relate to weight gain and adiposity? *Proc Nutr Soc*. 2011;70:485–493.
11. Wright CM. Implications of childhood obesity for adult health: findings from thousand families cohort study. *British Medical Journal*. 2001;323:1280–1284.
12. Wardle J. Parental feeding style and the inter-generational transmission of obesity risk. *Obes Res*. 2002;10:453–462.
13. Bouchard C. Genetics of obesity: what we have learned over decades of research. *Obesity*. 2021;29:802–820.
14. Dubois L. Genetic and environmental contributions to weight, height, and BMI from birth to 19 years of age: an international study of over 12,000 twin pairs. *PloS one*. 2012. doi:10.1371/journal.pone.0030153
15. Garn SM. Trends in fatness and the origins of obesity. *Pediatrics*. 1976;57:443–456.
16. Whitaker KL. The intergenerational transmission of thinness. *Arch Pediatr Adolesc Med*. 2011;165:900–905.
17. Eisenmann JC. Growth and overweight of Navajo youth: secular changes from 1955 to 1997. *International Journal of Obesity*. 2000;24:211–218.
18. Ryan AS. An evaluation of the association between socioeconomic status and the growth of American children: data from the Hispanic Health and Nutrition Examination Survey--NHANES 1982-1984. *American Journal of Clinical Nutrition*. 1990;51:944S–952S.
19. de Wilde JA. Tracking of thinness and overweight in children of Dutch, Turkish, Moroccan and South Asian descent from 3 through 15 years of age: a historical cohort study. *Int J Obes (Lond)*. 2018. doi:10.1038/s41366-018-0135-9
20. Gerards SM. Parental perception of child's weight status and subsequent BMIz change: the KOALA birth cohort study. *BMC public health*. 2014. doi:10.1186/1471-2458-14-291
21. O'Connor EA. Screening for obesity and intervention for weight management in children and adolescents: evidence report and systematic review for the US Preventive Services Task Force. *JAMA*. 2017;317:2427–2444.
22. Robinson E. Parental perception of weight status and weight gain across childhood. *Pediatrics*. 2016. doi:10.1542/peds.2015-3957
23. Ice CL. Morbidly obese diagnosis as an indicator of cardiovascular disease risk in children: results from the CARDIAC Project. *International Journal of Pediatric Obesity*. 2011;6:113–119.
24. Abraham S. Relationship of childhood weight status to morbidity in adults. *Int J Epidemiol*. 2016;45:1020–1031.

25. Llewellyn A. Childhood obesity as a predictor of morbidity in adulthood: a systematic review and meta-analysis. *Obes Rev*. 2016;17:56–67.
26. Vergnaud AC. Weight fluctuations and risk for metabolic syndrome in an adult cohort. *Int J Obes (Lond)*. 2008;32:315–321.
27. Sanaya N. The physiological effects of weight-cycling: a review of current evidence. *Curr Obes Rep*. Mar 2024;13:35–50.
28. Freedman DS. Tracking of BMI z scores for severe obesity. *Pediatrics*. 2017;140. doi:10.1542/peds.2017-1072
29. Satter Eating Competence Model (ecSatter): Evidence-based research. *https://www.needscenter.org/resources/satter-eating-competence-model-ecsatter/*
30. Hample SE. Executive Summary: clinical practice guideline for the evaluation and treatment of children and adolescents with obesity. *Pediatrics*. 2023. doi:e2022060641

CHAPTER 5

Discover the Joy of Eating

Your child will grow up to have your eating attitudes and behaviors, so consider what you want for them. Do you want them to feel confident and positive about food and their eating? Do you want them to feel accepting of and loyal to their body? That would be the trust paradigm. Or do you want them to debate about good-food/bad-food, worry about what to eat and not eat, anguish over the bathroom scale, and be critical of their weight? That would be the control paradigm.

The trust paradigm seems an obvious choice, but it is not so obvious at all, because negative feelings about food, eating, and weight are the norm in our control-paradigm-based culture. Guilt and uncertainty about eating and weight is the soup we swim in. We are so surrounded and influenced that those negative attitudes are invisible to us and seem normal. We go along with conventional expectations in the name of health, but, as is pointed out in the Chapter 1 section, "Why you don't have to be afraid of food," page 17, those health outcomes are more of a wish than a guarantee.

IN THIS CHAPTER

This chapter addresses your eating attitudes and behaviors in the context of the Satter Eating Competence Model (ecSatter). It gives guidance on how you can discover the joy of eating based on ecSatter and apply that joy to eating during pregnancy. It tells you how you can use the principles of Eating Competence to address the challenges of food insecurity, eating disturbances, weight concerns, picky eating, and medical conditions.

CONSIDER EATING COMPETENCE

The control paradigm has a lot to answer for. Consider the young woman whose pregnancy was being spoiled by being told not to diet but to gain only so much weight. Consider the young man who would—and could—only eat at certain fast-food restaurants because that is where his parents fed him in order to get him to eat. Consider the young woman who worried so much about what to eat that she spent hours in the grocery store reading food labels and could not join her friends when they ate out. Consider the young father whose on-again, off-again high-protein, low-carbohydrate dieting for his up-and-down weight created no end of misery for him and undermined family meals. Consider the university student who simply couldn't help binge-eating once she got away from her parents' rigid control. Or her classmate, who was so overwhelmed by the amount and variety of food in the school cafeteria that she couldn't begin to choose for herself.

These are all people who were handicapped by our culture's good/bad approach to food, not only with their eating but with their attitudes about themselves and the world. They are also people who freed themselves from their eating struggles by becoming Eating Competent and in the process gained self-confidence, self-respect, and the joy of eating.

Consider your eating attitudes and behaviors

If the eating struggles of people in these anecdotes resemble your own, know that you don't have to put up with all that conflict and anxiety about eating. It does way more harm than good: It creates barriers to your providing well for yourself as well as to your parenting with feeding. The struggles I just described emerged when young people did to themselves what their parents had done to them—or tried to do the opposite. You do not want that for your child.

Let's do a bit of consciousness raising to help you identify your own eating attitudes and behaviors. Answer yes or no to whether each item describes how you feel and what you do with eating.

- I set aside time to eat.
- I pay attention while I eat.
- I am comfortable about eating as much as I want.
- I trust myself to eat enough for me.
- I feel it is okay to eat food that I enjoy.
- I feel it is okay to enjoy eating, period!

If you answered *no* to any or all of these items, you have been infected by the prevailing negativity with respect to food and eating. Let's see if we can heal that negativity.

WHAT IT MEANS TO BE EATING COMPETENT

These six items in our little quiz are the essence of the ecSatter. The first two items have to do with feeding yourself faithfully; the last four have to do with giving yourself permission to eat.

As I told you in the Preface, the ecSatter grew out of my frustration with what I had been trained to do as a registered dietitian. I observed far too often that trying to follow special diets spoiled my patients' eating. They first came to see me feeling relaxed and comfortable with eating, looking forward to the next meal, and enjoying the process of planning and cooking. They were also wary, expecting to have their eating criticized. I did not disappoint. At the same time as I tried to be positive and supportive, I still gave eat-this/don't-eat-that guidance, and their eating became a guilt-ridden chore and bore. Surely this wasn't helping them!

Where ecSatter came from

I went back to the drawing board. I began to think in terms of trusting my patients to manage their own eating the same way I expected parents to trust their children's eating. I defined attitudes and behaviors that allowed adults to eat well. Working with Dr. Barbara Lohse, my research partner, we labeled those qualities the Satter Eating Competence Model (ecSatter). Eating Competence is being positive, comfortable, and flexible with eating and matter-of-fact and reliable about getting enough to eat of enjoyable and nourishing food. Clinically I developed a test for effective eating attitudes and behaviors that later came to be called ecSI 2.0, and Dr. Lohse and I collaborated on validating it. That is, we made sure it tested what we said it tested. Once we demonstrated ecSI 2.0 was valid, we and others began the ongoing process of gathering evidence.

That evidence has been more persuasive than in my wildest dreams: People who are Eating Competent are healthier in all ways.[1] They have better diets, lower BMIs, fewer indicators of distorted eating and behaviors, better lab tests, and are more active. Not only that but they feel better about their bodies, themselves, and other people. In other words, adults who are positive and trusting in the way they feed themselves are more confident and joyful *people*. I paraphrased the six items on our consciousness-raising quiz (above) from ecSI 2.0. Those six items do not substitute for ecSI 2.0. Search the ESI website for *ecSI 2.0* and *sDOR.2-6y* to find out how you can get permission to use it.

Eating Competence combines pleasure and health

When you are Eating Competent, you can have both pleasure and health. In fact, our research with ecSatter and with sDOR indicate that pleasure is *essential* for health. The same as in sDOR, there is absolutely nothing in ecSatter about eating certain amounts and types of food. Only one of the 16 ecSI 2.0 items addresses food selection: "I consider what is good for me when I eat." In the context of Eating Competence, "good for me" food is food I enjoy and eat because I *want to*, not because I *should*.

The same as with sDOR, the positive eating attitudes and behaviors of ecSatter are the *endpoint*, not the means to the end of eating "right" and/or weighing "right." For both ecSatter and sDOR, all good things flow from positive eating attitudes and behaviors. Period.

Eating Competence can feel like a miracle

For my patients who struggled so much with eating that their quality of life was impaired, the experience of Eating Competence seemed like a miracle. As one of my patients said, "If I have to count it, measure it, or weigh it, it makes me crazy." Instead, she discovered she could eat as much as she wanted without going out of control and eat what she wanted without feeling guilty. Many others shared her experience. Instead of having eating be an ordeal where they restricted and deprived and scrutinized and doubted practically everything they ate, they learned to provide. Instead of having to throw away all controls and tolerate guilt and shame in order to eat as *much* as they wanted of *what* they wanted, they could eat enough, eat food they enjoyed, all the time, in an orderly and self-respecting fashion. While improving self-esteem and body image wasn't a focus, people who became positive and self-trusting with eating felt better about themselves overall and were more comfortable with their bodies.

Let's contrast the stuck-with-eating examples I shared with you earlier in this chapter with some stories about people who became Eating Competent. Consider Sarah, who was ashamed of how much she enjoyed bakery-fresh bread. Sarah gave herself permission to eat bread at every single meal. That lasted for a month, and then she discovered she still enjoyed bread but now she was hungry for fresh tomatoes and avocados.

Consider Joseph, a foodie who developed type 2 diabetes as an adult. He blamed his diabetes on his love of good food, but there was really no relationship. Any relationship between his eating and diabetes probably had more to do with his yo-yo dieting. Joseph struggled constantly with his weight and didn't dare let himself eat what he enjoyed for fear of going out of control. In treatment, he learned to feed himself faithfully and give himself permission to eat. He got so he could comfortably eat the delectable, beautifully prepared food he enjoyed. His weight stabilized and his blood sugars improved.

Along the lines of miracles, consider Amanda, who had been on diets since her parents first took her to Weight Watchers when she was eight years old. Amanda had been truly traumatized about her eating and weight by her brothers' relentless teasing. In treatment, Amanda let go of her shame about her eating and weight. Her epiphany came when she found her stopping place halfway through a second piece of pie. She was ecstatic: "Do you know how good it feels to look at a piece of pie and truly not want it?" Amanda discovered that the "shameful" part of herself that loved to eat was not shameful at all but only natural.

What about food selection?

I don't talk about food and nutrition in this chapter except for when it is necessary to get the job done with respect to supporting your Eating Competence. You have enough to think about right now. When you feed yourself faithfully and give yourself permission to eat, you will eat the variety of food that you need. Until we get to the last few chapters I stay away from discussing food selection because I don't want to dump you into the attacks of conscience that can suck you into an eat-this/don't-eat-that mindset. When you are first discovering Eating Competence, food and nutrition information can turn against you.

If and when you are really, *really* ready for it, the Chapter 11 section, "Celebrate food," page 395, addresses the topic in more detail and ever-so-gently from the perspective of "why it is okay to eat this." Wait to read that section until you have settled down to the long haul of feeding your family. The food selection information is presented in a positive and permission-giving way, but it is still all too easy to drag yourself back into dos and don'ts.

To start with, dietitians are enslaved by food biases the same as I was, and I have tried to free them. During my presentations I would tell them, "Plan a reprehensible menu." I expected them to plan a menu that offended conventional nutrition standards, and they did not disappoint. Whatever they proposed, I pointed out its nutritional value and reminded them that the point of eating is *seeking* food, not *avoiding* it.

I often heard about Spam: not unsolicited messages but the canned meat product made mostly from ham. Ask your grandmother about it. Back in the day it was fast food, and it is still a mainstay for people who don't have much refrigeration. In southern Illinois, I heard about chicken-fried Spam. Since Spam is made in Minnesota, you find Spam on Minnesota restaurant menus. On Manitoulin Island in Ontario, I heard about Indian tacos made with fry bread and slices of Spam. In Hawaii, I was reminded that Spam is a favorite food, rivaled only by pineapple.

My colleagues objected to Spam because of its relatively high fat and sodium content and, truth be told, because it isn't "fresh." Of course it isn't! That's the point, and that's why Spam became popular in the first place. You can keep Spam in the pantry and haul it out for a sandwich or main dish or even a pineapple-Spam-chunk kebab. Is there a point to my rambling? I think so, and it this: *Eat what you enjoy and what is available to you*. Don't let anyone else tell you that your food is reprehensible.

ecSATTER CAN WORK FOR YOU

ecSatter works because you cooperate with your body rather than struggling against it.

DETERMINING *WHAT* TO EAT

- Provide regular, reliable, and rewarding meals.
- Depend on your food-acceptance capabilities to know what to eat.

We talked about your child's Eating Competent food-acceptance skills in Chapter 2. The same for you as for your child, food acceptance is all positive: You can comfortably participate in family meals, be around food you don't enjoy without getting upset or feeling obligated to eat it, let yourself eat only the parts of the meal that appeal to you and comfortably ignore the rest, and be polite while you do it all. Saying, "yes, please," and "no, thank you," and refraining from commenting on the food keeps you from yucking on someone else's yum.

DETERMINING *HOW MUCH* TO EAT

- Provide regular, reliable, and rewarding meals.
- Depend on your food regulation capabilities to know how much to eat.

We talked about children's food regulation skills in Chapter 3. Many parents have said they learned about internally regulated eating from watching their child. Children know how much to eat, and they instinctively trust their hunger, appetite, and satiety. The same as your child, you know how much to eat. However, you have likely ignored and overruled your hunger, appetite, and satiety for so long those sensations may seem to have disappeared. Not so. They are still there, waiting for you to rediscover them.

FIGURE 5.1: THE JOY OF EATING: BECOMING EATING COMPETENT (*sBEC*)

Becoming Eating Competent (sBEC) translates the routine plus trust of the Satter Division of Responsibility in Feeding (sDOR) into feeding *yourself.* Do the *what, when,* and *where* of feeding *yourself,* then let *yourself* eat *whether* and *as much* as you want.

Feed yourself faithfully.
Have regular and reliable sit-down meals and snacks made up of food you enjoy. Reassure yourself you will be fed. Take time to eat.

- Take time to eat.
- Eat what you eat now; add new food when you get interested.
- Eat at more-or-less predictable times.

Give yourself permission to eat.
At meals and snacks, eat what you enjoy and eat as much or as little as you want.

- Reassure yourself: "It's all right to eat this."
- Sit down and pay attention.
- Eat it if it tastes good, don't eat it if it doesn't.
- Trust that you can eat enough for you. Go to sit-down meals and snacks hungry (not starved) and eat until you truly feel like stopping.

Notice as you learn and grow.
As you combine feeding yourself faithfully with giving yourself permission to eat, you will find that your eating falls more and more into place.

- You feel good about your eating.
- You are comfortable with tuning in.
- You are reliable about seeing to it that you get fed.
- You trust yourself to eat enough for you.
- You are relaxed about eating food you enjoy, even including "forbidden foods" at meals and sit-down snacks.
- Big servings don't make you overeat. You eat it all if you want to, not if you don't.
- You enjoy more and more foods: You eat fruits, vegetables, whole grains, and other nutritious foods because they *taste* good, not because you *have* to.

HOW YOU CAN DISCOVER THE JOY OF EATING

Figure 5.1 summarizes what to do to let yourself be relaxed and confident with eating. Becoming Eating Competent (sBEC) guides you in being accepting and supportive of your needs by providing yourself with enjoyable food at structured meals and sit-down snacks, then trusting yourself with respect to whether and how much to eat. sBEC lets you experience the joy of eating by combining *feeding yourself faithfully* with *giving yourself permission to eat*.

Feeding yourself faithfully and giving yourself permission to eat means providing structure for your eating plus trusting your body to do the fine-tuning with respect to *whether* and *how much*. Feeding yourself faithfully is positive discipline: it is order, and freedom grows out of order. Chaos is enslaving because you spend so much time and energy coping. Combining permission and positive discipline puts your mind, feelings, and body in harmony. Together, the two even out the peaks and valleys in eating that grow out of grabbing, grazing, going on and off calorie restriction, and alternating between being "good" and being "bad" with food selection.

Free yourself to enjoy family meals

Achieving Eating Competence is somewhat nebulous, so I talk about it in a variety of ways. One discussion may be more helpful for you than another. Here, I talk about it from the point of view of freeing yourself to provide enjoyable family meals. Part 1, "How to Eat," in *Secrets of Feeding a Healthy Family* talks in more detail about understanding and achieving your own Eating Competence. It has helped many readers feed themselves in a kinder, gentler way. The 40-page booklet *Feeding Yourself with Love and Good Sense* coaches you step-by-step in becoming Eating Competent. The booklet helps you to learn Eating Competence with your body. It takes you through the motions and encourages you to feel what you feel. Eventually, you will find yourself being relaxed and comfortable with eating. On the other hand, the process could be so overwhelming for you that you need in-person expert help. Get in touch with the Ellyn Satter Institute for help finding a professional who has been trained in *How to Eat* treatment.

Giving permission leads to eating order

While many fear that giving permission to eat preferred foods in satisfying amounts will promote out-of-control eating, in practice quite the opposite occurs. Eating becomes more moderate, but don't let that scare you. Moderate in the conventional food world—from the control-paradigm perspective—means "don't eat so much; don't eat the food you like." Moderate in the context of Eating Competence—from the trust-paradigm perspective—means consistently eating what and as much as you want, not eating a lot and then compensating, no ricocheting between avoiding favorite foods and then eating them like there is no tomorrow.

Foods that are no longer forbidden become ordinary foods that can be consumed matter-of-factly without extremes of avoidance or excess. Large portion sizes become less appealing in the context of regular and reliable meals and snacks where you can eat as much as you want of food you enjoy. Healthful foods become foods you enjoy because you don't *have* to eat them. As it says in *What is normal eating* (Google it), "normal eating . . . is eating a lot sometimes and feeling stuffed and uncomfortable . . . and not eating much another and wishing you had more. Normal eating is trusting your body to make up for eating a lot or not eating much."

- Feed yourself faithfully
- Develop a meal and snack routine that works for you.
- Include foods you truly enjoy. Don't be ruled by lists of food-to-eat and food-to-avoid.
- Make eating times pleasant. Relax. Pay attention. Take your time.
- Experiment with new food if and when you are ready; take it slowly.

Make eating a priority. Have regular and reliable meals and snacks. Structure is the supportive framework for taking positive care of yourself with food.

The Chapter 1 section, "You need meals," page 18, advises you not to think "healthy home-cooked" but rather *possible, practical, familiar,* and *enjoyable.* Basing your family meals on food you enjoy will support you in hanging in there for the long haul: a lifetime of taking care of yourself with food. Eating when hunger or opportunity strike makes eating an afterthought. It is much too important for that. Eating is one of your most basic needs, and you must reassure yourself that you will be fed, just as you reassure your child. Make feeding yourself a priority as you do for your child.

The Chapter 2 section, "Master family meals," page 56, emphasizes going easy on yourself: starting where you are with respect to having meals. Build structure around the food you currently eat. Develop a meal and snack routine that works for you. Give yourself the opportunity to eat at more-or-less regular times. Hunger will follow: Once you establish a rhythm of providing yourself with food, your body's rhythms of hunger and appetite will respond.

That same Chapter 2 section reassures you that you won't get stuck where you start. Once you take the first step toward developing the meal habit—eating what you eat now at predictable times—other steps will follow. If you wish. Experiment with new food if and when you get ready—even if it takes a *long* time to get ready. Take it slowly, at your own pace.

The "How to Cook" section in my book *Secrets of Feeding a Healthy Family* gives easy and delicious recipes and offers how-to guidance for planning and preparing meals. The theme is "you can do this." Feeding yourself and your family is easier when you can cook, and you may as well be efficient and effective at it. *Secrets* is all about good food, joyful eating, rewarding food preparation, and emotionally gratifying family meals.

What I don't tell you in any of those places is *what* to eat. Telling you what to eat will put you in your head rather than in your body and undermine your Eating Competence.

Give yourself permission to eat

Reassure yourself, "It's all right to eat this. I just need to pay attention while I eat." Combined with structured meals and snacks that provide you with food you enjoy, giving yourself permission provides the formula for trusting your body to know how much to eat.

You can recover your internal regulation capabilities even if you have ignored them for a long time. At first, giving yourself permission and paying attention while you eat may feel like groping in the dark. As you persist, you may discover why you *haven't* been paying attention. At first you may get into self-talk about why it isn't okay to eat. Use the "it's all right" message to drown it out. That's the easy part. Coming to terms with feelings and memories takes longer.

Feel the feelings

Because the act of eating calls up associations from our very earliest times, it comes fully loaded with feelings and memories—some sweet, some bittersweet, some painful. When you start paying attention to your eating, you may get into treasured memories of people and places and maybe feel sad that those people and places are gone. You may feel upset and turned off without quite knowing why. You may discover negative memories of being shamed about your eating. Women who have grown up with food insecurity encounter the fear of not getting enough to eat at the same time as they are ashamed of wanting more than their parents were able to provide. People who have been put on diets as children feel the same fear and shame: fear of hunger and shame about wanting more food than their parents and, later on the broader culture, want them to have.

Feeling the feelings over and over takes away their painful edge so you can comfortably tune in on your eating. Trying to ignore the feelings keeps them fresh and upsetting forever. Tune out if it is too much. Tune back in when you are ready. Feeling and remembering, again and again, takes the painful edge off those memories and lets you comfortably integrate them into your life. Gaining comfort lets you tune in to your eating—to relax and enjoy it.

If you have been traumatized with eating, your feelings may be so strong that you just can't go there. Then, you will benefit from having a supportive and understanding person to help you work through the process. Get in touch with the Ellyn Satter Institute for help finding trained professionals who will guide and support you as you become Eating Competent.

Permission is nutritional judo

During my decades of clinical practice, I not only found out that my patients couldn't follow their prescribed diets, I found out *why*. Deep in their heart of hearts (or in their taste buds and stomachs), what most people *really* wanted and *needed* was eating food they genuinely enjoyed until they got enough of it. So why not, I reasoned, practice nutritional judo?

Judo means "the way of gentleness," and is an orderly and positive way of trusting and making use of one's own needs and the drive to satisfy those needs. With respect to eating, those needs are hunger and the drive to survive, appetite and the need for pleasure, the social rewards of sharing food, and the body's enormous tendency to maintain a stable weight range.

Feeding yourself faithfully and giving yourself permission to eat allows you to trust and respond to your wants and needs rather than trying to resist them. The same as my patients, you will do far better when you free yourself from eat-this-don't-eat-that guidelines. Consider the matter of "forbidden" foods. The cultural sense of being "naughty" when you eat certain foods is likely to make you periodically throw away self-awareness and eat more than you really want. Giving yourself permission and feeding yourself faithfully—including "forbidden" foods in meals and snacks—allows you to tune in to those foods and eat as much or as little as you are hungry for—just as you do any other food.

Forget about "bad" lists—whether they come from yourself or from somebody else. "Bad" lists ignore nutritional principles. Mashed potatoes, French fries, hashbrowns, and tater tots are still potatoes, and potatoes are nutritious. Fried chicken is still chicken and tastes great with mashed potatoes and green beans, broccoli, bread, or other foods—foods that might be low in fat but might not. Trust your appetite. The appetite gets weary of all high-fat food and craves some food that is lower in fat. The same happens in reverse: Eating generally low-fat food makes you crave foods that contain fat.

"Bad" lists are riddled with unfounded assumptions. Hamburgers have nothing whatsoever wrong with them—they are grilled, not fried—and depending on your preference can even come with lettuce and tomatoes. Oh, wait, the nutrionistas say you aren't supposed to eat too much red meat! As the Chapter 11 section, "Celebrate food," page 395, tells you, beef is highly nutritious, and current research shows eating beef doesn't increase blood lipids.[2] Including it in your diet makes it just one of many foods you depend on to keep you nourished.

You need both permission and routine

In becoming Eating Competent, some people have more trouble with permission, some with the routine of feeding themselves faithfully. The ones who hang in there discover that they need both permission and routine to find peace and comfort with eating. Other non-dieting methods tend to be strong on permission, weak on routine. Mindful eating is all permission. Intuitive eating is permission, some discipline in the form of paying attention to eating, but no routine.

Methods that claim to be non-dieting make negative and controlling use of routine by complicating eating so much that people eat less.

Those who gain Eating Competence reap the benefits described in the research literature: Life gets better, moods improve, and nutritional status is good. Those quality-of-life outcomes improve wellness. The medical world prioritizes weight and laboratory tests, so researchers keep track of those as well: BMIs remain about the same or a little lower; lab values are better.[3]

It is absolutely understandable that folks in the weight-activist world object to our reporting BMI. To them, it means that we are going over to the dark side. They flinch at the mention of BMI because they have so often been shamed for having high BMIs. We are not abandoning them; in reality, we are supporting them. Reporting BMI reassures folks in the nutrition and health worlds that giving permission to eat does not promote out-of-control eating, lab values, and weight. Professionals need this evidence to support weight neutral approaches to health.

THE JOY OF EATING DURING PREGNANCY

I hope you are reading this before your baby comes. Pregnancy in general and eating during pregnancy in particular give you a priceless opportunity to gain respect for your body and for the miracle of giving birth. There is no better foundation for feeding your family than feeding yourself faithfully and giving yourself permission to eat. All too often pregnancy is spoiled by its own particular version of the weight dilemma: being simultaneously advised not to diet and not to gain too much weight. Let permission plus discipline resolve that weight dilemma, as well.

Ordinary food prepared in ordinary ways does just fine with respect to supporting your pregnancy. Take your multivitamin mineral supplement: You and your baby particularly need the insurance that you are getting enough folic acid and iron. Have meals you enjoy. Go to meals hungry, eat as much as you want, then stop, knowing another meal or snack is coming soon and you can do it again.

Trust your body to gain the amount of weight it needs. Your hunger, appetite, and weight gain will be different from those of other women and will vary month to month and in your first, second, and third trimesters.

Learn to trust your body

If eating has been a challenge for you, now is a good time to learn to trust your body. From the sBEC point of view, learning to trust your body is quite different from using pregnancy and "eating for two" as a reason for throwing away controls with eating. In fact, trusting your body may be the main and only anchor you have as you deal with unpredictable variations in hunger, appetite, and even nausea. Feeding yourself faithfully (to the extent that you can) and giving yourself permission (ditto) reassures you that you can eat what and as much as you want without having to go out of control to do it.

Get into the meal routine, pay attention to what goes on inside you, and let your self-trust guide you in what and how much to eat. In short, let yourself enjoy eating rather than worrying about it. Don't spoil your pregnancy by dieting or worrying about your weight! Trusting your body now will support you in the early months, whether you breast- or formula-feed, and let your body go back to weighing what is right for it. Trusting your body will, in fact, support you in the years to come.

A past or active eating disorder can make eating during pregnancy a particularly challenging ride. Many manage to control their eating extremes during pregnancy, but it is challenging to get into the meal habit, and trusting internal regulators may seem impossible. For established eating problems, consider engaging with your therapist and an Eating Competence savvy dietitian. I have helped pregnant women recover from extreme distortions in eating attitudes and behaviors, and it was some of the most rewarding work I have ever done—both for them and for me.

ADDRESS FOOD INSECURITY

Do you worry about having enough money for food? If so, you are experiencing food insecurity, and you have lots of company. An estimated 13 percent of U.S. households experience food insecurity, and 17 percent of children live in households experiencing food insecurity. Most of those households are headed by women. Food insecurity isn't confined to low-income households: Children in higher-income households experience food insecurity when parents have difficulty managing their finances to buy food or are inconsistent about feeding them.

Running out of food money before the end of the month is so miserable that it is hard to imagine. Professor Christine Olson from New York's Cornell University asked women who had grown up with food insecurity to share what it was like for them. They talked of being constantly afraid of going hungry, feeling panic when there wasn't enough food, and being likely to binge-eat when food again became available. Feeling particularly afraid made them reach for particularly high-calorie food, such as potato chips, dip, soda, and cheesecake. And they felt guilty about it all.[3]

Eating Competence supports getting enough to eat

Dr. Olson's women scolded themselves for eating high-calorie food, but from the point of view of Eating Competence, it makes all kinds of sense. The women were practicing nutritional judo: To get enough to eat, they were instinctively eating the higher-calorie, higher-fat food they found appealing. The missing piece—and it was a huge one—was that they weren't giving themselves *permission*. They were seeing their food choices as bad and therefore feeling ashamed of themselves for "breaking down" and eating "bad" food.

People who are hungry naturally prefer higher-calorie, higher-fat food—their bodies have wisdom that is best to obey. sBEC says to provide rather than deprive: to eat food you enjoy in amounts you find satisfying. When you are particularly hungry, you are likely to prefer higher-calorie foods that taste good, fill you up, and keep you satisfied for a while. It is the same if you are on a weight-reduction diet, or on an airplane with no food stash. When you get off that plane, you are more likely to think "fries" than "salad."

If you worry about having enough money to buy food, consider making use of the Special Supplemental Nutrition Program for Women, Infants, and Children (WIC) and the Supplemental Nutrition Assistance Program (SNAP), as well as food pantries. To make your food dollars go farther, maintain the structure of meals and snacks. Respect your body's wisdom by routinely choosing higher-calorie foods. Choose whole milk; use gravies and sauces with potatoes, rice, and noodles; use higher-fat meats, poultry, and fish; put butter, margarine, or other culturally preferred fats in beans (yes, bacon, fatback, or lard!), on vegetables and at the table; use canned fruit in heavy syrup and/or baked into desserts.

Discourage random snacking by including "forbidden food" at meals and sit-down snacks. Have cookies and allow chips and even (gasp) soda for sit-down snacks, if you enjoy soda. By providing yourself with regular, reliable, and attentive access to those foods, you will likely drink less soda than if you sip along throughout the day; you will certainly be kinder on your teeth! Make use of "forbidden" foods often at meals and snacks to provide calories and enjoyment. Your appetite will tell you when you have enough high-calorie food and you will automatically eat other food that is lower in calories. Ration the expensive food—say have one pork chop or only so many strawberries for each person—but reassure your eaters that there is enough of the other food so everyone can get filled up.

Worrisome advice? Too many calories? From the control-paradigm perspective, those who are food insecure tend to have higher body weights because they eat the wrong food. From the trust-paradigm perspective, their body weights are higher because they are afraid of going hungry. That fear of hunger persists and drives eating a lot when food becomes available. Having higher calorie food allows getting enough to eat and neutralizes the fear. Too much of the wrong kind of fat? The "healthy eating pattern" says to keep animal fats to a minimum, presumably to limit saturated fat intake. However, all animal fats contain monounsaturated fat as well as stearic acid, a saturated fat. Monounsaturated fat raises good cholesterol. Stearic acid neither raises nor lowers blood cholesterol. The Chapter 11 section, "Enjoy fats and oils," page 400, discusses fat chemistry and frees you to use animal fats as well as vegetable fats.

Being Eating Competent helps address food insecurity

ecSatter offers no particular guidance on budgeting or food resource management. However, people with low incomes who take the lead with family food management and are also Eating Competent tend to see themselves as food secure. Equally low-income people who are not Eating Competent are more likely to characterize themselves as food insecure. Low-income Eating Competent homemakers likely gain a sense of food security from being able to manage limited food resources. They are least likely to run out of food before the end of the month, most likely to feel confident about managing food money, plan meals, shop with a list, and cook from scratch.[1]

Eating Competent parents are experts at *faithful feeding*: They depend on structure to make their food money stretch to cover. They provide filling and satisfying food at regular meals and sit-down snacks and don't allow raiding the refrigerator and cupboard for between-time snack foods. Instead, they include those snack foods at meals and sit-down snacks. Since family members get as much as they want of the food they enjoy at regular eating times, they are less likely to seek out food at odd times.

Food insecurity and weight

Being confident you can give your family enough to eat, unhindered by good-food/bad-food expectations, is critical for your child as well as for you. Parents who experience food insecurity are more likely to be concerned about child "obesity" and therefore more likely to restrict some foods and pressure children to eat other foods.[4] As we discussed elsewhere, such crossing of the lines of sDOR offers a perfect recipe for child weight acceleration.

The same for adults as for children, fear of hunger is the weight-destabilizing factor, not poor food selection. Not having enough money to buy food creates a repeated pattern of going without, then eating a lot when food is available. Because it is expensive and doesn't give enough calories, trying to follow the "healthy eating pattern" contributes to feast and famine.

As many of my patients over the years have lamented, "I know what to do. I am just not able to do it." Little wonder! It didn't work for them or their families to eat unadorned fruits and vegetables, breads and cereals, low-fat dairy and other protein sources, and avoid sweets, chips, and other high-calorie snacks. The same as Dr. Olson's Cornell women who had experienced food insecurity, they instinctively ate higher calorie foods to get enough to eat. The problem, and it was a serious one, was that they were ashamed of eating those foods, and that created repeated patterns of restriction and overcompensation.

In contrast, ecSatter works because it is consistent: Rather than having peaks and valleys in eating in response to economics and impulse, being

Eating Competent supports eating as much as desired of enjoyable food—all the time.

Think in terms of Eating Competence when you solve eating problems: when you address your weight concerns, picky eating, medical issues such as diabetes, celiac disease, and food allergies, and eating disorders.

THE WEIGHT DILEMMA

Eating Competence is weight neutral: It focuses on positive eating and health attitudes and behaviors and trusts the body to weigh what it will in response to those attitudes and behaviors. Weight neutral approaches set aside weight loss as a medical intervention and instead focus on well-chosen treatment for specific ailments. Eating Competence is based on the trust paradigm, in contrast to the societal control-paradigm-based insistence on weight loss as a prerequisite to health. ecSatter is consistent with the Health At Every Size® (HAES®) philosophy.

That control-paradigm insistence on weight loss as a medical intervention—often the first and only intervention—creates a dilemma. The reality is that the chances are very low of achieving lasting weight loss, but both professionals and the public keep trying. Why? Three of the big reasons are money, aesthetics, and weight stigma. Weight loss is a multibillion-dollar industry. Being thinner is considered more attractive. People of size can experience discrimination. Weight loss for health could be number four on the list, but it isn't. Weight loss is an ineffective medical intervention and only rarely achievable.

The logic of weight

In our thinness-worshipping culture, resolving the weight dilemma by setting aside striving for weight loss is a *really* big ask that involves no less than being able to accept your body. You can't resolve that ask with logic, but let's get logic out of the way by examining the evidence. The control-paradigm interpretation of this evidence is that any amount of weight above cutoff points is bad and must be addressed with weight loss. The trust-paradigm interpretation is that wellness comes in all sizes and that weight loss attempts do more harm than good. Definitions of adult "overweight and obesity" no more logical and helpful for adults than they are for children.

- Compared with "normal" weight (BMI 18.5 to 25), mortality rates are lower for individuals who are "overweight" (BMI 25 to 30) and have "Class 1 obesity" (BMI 30 to 35).[5] You read that right: I said "overweight" and "obese" people have lower mortality rates. Despite that extraordinarily strong data, BMI 18.5 to 25 continues to be defined as "normal" weight.

For an example of how fiercely prevailing paradigms are defended, read author Katherine Flegal's article, "The obesity wars."[6] After publication of her 2013 article that I just cited, Flegal was professionally attacked. She and her research were targets of an aggressive campaign that included insults, errors, misinformation, social media posts, behind-the-scenes gossip and maneuvers, and complaints to her employer. Flegal's publication was evidence-based. Her detractors were belief-based.

- Weight loss is an unachievable and ineffective medical intervention. A tiny percentage of people who lose weight keep it off; there is little to no data correlating weight loss with improved medical outcomes.
- Weight loss attempts contribute to yo-yo dieting: a repeated pattern of weight loss and regain to a higher level. Such weight instability does have negative health consequences.[7]
- Weight-neutral approaches to health such as ecSatter have considerably more positive outcomes than weight loss approaches.[8]
- Eating Competence[1] and being physically active[9] are correlated with wellness at *any* weight level.

The Chapter 4 discussion of weight and health issues for children applies to adults as well. Those health issues were summarized in the section, "Are 'extremely obese' children unhealthy?" page 123.

The dream of weight loss

Sharing the logic didn't help my patients resolve their weight dilemma. They were only able to consider giving up their dream of weight loss after they had been defeated by their failed attempts. For them, doing and being all they wanted to do and be depended on being thinner. The amount of weight didn't matter—at times it was imaginary. Their self-loathing was strongest and most insidious when it came from childhood, especially early childhood: Their parents saw them as being "too fat" and had tried repeatedly to get them thinner. Children don't compartmentalize: If part of them is unacceptable, they are unacceptable all over, and those feelings of being unacceptable persist in adulthood. Typically, as preadolescents my patients applied the slimming regimen to themselves, and they had been yo-yo dieting ever since: forcing their weight down, then regaining to a higher level.

My colleagues and I have found that most of our patients were in their thirties and forties and even older before they were defeated by their weight-loss efforts. There are exceptions. My Ellyn Satter Institute colleague Anne Blocker works with university students who are so freaked out and miserable about their eating that they are ready to discover Eating Competence. My colleague Alexia Beauregard works with soldiers who are relieved to give up dieting. Their weight dilemma is the military's expectation that they "make weight" and their reality of yo-yo dieting and being so exhausted from undereating that they have trouble passing their fitness tests.

Understand the eating and weight backstory

Part of giving up the weight-loss dream is forgiving ourselves for our weight. The same as I did for Marcus, my colleagues and I consider our patients' backstories. Often their weight acceleration began with the first weight-loss attempt, whether that attempt came from parents or from themselves. A few didn't gain weight in response to food restriction: When parents kept the upper hand with their child's eating, they forced the child's weight to remain at a certain level and kept it under strict control. They did, that is, until the child was able to be out on their own. At that point they sneaked to eat the food their parents didn't want them to eat—and they were ashamed. The Chapter 3 story of Mary, page 81, tells of feeding intentions gone *very* wrong: Mary developed bulimia in her fruitless efforts to impose on herself the restrictions her parents had imposed on her.

Reviewing the backstory makes it clear: Still another weight reduction effort is unlikely to be successful. That harsh reality introduces hope in a different form: that of setting aside weight loss as an outcome goal and learning to be orderly, positive, and self-respecting with eating.

Find peace with eating

I developed the *How to Eat* intervention to work clinically with the people I just described—I called them dieting casualties. Many today are dieting casualties not just because of a constant and futile struggle with weight, but because they are stuck with eating in other ways. They are conflicted about good-food/bad-food and experience eating as unrelenting misery and shame. At the same time as they strive to live by the credo "don't eat so much; don't eat the foods you like," today's dieting casualties most often aren't even *aware* that they have been enslaved by food restriction. Their often vague but cruel self-expectations about eating leave them so insensitive to and mistrustful of their wants and needs with food and eating that they can only respond to extremes of hunger, food craving, and fullness. While their struggle with eating plays a central role in life, they aren't eating disordered: They do not use food and their struggle with eating to try to solve their other problems.

The Ellyn Satter Institute trains health and mental health professionals in the *How to Eat* method. It is an eight- to ten-week, step-by-step approach that helps replace negative and chaotic eating with Eating Competence: with orderly, positive, and dignified eating. Becoming aware of and resolving conflict and anxiety about eating makes it possible to discover and trust the internal regulators of hunger, appetite, and satiety.

Typically, in about the fifth week our patients discover their stopping place. It is like watching them be reborn. As one of my patients exclaimed, "It's like sanity in the midst of all this insanity." To fully understand what it means to them to become Eating Competent, you have to have experienced both: the misery, torment, and self-shaming that go along with relentless struggles with eating and/or weight, and the joy, freedom, and self-acceptance that go along with being relieved of the struggles.

Becoming Eating Competent helps with respect to giving up the dream of weight loss. Until our patients experienced positive and self-trusting eating, they couldn't possibly know what it had been costing them to be so negative and controlling. Being able to trust their eating also allows our patients to trust their bodies and be more accepting of their weight.

Being Eating Competent takes on a life of its own because the rewards of positive, sustainable eating are built right into it. For some, that isn't the happily-ever-after end of the story. When life circumstances pile up, they go back to being chaotic with eating. Those times pass, and they go back to feeding themselves faithfully and giving themselves permission to eat. Others give in to internal and external pressure and try again for weight loss. That's too bad, but at least they are able to tell what the effort costs them. Sometimes they choose to go back to being Eating Competent. Sometimes they don't.

Make your decision

Which brings us to you. Will you let yourself become Eating Competent—have the joy of eating—and let your body weigh what is right for it? Or will you adhere to rigid dietary expectations in pursuit of weight loss and pay the price of struggles with eating and body self-loathing that accompany the effort? Your choice affects your family as well. It is extraordinarily difficult to raise Eating Competent children if you are not Eating Competent yourself.

Becoming Eating Competent —feeding yourself faithfully and giving yourself permission to eat—may be relatively easy for you. It depends on your level of conflict and anxiety about eating. Many have been able to do it based on reading my books or browsing the Ellyn Satter Institute website. Or you may need someone else to help you. Get in touch with the Ellyn Satter Institute for help finding a professional who can work through *How to Eat* with you.

PICKY EATING

Do you consider yourself a picky eater? Keep in mind that everyone has food preferences. Even adults have foods they don't enjoy and don't eat and that's just fine. Foods you don't enjoy are unlikely to show up at family meals. That too, is fine. Some adults are especially reluctant to eat unfamiliar food, and their food variety is low. Also fine. As long as adults and children enjoy family meals and feel positive about food, children of selectively eating parents can push themselves along to eat unfamiliar food at school, at the grandparents, and at the neighbors.

Extreme food selectivity

There is nothing wrong with being a picky eater, as long as you have good social skills and don't beat up on yourself about it. Garden-variety picky eating morphs into extreme food selectivity when it is accompanied by being *upset and anxious* about being a selective eater—or perceiving yourself as one. You might actually eat a fair variety of food but still feel ashamed that you don't eat more: It depends on your upbringing. If your parents have been relaxed and accepting about your food selectivity, you will be too. If they have seen your selective eating as being negative and tried to change it, you will likely experience conflict and anxiety about what you see as your limited food acceptance. It's about eating attitudes and behaviors, not about what is and isn't eaten.

If you are an upset and anxious selective eater, meals are likely stressful for you: You might react strongly and negatively to certain smells and textures, feel that if you are persuaded to serve yourself a food you have to eat it all, and be ashamed of your inability to eat from more than your short list of acceptable foods. Extreme food selectivity could limit your social life if you are not comfortable eating with others for fear that your eating will attract attention and even ridicule.

Weight loss or nutritional deficiency added on to food selectivity can take you into the realm of Avoidant Restrictive Food Intake Disorder (ARFID). Marked interference with your psychosocial functioning can indicate Other Specified Feeding or Eating Disorder (OSFED). To find someone well-versed in Eating Competence to help you address such an established eating problem, email *support@ellynsatterinstitute.org*.

Start with your feelings

From the Eating Competence point of view, the solution is not getting yourself to eat a greater variety of food but letting yourself feel positive about eating the food you currently enjoy. Trying to get yourself to eat more foods is likely to duplicate the growing-up pressure criticism that created your food selectivity in the first place. Do you currently eat without eating—that is, eat without paying attention? That grows out of conflict and anxiety about eating. Resolve your conflict and anxiety by feeding yourself faithfully and giving yourself permission to eat. Tune in while you eat and feel the feelings. At first those feelings could be strong and even scary. As you continue to feel the feelings they will mellow and you will get to the point where you can tune in to your eating.

Learn social skills

Once you get permission and discipline under your belt, so to speak, learn the social skills you need to eat with others. In the process of defending yourself against unwanted food, you may have developed some negative behaviors. It is okay to pick and choose from what is on the table, to decline to be served, to take moderate portions, to eat only one or two food items, to leave unwanted food on your plate, and to take more of one food without finishing another. Don't complain and don't explain. Master the broken record technique for when food is repeatedly pressed on you: "No-thank-you-no-thank-you." At the same time, be careful not to do anything that draws attention to your food refusal, such as criticizing food, asking for food that is not on the menu, or taking a lot of food and then not eating it.

Increasing food variety is optional

Eating new food will come last if it comes at all. Do you want to eat new food, or do you want to want to? Once you gain peace and comfort with your eating, you are likely to ever-so-gradually and naturally begin to take an interest in new food—or you might not. Either is okay. In either case, you do not have to be miserable about your eating.

It's all a tall order, and you might need help working your way through the process. Get in touch with the Ellyn Satter Institute for help finding trained professionals who will guide and support you as you discover your freedom and joy of eating.

FOOD ALLERGIES

For you as for your older baby, toddler, or preschooler who has food allergies, eating need not be painful or disappointing. It is important for you to be able to look forward to eating and your mealtimes need to continue to be a relaxing and enjoyable part of the day. You can still feed yourself faithfully and give yourself permission to eat. I realize it is easy for me to say, but giving yourself permission is important. Put the emphasis on providing rather than depriving. Work with an allergist to be sure your list of foods-to-avoid is as short as possible.

DIABETES

This section is not to tell you how to manage your diabetes. It is to introduce you to the possibilities of integrating Eating Competence principles into managing your diabetes. Stated another way, you do not have to give up the joy of eating to successfully manage your diabetes. You can continue to focus on feeding yourself faithfully and giving yourself permission to eat as we have been discussing in this chapter. Your cues of hunger and satiety still work, whether you are taking an oral hypoglycemic agent or injecting insulin. As you know from reading this far in *Ellyn Satter's Child of Mine*, Eating Competence isn't willy-nilly eating-whatever-you-want, whenever-you-want. It is the positive discipline of having satisfying meals and sit-down snacks at more-or-less predictable times.

Eat to balance available insulin

With type 1, type 2, or gestational diabetes, your pancreas doesn't produce enough insulin at any one time to metabolize the glucose your body makes from what you eat. With type 1, insulin is injected; with type 2, medication stimulates your pancreas to make insulin. Gestational diabetes is managed primarily with diet. Type 2 diabetes can also be caused by insulin resistance: You make enough insulin but your body can't use it. Being active can make body cells more receptive to insulin.

Spacing out regular meals and snacks throughout the day helps keep you from exceeding your insulin availability at any one time. Having protein, fat, and carbohydrate at each meal or snack, with particular emphasis on including fat, slows down the rate at which nutrients get into your system so your available insulin can match it. That is why you can even include sweets in a meal or snack that includes protein, fat, and carbohydrate.

Food first or insulin first?

Carbohydrate counting works with Eating Competence: You eat as much as you are hungry for, then count carbohydrates after the meal. My colleague Anne Blocker, a certified diabetes specialist, refers to this as post-dosing.

Alternatively, you can manage your diabetes by figuring out your eating ahead of time with food portions and an eating pattern. Your health care provider may teach you that management system, and you may feel most comfortable with it. That pattern will give you enough to eat to satisfy your hunger and your weight may stabilize, but it might not satisfy your appetite.

With an eating pattern, medication leads the way: You try to balance your available insulin with your food intake. With Eating Competence, eating leads the way: You eat as much as you want of food you enjoy at regular eating times. Then you balance your eating with your available insulin. Some people do a pre-dose and a post-dose. Work with your health care provider to adjust your insulin to metabolize what and how much you eat.

Monitoring blood sugar

Monitoring your blood sugar can help you develop your awareness of how you physically feel: Too-low blood sugar can make you feel shaky; too-high blood sugar can make you feel listless, nauseated, and even hungry. If your blood sugar is consistently too low or too high, talk with your health care professional about adjusting your insulin or medication. Your blood sugar will vary from day to day and throughout the day. Work with your diabetes educator to find a comfortable range for you. Often, a blood glucose range that is a bit wider and more flexible is easier to manage and supports your overall well-being more than one that is relatively narrow.

Physical activity

Pursue enjoyable and sustainable physical activity to help normalize your blood sugars, make your available insulin work better, and give you other health benefits. Regular activity helps enhance sensitivity to food regulation cues and thereby helps keep your food intake and insulin in balance.

CYSTIC FIBROSIS

Take a look at the Chapter 11 section, "The toddler with cystic fibrosis," page 384. The same for you as for your toddler, you can cooperate with your body rather than struggling against it when you have cystic fibrosis (CF). Your capabilities with food acceptance and food regulation still work when you support them with regular, reliable, and rewarding means.

Standard guidelines recommend that individuals with CF consume up to 110 to 200 percent of the general population's daily energy intake, with 35 to 40 percent of energy from fat and 15 to 20 percent of energy from protein.[10] The idea is to eat more to compensate for losing poorly absorbed nutrients through the digestive tract. Following those recommendations will take you right into the control paradigm.

Protect yourself by considering the logic behind such recommendations—or the lack of it. The body regulates food intake based on the calories and other nutrients that get into your *bloodstream*—what you actually *absorb.* You *automatically* compensate for calories that get lost through your digestive system. Unless you have a lung infection accompanied by poor appetite, your body even compensates for breathing problems. You have greater hunger and appetite to support the increased metabolic work of lung inefficiency.

I realize some people with CF are advised to keep their weight down. It's not my recommendation, so I won't try to explain it. I only know that struggling with weight loss with resultant unstable body weight is particularly negative for you when you have any kind of medical condition. Your body is working hard enough already; it doesn't need the additional stress of coping with unstable body weight.

EATING DISORDERS

Almost everyone feels some conflict and anxiety about what and/or how much they eat. Almost everyone repeatedly or continually restricts the amount or type of food they eat to be "healthy" or to keep their weight down. Almost everyone talks about it in tedious detail! The distorted eating attitudes and behaviors that go along with food restriction always take a toll, but they take a *big* toll and start to look like an eating disorder when eating and/or not eating become your life's focus. You cross the line to having an eating disorder when you start to use your eating and/or not eating as a way of addressing your other life problems.

An eating disorder—or not?

We all have life issues. You have an eating disorder when you use your eating or not eating in the *service* of your life issues: Trying to lose weight to be more comfortable in the world; eating "right" to control your anxiety. If your eating problems exist side by side with your other life issues with no crossover, you don't have an eating disorder. You might need *help* with your life issues and with your eating, but resolving one does not depend on resolving the other.

Some behaviors are right on the cusp of being an eating disorder. Restricting your food intake and periodically overeating can look and feel like binge eating disorder. Even if your weight is high or in the "normal" range, keeping it artificially low *for you* can look and feel like anorexia nervosa. Extreme food selectivity and aversion to unfamiliar food tastes and textures can feel like an atypical eating disorder. So can restriction and preoccupation with eating only "healthy food," anxiety about eating to maintain wellness, dread of choking or vomiting, or fear of eating foods that could cause an allergic reaction.

When to seek help

Whether or not you have an eating disorder, such extreme and negative eating attitudes and behaviors cause you pain and impair your quality of life. Seek help from a professional who is proficient with Eating Competence and who has helped people who struggle with extreme distortions in eating attitudes and behaviors. If one or more of these bullet points applies to you, you do need help—and you are entitled to it.

- Your concerns about your weight or about what to eat/not eat affect your relationships with other people.
- You see "successfully" managing your eating and weight as central to your life satisfaction.
- The feelings that come up when you tune in to your eating are so scary and upsetting that you just can't tolerate them on your own.

BON APPETIT

Celebrate eating. Eating is okay. Eating *enough* is okay. *Enjoying* eating is okay. Eating what you *like* is okay. Taking *time* to eat is okay. Making eating a *priority* is okay. To be consistent and effective in feeding yourself and your family, build on *enjoyment*. Optimism, pleasure, and self-trust are good motivators. Pessimism, avoidance, and self-doubt are poor motivators.

Are you waiting for the other shoe to drop? It won't. That's all there is to it. I think it's enough. In fact, it wouldn't be surprising if you were feeling a bit overwhelmed right now. Overhauling eating attitudes and behaviors is major. Eating is complex, and patterns of thinking, feeling, and behaving relative to eating are deeply embedded.

It may not be as difficult as you fear because Eating Competence works *with* your body rather than *against* it. It taps into your inborn capabilities and supports you in rediscovering what is natural. Clinically, I am continually astonished at how working toward natural eating allows even the most negative, conflicted, out-of-control eater to rapidly bring order and comfort into eating.

Your Eating Competent attitudes and behaviors may grow to feel so familiar that, until you stop to think about it, you may not realize that anything has changed. Why not again take that little self-test we started with:

- I set aside time to eat.
- I pay attention while I eat.
- I am comfortable about eating as much as I want.
- I feel it is okay to eat food that I enjoy.
- I feel it is okay to enjoy eating, period!

Are your yes or no answers the same as at the beginning? Are they different? Do you *want* to answer yes to all the items? Give yourself time and let yourself grow.

REFERENCES

1. Satter Eating Competence Model (ecSatter): Evidence-based research. *https://www.needscenter.org/resources/satter-eating-competence-model-ecsatter/*
2. Sanders LM. Beef consumption and cardiovascular disease risk factors: a systematic review and meta-analysis of randomized controlled trials. *Current Developments in Nutrition*. 2024. doi:10.1016/j.cdnut.2024.104500
3. Olson CM. Growing up poor: long-term implications for eating patterns and body weight. *Appetite*. 2007;49:198–207.
4. Adams EL. Food insecurity, the home food environment, and parent feeding practices in the era of COVID-19. *Obesity (Silver Spring)*. 2020;28:2056–2063.
5. Flegal KM. Association of all-cause mortality with overweight and obesity using standard body mass index categories: a systematic review and meta-analysis. *JAMA*. 2013;309:71–82.
6. Flegal KM. The obesity wars and the education of a researcher: a personal account. *Progress in Cardiovascular Diseases*. 2021. doi:10.1016/j.pcad.2021.06.009
7. Park SY. Weight change in older adults and mortality: the Multiethnic Cohort Study. *Int J Obes (Lond)*. 2018;42:205–212.
8. Eaton M. A systematic review of observational studies exploring the relationship between health and non-weight-centric eating behaviours. *Appetite*. 2024. doi:10.1016/j.appet.2024.107361

9. Barry VW. Fitness vs. fatness on all-cause mortality: a meta-analysis. *Prog Cardiovasc Dis*. 2014;56:382–90.
10. Thornton RR. Dietary intake and quality among adults with cystic fibrosis: a systematic review. *Nutr Diet*. Sep 2024;81(4):384–400.

PART II

How to Feed: The Early Months

CHAPTER 6

Your Feeding Decision: Breastfeeding or Formula-Feeding

In today's newborn-parenting world, you have decisions within decisions about feeding. What will you feed your baby? Will it be breastmilk—by which I mean human milk—or formula, or a combination of the two? Having made that decision, what will be your mode of delivery? Will it be breastfeeding—by which I mean breastmilk fed directly from the breast—or bottle-feeding—expressed breastmilk and/or formula fed from a bottle or from a supplemental nursing system? Those systems trickle breastmilk and/or formula from a reservoir through thin tubing onto your nipple as your baby nurses. Along with consideration of the supplemental nursing system comes the consideration of *chestfeeding* and the possibility of either parent's feeding the baby using that mode of delivery. Of course, any decision you make before your baby is born has to be tentative. You can't know what your baby will need and how they will be able to eat, and you can't predict if you are in the tiny number—1 to 5 percent—of women (those declared female at birth) who can't breastfeed.[1] Do you see what I mean about decisions within decisions in today's world?

Of all the considerations, the most important is the feeding relationship. When you follow the Satter Division of Responsibility in Feeding (sDOR) babies get their nutritional and emotional needs met with breastfeeding, bottle-feeding, and any variation and combination *with which you feel comfortable.* With all, babies grow up to be healthy, well-adjusted, intelligent, and thin, fat, or in between. I support breastfeeding for its built-in feeding-dynamics advantages. I support providing babies with unpasteurized breastmilk because it contains *living* components uniquely adapted to the human child. However, I support *more* your making the feeding decision that is right for you. It is my absolute conviction, supported by my long experience and research on parent-infant interactions around feeding, that to support your baby's nutritional needs and both your and your baby's emotional needs, you must be comfortable with your method of feeding. Breastfeeding can help you tune in to your baby. But if you find it unpleasant, it can spoil your feeding relationship.

Don't let anybody else decide for you. You know yourself and your circumstances best, and you will soon know your baby best: You can rely on your own judgment. Breastfeeding is currently strongly favored. Because of its advantages, it is worthy of consideration. To help you decide, learn about breastfeeding. Talk with someone you trust who has breastfed. Try breastfeeding at first and give yourself an out. If you and your partner or the person you depend on feel positive about it (or even if it is just okay) and if breastfeeding works with you and your baby, breastfeed. Get help if you need it.

Consider other modes of delivery of human milk: expressing and bottle-feeding, supplemented or not with formula. If breastfeeding or other breastmilk-milk delivery options don't feel good to you, you don't have to pursue them. Doing a trial run means you have given it your full consideration, and providing your baby with breastmilk for even a few days or a few weeks benefits you and your baby.

Whatever nutritional source or mode of delivery you choose, you are entitled to support from your health care providers and help with establishing a positive feeding relationship with your baby.

QUESTION BREASTFEEDING RESEARCH

Breastfeeding research tends to be viewed through rose-tinted glasses. Breastfed babies do have a lower risk of ear infections, respiratory infections, and diarrhea. However, research does not support claims that breastfed babies are more intelligent, less likely to become "overweight" or "obese," or develop degenerative diseases in later life.

Research has difficulty defining what breastfeeding *is*, let alone what outcomes correlate with it. To me, breastfeeding is 24/7 feeding an infant from the breast, with the occasional relief bottle of expressed breastmilk or formula, with no value judgment intended. But what about the variations? For the purposes of research, is primarily feeding expressed breastmilk from the bottle still breastfeeding? Many researchers accept that definition. UNICEF seems to agree, as it defines exclusive breastfeeding as feeding nothing but breastmilk, not necessarily from the breast. By that definition, UNICEF data on breastfeeding show 26 percent of North American babies are exclusively breastfed. How old were those babies? Were they breastfed from the breast, the bottle, or a supplemental nurser, or what? And for how long? We don't know.

Breastfeeding research provides incomplete information

Breastfeeding research concerns itself only with nutritional issues[2,3] and is often difficult to interpret. Numbers of subjects are small, data-gathering methods are questionable, distinctions aren't always clear among "exclusive" or "any" use of human milk or the duration of such usage. Most concerning of all, studies may or may not distinguish among other factors that can affect child outcome, such as parent socioeconomic status and education.

The data is strong enough to suggest that exclusive breastfeeding for the first six months can protect a baby against ear and respiratory infections, and possibly from dermatitis and eczema. Again, does that "breastfeeding" mean human milk delivered from the breast? Or can it be delivered by bottle? Babies' patterns of suckling are different between the two and can have an impact on their respiratory system.

The data is *not* strong enough to support other reasons to breastfeed. If you do a search for *breastfeeding and child obesity*, you will see that agencies, health-care firms, and researchers promote breastfeeding on the grounds that it protects against "overweight" or "obesity" in later life. It is unclear whether that means breastfeeding 24/7 from the breast or delivery of human milk, in any amount or duration, by any means. The same applies to saying that breastfed babies are more intelligent in later life. A Scottish study of nearly 200,000 child, so huge that almost any correlation was statistically possible, claimed to demonstrate a connection with protection against disability. *Some* breastfeeding at age six to eight weeks correlated with a lower incidence of special educational needs in primary and secondary school![4] As with the "overweight/obesity" correlation, outcome-influencing variables between infancy and later life, such as parents' education and economic status, boggle the mind.

Feeding dynamics is not examined

Research addresses itself with *what* infants eat, not with the *manner* in which they are fed. That is, research does not address the feeding relationship: The degree to which the parents calm and organize their baby and feed based on information coming from them. That's too bad, because if there are correlations between breastfeeding and child weight and intelligence, they are likely related to the feeding relationship. By its very nature, breastfeeding—feeding your baby from your breast—encourages your following sDOR, thereby connecting with your baby. Doing your jobs with feeding and understanding and supporting your baby's doing their jobs with eating supports their eating and growing in the way that is right for them. The same thinking applies to intelligence. All babies long to be understood. Paying attention to what your baby "tells" you encourages them from the first to communicate with you and thus supports their intellectual development.

In order to successfully breastfeed, you *must* listen to and understand your baby. Overriding babies' cues is difficult but possible and is likely to undermine breastfeeding. With bottle-feeding it is easier to override babies' feeding cues. The Chapter 7 section, "Feed the way your baby tells you," page 183, discusses how to get on your baby's wavelength with feeding.

Breastfeeding in developing countries

Speaking of UNICEF, the health implications of breastfeeding in developed countries are quite different from those in the developing world. Without breastfeeding, developing world circumstances with respect to income, sanitation, and access to clean drinking water make it extraordinarily difficult to feed babies enough safe and nutritious food. In those settings, UNICEF estimates that optimal breastfeeding is so critical that it could save the lives of almost a million children each year. I certainly don't argue with their conclusions.

AGENCIES PROMOTE BREASTFEEDING

Based on their interpretation of the available research, the American Academy of Pediatrics (AAP), along with other public health agencies, recommend "exclusive breastfeeding for about 6 months . . . and support continued breastfeeding along with appropriate complementary foods introduced at about 6 months, as long as mutually desired by mother and child for 2 years or beyond."[2] Such recommendations and support can morph into such enthusiastic promotion and relentless encouragement that parents can feel that bottle-feeding is failing their baby. Rather than promoting breastfeeding, I promote informed decision making. I wonder if agencies would get more breastfeeding takers if they did the same thing—and really meant it. It would be kinder to parents.

I consider a positive parent-child feeding relationship to be critical enough to be a public health issue, and basic to that relationship is feeding in a way you are comfortable with. I bring in public health because AAP considers breastfeeding and/or the provision of human milk a "public health imperative." Their point of view is that your providing your baby with breastmilk impacts the health and protection of society as a whole. Is the evidence supporting human milk feeding as strong and important to society as clean drinking water, safe food additives, and immunization against disease? I don't think so, but you might disagree.

Formula-feeding parents are ashamed

The current climate of promoting breastfeeding is hard on parents who choose to bottle-feed. Formula-feeding parents experience guilt, dissatisfaction, and stigma relative to their feeding choice. Parents feel bad when they cannot or don't want to conform, and feeling bad interferes with their relationship with their baby. Formula-feeding parents report receiving little information and support from health professionals, and what information they do get frames bottle-feeding as being second-best to breastfeeding. There is a reason professionals are weak on formula-feeding education. Australian hospital nurses reported having little access to bottle-feeding information and some had the idea that they were not supposed to give that information.[5]

It is unclear whether or not the ongoing campaigns by health and nutrition agencies have increased breastfeeding and/or the provision of human milk. According to the Centers for Disease Control and Prevention figures released every two years, 63 percent of babies are exclusively breastfed at birth, dropping to 25 percent at six months. The figures for "any breastfeeding" are 83 percent at birth, 56 percent at six months, and 36 percent at one year. Of course, those figures include the exclusively breastfed babies who by one year are likely eating solid foods. For updates, do a web search for *Breastfeeding report card.*

It is clear, however, that breastfeeding campaigns have increased guilt, and guilt is a poor reason for doing anything. Hanna Rosin, then-breastfeeding mother and *Atlantic* writer, says, "In certain overachieving circles, breast-feeding is no longer a choice—it's a no-exceptions requirement, the ultimate badge of responsible parenting."[6]

Interference? Or support?

Because I do not *promote* breastfeeding and or the use of human milk, I am known in some circles as being anti-breastfeeding. In my defense, Baby-Friendly USA, which assesses hospitals, clinics, and teaching materials for consistency with breastfeeding, considers my writing to be supportive in that I say breastmilk is best for human infant nutrition. Moreover, I discuss breastfeeding before formula-feeding and provide no images of bottle-feeding parents. I would love to see that image guideline changed to "there are a roughly equal number of images of breastfed and bottle-fed infants." I have wonderful, touching images of exquisitely tuned-in parents bottle-feeding and others of parents doing the same with breastfeeding.

Baby-Friendly USA considers human milk provided by direct breastfeeding to be the biologically normal way to feed infants. I agree with them in reserving the word "breastfeeding" to mean human milk delivered directly to the infant from the breast. However, I consider saying it is "biologically normal" to be a value judgment that is disapproving of parents who choose to feed other ways. Beyond that, Baby-Friendly USA states that facilities providing maternity and newborn services have a responsibility to promote breastfeeding, but they must also respect the mother's preferences and provide her with the information needed to make an informed decision about the best feeding option for her and her infant. The facility needs to support mothers to successfully feed their newborns in the manner they choose.[7]

I am glad to see the statement about respecting parents' preferences and supporting them no matter what, but I am leery of the practice of providing that support only after parents are served a liberal dose of breastfeeding promotion. I consider *promote* to be a taking-away-choice word, the same as *should*, *ought*, and *get* (as in *get* your child to eat). I have seen the harm such promotion can do. Lillian, a WIC nutritionist, was herself doing breastfeeding promotion. During her pregnancy, her colleagues gave her much approval, encouragement, and information, and she looked forward eagerly to breastfeeding her baby. But she couldn't do it. She did all the right things, but she was one of that tiny percentage of women who simply cannot breastfeed.[1] She was devastated, and her disappointment made her unhappy and miserable during the first precious and formative weeks of her baby's life. She had been exposed to such breastfeeding fervor that she felt downright humiliated and inadequate.

Interference from hospital routines

Since hospital routines that support breastfeeding support mother-infant bonding, those routines apply just as much to parents who feed in other ways. They also apply to fathers as well as mothers. Best birthing practices as defined by the American Academy of Pediatrics include direct skin-to-skin contact, delaying procedures (weighing, bathing, medical procedures) until after the first feeding, and encouraging having the baby in the room with the parents. Errors in routines that have been shown to lower breastfeeding rates and duration include advising mothers to limit suckling at the breast to a specified length of time, routinely giving pacifiers, and giving infant formula or glucose water, except as needed for hyperbilirubinemia and hypoglycemia.[2]

Interference from formula companies

Interference with respect to your feeding decision can come from the formula companies as well. Formula marketing is formidable and versatile, with efforts ranging from professional journal articles to popular magazine articles and advertising to television and web-based advertising. The formula companies are obligated to put a disclaimer on their packages and feeding booklets, and they do. But at the same time as they say breast is best, they advertise "our formula is most like breastmilk." Formula manufacturers take turns providing the formulas for take-home packages from the hospital. Do those packages encourage or undermine breastfeeding? Formula in your hospital take-home package can make you prone to reach for it when you can't seem to fill your baby up. On the other hand, having an alternative way to feed your baby can make you braver about continuing to breastfeed. You get to decide.

CONSIDER INFANT NUTRITION

Human milk has nutritional and biological advantages, especially during the early months. Human milk is nutritionally very nearly complete, lacking only vitamins D and K. Beyond that, we have to admit that we don't know all there is to know about nutrition. Attempts by nutritionists and formula manufacturers to duplicate nature (i.e., human milk) are constantly improving, but all must still acknowledge that there is more to be known. Because human milk is high in whey protein and low in casein, it is digestible for the human infant. (Cow's milk protein composition is the opposite.) Colostrum, the yellowish fluid produced before mature milk comes in, and early human milk are relatively high in zinc. This high zinc level is provided at a time when the newborn has particular needs for zinc as a building block for zinccontaining enzymes. Nutritionists debate the right levels of zinc to put in formulas.[3] Colostrum and early human milk also contain proteins that give the newborn immunity from organisms that enter through the intestine. Human milk monoglycerides and free fatty acids of a particular chain length appear to destroy certain viruses and bacteria by dissolving the fatty sheath around them.[8]

Human-milk-fed infants get enough iron for their needs, but not too much. That balance is important to preserve the unique diarrhea-combating bacteria in their large intestines, *lactobacillus bifidus*. The relatively small amounts of iron in human milk are absorbed almost totally.[9] In contrast, iron in formula is only about 10 percent absorbed. Unabsorbed iron nourishes less-desirable bacteria in the colon, such as *Escherichia coli*, a bacterium that can overgrow and cause diarrhea.[8]

Feeding human milk may or may not help prevent allergies, depending on a host of factors including genetics of the mother and other food in the infant's diet.[10] Human milk seems to exert an immunoprotective effect, in that the baby fed totally on human milk may be protected from allergies or sensitivities to food. For instance, fully breastfed babies are less likely to develop celiac disease in response to gluten exposure. Human milk's immunoprotective effect provides support for the American Academy of Pediatrics recommendation to continue fully breastfeeding for the second six months while solid foods are being introduced.[2] On the other hand, feeding of human milk does not provide full protection against allergies. A very small group of extremely allergic human-milk-fed babies react to even minute amounts of food substances in their mother's milk and have to be put on an extensively hydrolyzed or amino acid formula. To continue providing their babies with breastmilk, mothers of those highly allergic infants have to avoid so many foods that their diets become incomplete nutritionally. Nutritional harm to the mother can impair her energy level and thereby have a negative impact on the mother-infant relationship.

Human milk is living and changing

The idea that human milk is living may conjure up visions of little creatures swimming busily around—and possibly gross you out. By "living," I mean human milk contains beneficial components that can be destroyed by the heating to which formula is subjected. Human milk's living components support immunity, gastrointestinal tract health, and the functioning of the immune system. Since it is living, human milk can contain active substances that even help it digest itself. For instance, human milk contains lipase, an enzyme that helps the infant's immature intestine digest fat, and amylase, which digests carbohydrate. Non-digestible sugars, oligosaccharides, protect against GI tract pathogens by acting as decoys, binding those pathogens and keeping them from attaching to the intestine.[3]

Human milk continually changes. Human milk for the newborn is different from that for the child a few months old; a specific example would be the variation in zinc levels. Also, within each breastfeeding, the first milk is quite low in fat and looks thin and bluish. Then as the feeding progresses, breastmilk contains more and more fat, until most of the fat is produced in the last minute of nursing. The infant then stops nursing and will only resume with the lowerfat milk from the other breast.[2, 3]

Commercial formulas are good imitations of human milk

Commercial formulas are digestible, we can generally keep them sanitary, and we are able to give enough of them to infants to allow appropriate growth. Of course, formula shortages in 2022 attributed to manufacturing problems have left us all wondering about that manufacturing and unsure about being able to get enough baby formula. Keep in mind, however, that careful infant formula inspection and testing uncovered the manufacturing errors in the first place. While that period of shortage created no end of problems, it still demonstrated that formula production is strictly regulated and monitored.

Formula's nutritional adequacy is demonstrated by healthy formula-fed babies who grow well. Commercial formulas are complete to the limits of present knowledge—no supplements are necessary. Formula manufacturers respond to research on human milk by duplicating as much as possible human milk components. However, when manufacturers boast in their advertising of some new breakthrough in formulation and claim that their formula is "more like mother's milk," that does not mean that the nutritional gap between human milk and formula has closed. Such formulas may contain protein, fat, and/or other ingredients in a form similar to that in human milk. Recently, for instance, formula manufacturers have been experimenting with nucleotides to try to duplicate the immunity-conferring properties of human milk. The nucleotides have helped, but babies even partially fed human milk still show superior patterns of immunity to respiratory diseases.

I still support your feeding choice

By now, this information about human milk may feel to you as if I am dropping the other shoe—taking back what I said earlier about supporting your feeding choice. That has not changed. Your choosing food and a feeding method that are right for you and your baby and your having a good feeding relationship are still more important than breastfeeding. That holds true for what I just said as well as for what I am about to say.

CONSIDER YOUR BABY'S MEDICAL CHALLENGES

You can breast- or bottle-feed your baby with medical or developmental challenges, fully or in part. For more, read the Chapter 7 section, "Babies who require tube feeding," page 212. Feeding from the bottle is seen in some circles as being less challenging for a vulnerable baby than establishing and maintaining breastfeeding. However, breastfeeding authority Ruth Lawrence argues otherwise. Using the definition of breastfeeding to mean feeding the baby directly from the mother's breast, she points out that breastfeeding can moderate the medical impact of many conditions, and that some of the advice you may be given is a holdover from less-informed times. For instance, parents of babies with heart defects may be discouraged from breastfeeding on the grounds that the baby doesn't have enough energy to take on the extra work of breastfeeding. In reality, the work required to breastfeed is less than that required to bottle-feed. Heart rate and breathing remain stable during breastfeeding: Babies who breastfeed have higher oxygen saturation rates, meaning their lungs work better. The chapter Breastfeeding Infants with Problems, in the Lawrence book *Breastfeeding*, is an often-updated resource that can guide your health professional to the latest research about managing breastfeeding for an infant with medical conditions.[11]

I certainly support Lawrence's assertion that breastfeeding moderates the impact of medical or developmental conditions. However, don't rule out the beneficial effect of accepting and supportive feeding from either the breast or bottle. Particularly for the vulnerable baby, it is critical to feed by paying careful attention to the baby's sleep rhythms, helping them be calm and awake during feeding, and depending on their hunger and fullness signs to determine how much to feed them. Chapter 7 addresses all those issues.

CONSIDER HOW YOU FEEL

Which brings us back to modes of delivery. We'll minimize the confusion in this section if we recall the definitions from early in this chapter: Breastfeeding is human milk fed directly from the breast; bottle-feeding is expressed human milk and/or formula fed from a bottle and/or from a supplemental nursing system.

They say in the real-estate world that the three important considerations in buying a house are location, location, and location. The three important factors in your feeding decision are feelings, feelings, and feelings.

Of course, there *are* situations that force you to choose formula: the rare condition of being physically unable to produce breastmilk, a severely allergic baby, certain illnesses, or your having to take a medication that comes through in your breastmilk and isn't good for your baby. Otherwise, it is all about feelings.

Emotional issues relative to breast- or bottle-feeding

Some women get a real emotional and physical high from breastfeeding. Others see it as all in a day's work. Some parents are turned off by breastfeeding and can't imagine doing it. Some partners are moved and inspired by watching their child being breastfed. Others are fine with it but not particularly touched. Still others find it off-putting. You can't anticipate how you and your partner will react until you are doing it. Both of you are entitled to consider and respect your feelings in making your feeding decision. If you don't agree, keep talking until you do. Get help if you need it—it is *that* important and will give you a foundation for addressing the many other issues that crop up with parenting.

It is difficult to express negative feelings about being a parent in general or breastfeeding, in particular. Negative feelings such as distaste, anxiety, jealousy, and entrapment are challenging to reveal and discuss, but it must be done. Otherwise, those feelings get stuck and make you act in ways you don't want to. Having negative feelings doesn't mean that you can't choose to breastfeed. Your feelings might or might not change, but awareness gives choice. When you know how you feel, you can make reasonable choices.

Working and/or taking occasional breaks from parenting are obviously easier with bottle-feeding. You might welcome the freedom, or you might be so besotted and involved that you can't stand to leave your baby. Your baby will have a lot to do with your needing to get away. They may be so placid, easy to satisfy, and predictable that you can even take them to a party, or they may be so high maintenance that you *must* have a break. Here's a hasty word of encouragement: children change. That's the point of helping them get organized. Keep in mind that those first few months are fleeting and taken in the context of your life with your child, they last all too short a time.

Many part-time workers or the fortunate ones who have nearby child care can continue to breastfeed. Other working parents pump and feed their baby stored breastmilk. It is quite a commitment, not everyone can do it, and you have to feel comfortable doing it. Some don't mind pumping. Others find it downright uncomfortable and even icky. *New*

York Times columnist Judith Warner made no bones about hating it. She first stated her commitment to providing her breastmilk for her baby, then described her view of pumping: "The grotesque ritual carried out behind closed office doors nationwide by beleaguered working mothers who are fully 'committed' (as the lactation counselors put it) to the goal of long-term, exclusive breast-feeding."[12] Note Warner's definition of long-term, exclusive breastfeeding: providing her baby only with her breastmilk, delivered by breast or bottle.

Connecting with your baby

Whether you breast- or bottle-feed, you connect with your baby when you respect their sleep rhythms, help them be calm and awake during feeding, and guide feeding based on their hunger and fullness signs. Connecting with your baby lets them feel understood and good about you and about themself. Breastfeeding gives you more help connecting, because in order to make enough breastmilk to provide for your baby, you *have* to connect. Since bottle-feeding allows you to impose schedules and amounts, you may have to make a particular point of going by your baby's feeding cues. It is a real issue and important for you to consider: Research indicates that bottle-feeding parents are less likely than breastfeeding parents to feed in response to their baby's cues. It doesn't have to be that way for you, but you do have to be aware of the possibility.

Your physiological responses to breastfeeding can help you be warm, close, and tuned in to your baby. But if you don't like breastfeeding, it can go the other way: Breastfeeding can make you remote, disconnected, and abrupt. You and your breastfed baby are a twosome, except for the occasional relief bottle. You can be a twosome with your bottle-fed baby when you do most of the feeding yourself, which your baby prefers anyway. Bottle-feeding lets your partner get in on the endless task of feeding and gives them the reward of knowing your baby well and responding sensitively to their cues.

To your baby, parents are the most important people in the world. Your baby is born knowing you and brightens up and turns toward you when they hear your voice. Your baby eats best and feels most nurtured with feeding when you do the feeding. You wouldn't feel comfortable eating with just any old body who comes along, and your baby doesn't either. Breastfeeding lets you keep your baby all to yourself for feeding. Not so with bottle-feeding, but don't let others press you to let them feed your baby if you don't want them to. Find ways of kindly saying, "This is my job." There will be other times to share your baby, but feeding need not be one of those times.

You need support with both breast- and bottle-feeding

Whether you breast- or bottle-feed, you need support. Try to get help and give your help some guidance about what they can do: take care of you and let you take care of your baby. Ask them to cook, clean, do laundry, provide moral support, give encouragement, and provide another set of eyes and ears as you try to understand what your baby is telling you. In fact, let's turn that sentence around and put cooking, cleaning, and doing laundry at the end of the list. New mothers say what they need most is moral support, encouragement, and help understanding their baby. Even the most inexperienced helper can be a calming presence while you get used to being parents. My mother came to stay with me when my children were born, and her help was worth more than rubies. I had the great privilege of being a new baby helper for two or three weeks when each of my grandchildren was born.

I didn't do much infant care and I certainly didn't know the answers, but I did help their parents to settle down so they could do their own thinking. After the birth of my first grandchild, Emma, my daughter and son-in-law were both in that mild state of shock that many of us experience when we realize how much responsibility we have taken on. When the twins, Adele and Marin, were born, it took all three of us to observe and understand their feeding behaviors. We had a running joke that started, "I have a theory . . . ." That meant that we had been observing the action and thought we could explain and supply a solution for the dilemma of the moment.

It will help a great deal with both breast- and bottle-feeding your baby to have other people to back you up. Think about this ahead of time, because it is important, and it does take some organizing. See the Chapter 8 section, "Consider support," page 220.

With respect to feeding, given today's emphasis, you are likely to have more access to encouragement, help, and information if you are breastfeeding than if you are bottle-feeding. Hospitals and pediatric clinics have on-staff lactation counselors who are well-trained, certified, and experienced, and can help you. The best counselors help solve problems and do not insist that you continue breastfeeding no matter what. They keep you from going on guilt trips, encourage you to use an occasional relief bottle if they think it is called for, and help you keep in perspective that you are doing well even when it seems like you aren't. Find a counselor you like and respect, who can give you advice in a way that you find helpful and supportive.

My only trouble with lactation counselors is that they may confine their work to breastfeeding parents! The attitude toward bottle-feeding seems to be that there is nothing to it: You put the nipple in the baby's mouth and that's the end of it. Not true. Bottle-feeding parents need help and support, too. Not only do they have to get on the same feeding wavelength with their baby, they have to understand the basics of infant formulas and master the mechanics of preparing and giving bottles.

Consider your sex life

Having a baby changes your personal relationship and sex life. Breastfeeding may change it more than bottle-feeding because of the exclusive mother-baby relationship that seemingly excludes the partner. Breastfeeding and sexuality are closely associated. It can be disturbing for a partner to see their mate's breasts, which they associate with their own erotic pleasure, used for feeding an infant. Masters and Johnson, pioneering and long-term researchers on human sexuality, found that women who breastfeed return more quickly to nonpregnant levels of sexual interest. Some women experience sexual arousal from nursing, some don't. Some enjoy that arousal, others don't.

With the initiation of suckling, the body releases prolactin from the pituitary gland, which causes uterine contractions during the feeding and for about 20 minutes afterward. This is one of the advantages of breastfeeding, as it enhances the return of the uterus to a more nearly prepregnant size. Some women experience the contractions as sexual, some do not, and others are not even aware of them. All are normal perceptions. Because breastfeeding and sexual arousal use the same nerve pathways and hormones, milk often drips from the breast during sexual arousal and orgasm.

The possibility of having nursing stimulate you erotically may be perfectly acceptable to you. On the other hand, it may be alarming and disagreeable. Having milk drip from your breasts while you are making love may be a real turnon for you—or a real turnoff. It's hard to know how you will react. Consider adopting a waitandsee attitude: Try out breastfeeding, let yourselves feel what you feel, and discuss it.

Consider your appearance

Most women are eager to return as quickly as possible to their pre-pregnant weight and shape and wonder how lactation—breastfeeding or providing human milk for their baby—will affect that. Many women find that even if they lose weight while lactating, their bodies only go back to pre-pregnant size and shape when lactation ends. You may have heard that you have to gain weight to breastfeed. You don't. You may or may not lose weight during lactation, but you may become leaner because breastfeeding draws on the calories stored in body fat.

Producing human milk uses calories from your body as well as from your diet, drawing on the fat you stored during pregnancy in preparation for lactation. In fact, about a third of your weight gain during pregnancy is fat, which represents an immense calorie store—on the average about 28,000 calories. Lactation allows you to make use of this calorie store: The calorie demands for a newborn usually start at around 400 calories per day. If you didn't gain much weight during pregnancy, you will have to be particularly careful during early lactation to eat enough.

Dieting to try to lose weight, especially strict dieting, can impair your milk supply. Generally, a weight loss of no more than ½ pound per week is safe, but the best indicator is how you feel and how your body performs. To maintain your spirits, your energy level, and your milk supply, you do need to eat enough.

CONSDER YOUR BREASTMILK SUPPLY

Making enough breastmilk, knowing your baby is getting enough, and getting enough to eat yourself are all issues to be considered. All impact your feelings.

Making enough breastmilk

At first you have to keep an eye on the newborn breastfed infant to know they are getting enough to eat. The American Academy of Pediatrics recommends that all newborn, breastfed babies discharged less than 48 hours after delivery be seen 2 to 4 days after discharge from the hospital, then seen again either 2 weeks or 1 month later. I think 2 weeks is better. The right-after-discharge visit is important to make sure of proper latch-on and positioning and that the infant is awake, alert, and eating well. It seems to me that considering the same issues is important for formula-fed babies, but those babies are routinely first seen at one month. However you are feeding, if you feel you and your baby need it, don't be shy about asking for a follow-up visit before the prescribed time.

Breastmilk is produced according to a law of supply and demand. Your baby's suckling and/or emptying your breasts by other means stimulates you to make breastmilk. During hungry days, your baby wants to eat often. Even if they don't get as much as they want from each nursing, their suckling stimulates your breasts to make more milk. After a day or two your supply catches up with their demand and you are in balance again—for a while. The more your baby suckles, the more breastmilk you are stimulated to produce. As babies get bigger and more active, they have hungry days when they want to eat more frequently and that stimulates you to make more breastmilk. After a day or two of frequent nursing, breastmilk production increases and the baby goes back to their usual regular or irregular pattern of eating.

Your ability to produce breastmilk has nothing to do with the apparent size of your breasts. You can be flat-chested and still have all the milk-producing tissue you need to make breastmilk. Larger breasts contain more fat and fibrous tissue than smaller breasts, but not necessarily any more milk-producing alveoli. Breast surgery, however, can have an impact on your ability to make and deliver milk to your baby. Breast implants can mechanically rearrange the milk-delivery apparatus in the breasts, but there is still a chance that the breast tissue will be intact enough to allow you to breastfeed. Breast reduction surgery can be planned ahead of time to leave enough ducts, sinuses, and nerve endings to allow breastfeeding.

As I said earlier, most women—people assigned female at birth—are physically able to breastfeed their infants. Most cases of breastfeeding failure come from anxiety, lack of understanding of the breastfeeding process, and/or lack of cultural and other support. Some of our best insights on this came from developing countries, where 40 years ago almost all mothers successfully breastfed their infants, even when they were poor and not eating well. I say *were* successful, because with the advent of western ideas and customs, ready availability of infant formula, and introduction of the idea that breastfeeding might not be successful, breastfeeding "failure" is on the increase. There are additional contributing factors, such as movement away from family support, mothers working away from their babies, and imitation of western patterns of infant feeding (that is, routinely relying on formula feeding). However, the fact remains that before those intrusions, a very high percentage of women breastfed successfully.

Knowing your baby is getting enough

You may decide to bottle-feed with expressed breastmilk or formula because you want to know how much your baby is eating. With the bottle-fed baby you can, of course, actually see how much is going in. With the breastfed baby, you can tell that something is going in from the tingling let-down sensation in your breasts and the drawing sound your baby makes as they take in breastmilk. You don't have to know how much your baby eats or needs to eat. Your *baby* instinctively knows, and their hunger and fullness cues are an accurate guide to how much they need to eat. With either breast- or bottle-feeding, your baby's consistent growth is the best evidence that your baby is getting as much as they need. You can trust even your newborn to know how much to eat. Your breastfed baby might eat a little or a lot and they might grow rapidly or slowly. The same holds true for your bottle-fed baby.

TAKING CARE OF YOURSELF WITH FOOD AND DRINK

Whether you breast- or formula-feed, you have to eat. You don't have to eat boring food, but you do have to eat. This goes for fathers as well as mothers. You need your strength, endurance, and emotional steadiness in order to be a good parent. When you are hungry or going without food, you will be worn-out, cranky, and discouraged. If you haven't already been taking care of yourselves with food, it's time to start. Read the Chapter 1 section, "You need meals," page 18. That section and all of Chapter 1 are about lightening your load rather than piling on more expectations.

Pay particular attention to Chapter 5, Discover the Joy of Eating. Trust your hunger and appetite to tell you how much to eat. Forget about the good-food/bad-food, healthy-food/unhealthy-food business. Eat what you eat and do it with enjoyment and reverence. Almost every food has some nutritional value. If you consider a food particularly nutritious, eat it because you enjoy it, not because you *have* to.

Breastfeeding—human milk production—requires, most of all, calories, particularly after the first month, and particularly if you haven't gained much weight during pregnancy. The quality of your diet comes after quantity, because with the exception of the water-soluble vitamins like the B vitamins and vitamin C, your body will sacrifice nutrients from itself in order to provide the nutrients in your breastmilk. Being Eating Competent keeps you from being nutritionally depleted.

CONVENIENCE, ECONOMY, SAFETY

Whether breast- or bottle-feeding is easier to manage depends on your perspective. In Chapter 8, Breastfeeding Your Baby, I spend a lot of time talking about mastering breastfeeding. In Chapter 9, Formula-Feeding Your Baby, I spend a lot of time talking about mastering equipment and choosing formulas. In both chapters, I emphasize getting on the same wavelength with feeding your baby. Either feeding method will give you much to learn and will require your intelligence, sensitivity, time, and effort.

Convenience

Is it more difficult to prepare bottles or to learn how to breastfeed? It seems to me a matter of individual judgment and preference. It saves pre-planning and packing to take the breastfed baby and a disposable diaper and be all set for an outing. For long trips, it's even better. On the other hand, you'll need to pamper yourself a bit more to help establish and maintain a breastfeeding relationship. Bottle-feeding has the advantage of letting you leave your baby for work or outings.

Are babies' eating patterns more predictable with bottle-feeding than with breastfeeding? It depends more on the baby than on the feeding method—some babies are just more regular than others. Eating times are perhaps a bit more widely spaced with formula-feeding because formula digests less rapidly than human milk. You can try to force a schedule with either method of feeding by trying to stave your baby off or waking them up to feed them. It probably won't work, and it isn't good for you or your baby. It also could spoil your breastmilk supply. Both breast- and bottle-fed babies gradually evolve a feeding routine, and both cluster-feed at times: They ask to be fed a half-hour after they get done eating and do it still again after that.

Breastmilk is ready to feed and just right for your baby's needs. My four-year-old niece Michelle had her first exposure to breastfeeding when she watched me feed my infant son Lucas. Michelle got the idea right away. Including her mother in her being-a-mommy play-acting, she lifted her shirt and plastered her doll's face to her flat little chest. "Yes, this is how I do it," she chatted. "All I do is hook him on right here. Isn't that just the handiest thing?" Breastfeeding is handy.

Will you be comfortable breastfeeding in public? Social custom varies a lot in this regard, so it really comes down to you. Good for you if you are adroit enough and comfortable enough to breastfeed in public. On the other hand, it may be a good thing for you to retire and retreat to feed your baby. Getting away from a crowd and having quiet personal time can be quite lovely. Some babies, in fact, need such quiet to eat well, so you may find yourself retreating whether you are breast- or bottle-feeding.

Economy

The direct cost of fully breastfeeding a baby in terms of your food and vitamin D for the baby is about a third that of standard formula-feeding. Special formulas cost two or three times more.[13] Additional direct breastfeeding costs include breastfeeding-convenient clothing, pumping and storage equipment, and furniture and gadgets to make breastfeeding easier and more comfortable.

If you stay home to breastfeed your child or even if you work and pump breastmilk, the cost picture changes drastically. Leaving your job means lost income. Working and pumping might also mean lost income.

Pumping your breastmilk can take three to four hours per day. If you figure your time at minimum wage, it brings the cost of breastfeeding up to three or four times the cost of formula.[13] There are lots of ins and outs relative to calculating the breastfeeding-associated cost of your time. Working remotely is a possibility, but pumping still takes time. Women who can afford quiet, hands-free breast pumps reduce that time by pumping while they make phone calls or do desk work.

For more, see the Chapter 8 section, "Breastfeeding in your absence," page 258.

Safety and sanitation

The U.S. Food and Drug Administration makes sure all formulas legally sold in the United States meet federal nutrition, labeling, and other requirements. Illegally imported formulas do not come under FDA control and may or may not be safe. The FDA specifies minimum amounts for all 30 nutrients that must be included in baby formulas and maximum amounts for 10 nutrients. In addition, any ingredient used in infant formula must be safe and suitable for such use. Manufacturing standards must control against contamination with bacteria, and water used in manufacturing must meet safety standards. Formulas must be labeled with directions for preparation and use, a pictogram showing the major steps for preparing infant formula, use by date, and instructions indicating whether water should be added. Some formulas state recommended amounts for babies to consume, which is unnecessary and destructive information. Only the individual baby knows how much they need to consume, and they communicate that via their feeding cues.

For the formula-fed baby, you need safe water, very clean nipples and bottles, clean hands, and a clean environment for preparing bottles. You need to mix the formula and water absolutely accurately and once mixed, formula must be fed right away or kept at refrigerator temperature. Pumped human milk needs immediate refrigeration. With exclusive breastfeeding, you don't have to worry about the safety of the water supply, keeping enough formula in the house, or having clean nipples or bottles. With partial breastfeeding, of course, you do.

To provide your baby with your breastmilk, you have to be as careful with alcohol and caffeine as you were during pregnancy, and it is best to stop smoking if you can. Whether you breast- or bottle-feed, keep smoking away from your baby.

A certain very small and variable percentage of every drug shows up in human milk. Certain antacids, anticoagulants, hormones, anticonvulsants, laxatives, and illegal drugs are absolutely contraindicated for use while breastfeeding your baby. Chemotherapy drugs for cancer are also out. Breastfeeding and/or providing your baby with your breastmilk may or may not be out if you have AIDS. Current studies show the risk of HIV transmission via breastfeeding from a parent with HIV who is receiving antiretroviral treatment and is virally suppressed is less than one percent.[14] Since the statement says *breastfeeding*, we can assume the combined transmission effects of close contact between mother and baby and substances in the human milk.

To find out whether the medications you take or the drugs you use will rule out providing your baby with your breastmilk, check with your physician and your pharmacist. The American Academy of Pediatrics regularly publishes updates on drugs and breastfeeding, and your counselors will have access to that information.

Women with active tuberculosis could give their baby the disease with the close contact of either breast- or bottle-feeding. However, after the mother has been treated for two or more weeks, close contact is okay and along with it, breastfeeding.

Also consider environmental contaminants. It is somewhat cold comfort to know that the newborn already has more insecticide stored in body fat from exposure before birth than they are likely to get from being provided with breastmilk. In other words, the exposure is unavoidable, and it is unlikely that you will exacerbate the problem with breastfeeding. Beyond that, certain chemical pollutants in the food chain are excreted in the fat of human milk. The insecticide DDT was banned from general use years ago but is still present in human milk, although the maximum your baby is likely to get is several hundred times lower than that known to cause acute intoxication in humans.

Polychlorinated biphenyls (PCBs) have caused more-recent concern. PCBs are heattransfer agents that are present in the food supply purely by accident. PCBs are carried in body fat and transferred to the fetus and to human milk. Most health authorities recommend no change in current usage of human milk, based on the absence of evidence of harm to infants from PCB levels. However, it is recommended that young women in general and pregnant or lactating women in particular limit their consumption of freshwater fish, which can be high in PCBs. Further, they recommend that if a woman has been exposed to known contaminants that she have her breastmilk analyzed and decide on an individual basis whether or not to continue to provide her baby with her breastmilk. If you fish, you can get up-to-date recommendations on fish to eat and not eat from the back of your fishing license and your state health department.

Cows' milk contaminated with PCBs is simply not allowed on the market. Formula does not contain PCBs because milk fat is replaced with vegetable fat in formulas.

DO WHAT IS RIGHT FOR YOU

All your logic may tell you that breastfeeding is the most desirable alternative, but your feelings may say you don't want to. Don't let anyone—not even yourself—tell you how to feel. They are *your* feelings and they are valid. If you would like to *change* your feelings, that's another matter. Think about how you feel and talk about it with the person you most depend on. Talk over your feelings with each other to see if you can discover where those feelings come from. Step back and try to get a broader perspective on the matter. Your feelings may have something to do with your history or the way you see yourselves in relation to each other or in relation to the world in general. Your negative feelings about breastfeeding do not mean that you don't love your baby or each other.

Consider getting professional help if you have difficulty talking with one another, you are very upset about making the decision, you react in a way that puzzles or distresses you, or you suspect you have been traumatized in a way that impacts your decision. The more comfortable you can be with yourself and with each other, the more you have to offer your baby. And the more likely you are to have a joyful experience with parenting, no matter how you decide to feed your baby.

REFERENCES

1. WHO. Health factors which may interfere with breast-feeding. *Bull World Health Organization*. 1989;67 Suppl:41–54.
2. Meek JY. Policy Statement: breastfeeding and the use of human milk. *Pediatrics*. 2022. doi:10.1542/peds.2022-057988
3. Martin CR. Review of infant feeding: key features of breast milk and infant formula. *Nutrients*. 2016. doi:10.3390/nu8050279
4. Adams LJ. Infant feeding method and special educational need in 191,745 Scottish schoolchildren: a national, population cohort study. *PLoS medicine*. 2023;20. doi:10.1371/journal.pmed.1004191
5. Kotowski J. Bottle-feeding, a neglected area of learning and support for nurses working in child health: an exploratory qualitative study. *Journal of Child Health Care*. 2022;26:199–214.
6. Rosen H. The case against breast-feeding. The Atlantic. Washington DC. April 1, 2009.
7. Baby-Friendly USA I. *Guidelines and Evaluation Criteria for Facilities Seeking Baby-Friendly Designation, Sixth Edition*. Baby-Friendly USA.
8. Work Group on Breastfeeding. Breastfeeding and the use of human milk. *Pediatrics*. 1997;100:1035–1039.

9. Tawia S. Iron and exclusive breastfeeding. *Breastfeeding Review*. 2012;20:35–47.
10. Danielewicz H. Breastfeeding and allergy effect modified by genetic, environmental, dietary, and immunological factors. *Nutrients*. 2022. doi:10.3390/nu14153011
11. Lawrence RA. Breastfeeding infants with problems. In: Lawrence RA, Lawrence RM, eds. *Breastfeeding (Ninth Edition)*. Elsevier; 2022:474–514.
12. Warner J. Ban the breast pump. *New York Times*. April 2, 2009.
13. Mahoney SE. No such thing as a free lunch: the direct marginal costs of breastfeeding. *Journal of Perinatology*. 2023;43:678–682.
14. Abuogi L. Infant feeding for persons living with and at risk for HIV in the United States: clinical report. *Pediatrics*. 2024. doi:10.1542/peds.2024-066843

CHAPTER 7

Understanding Your Newborn

Understanding your baby and feeding in the way they want and need lets you connect with them. Connecting with them lets them feel loved and cherished. As you take care of your baby day-to-day, your attachment will deepen, starting right after delivery. Hospital breastfeeding protocols, which are just as important for formula-feeding parents, say to postpone bathing and medical procedures until after the first feeding. Right after delivery is a magical time. Babies are wide awake for an hour or two, parents are excited, and it is a sweetly rewarding time before fatigue overtakes everyone. Particularly for parents who are coping with difficult life circumstances, those early moments of closeness can affect their relationship for a long time.

IN THIS CHAPTER

This chapter is about helping your baby achieve and maintain social and emotional homeostasis. Babies who have achieved homeostasis give understandable cues, remain calm in the presence of commotion, can transition with minimal fuss from waking to sleeping and back again, can eat smoothly and efficiently, and may even have the beginning of a routine with sleeping and eating. Babies who haven't achieved homeostasis are difficult to read, easily upset, rarely do the same thing twice, and may have trouble with eating and sleeping.

The first few topics in this chapter summarize the main points about understanding your baby and helping them achieve homeostasis: Feed the way your baby tells you; get on your baby's wavelength; play with your baby. Routine evolves from your baby's homeostasis, which is quite different from imposing a schedule.

After that, we get into detail. The "More about" sections addressing sleep, crying, and development help you understand and support your baby. The sections "Vulnerable babies; controlling advice" and "Babies with medial conditions" address challenging situations. Those sections reassure you that you can avoid interference and get on your baby's wavelength, even if they have to be tube-fed.

NEW BABIES ARE CHALLENGING

If it seems hard it is because it *is* hard. You will get things wrong and that is okay—you can keep trying until you get things right. It can take a while, because that new baby time is difficult. No sense blaming yourself for it. Don't get me wrong, I love babies and was sorry to stop having them. I love my grandchildren and took great joy in helping during their newborn-baby stages. But I am envious of people who are baby whisperers. While I was a nifty, calming presence for my adult children as parents, I was not the greatest at calming them down when they were babies. I find the newborn stage in parenting to be—well—challenging—alarming—exhausting. Kjerstin, my firstborn, was an easy-to-read and easy-to-satisfy baby but I found even her upsetting. I was afraid I couldn't get her to stop crying. I soon learned she only cried when she was hungry, but even then, it took hours and hours to attend to her every need and getting up at night to feed was exhausting.

Lucas and Curtis took newborn parenting to a whole new level. They were irregular in their eating and sleeping, wanted to eat unbelievably often, and were easily upset. It is hard to calm an infant when you are exhausted and stressed. I breastfed them the same as I had their sister and had to reassure myself over and over that they would have behaved the same had I been bottle-feeding. I said that Curtis learned to smile just in the nick of time. I was joking, but his becoming more sociable encouraged me and seemed to settle him down and make him more understandable. My heart goes out to parents of colicky babies, who experience all I did with hours and hours of their baby's inexplicable and inconsolable crying on top of it.

I learned more about what was going on in those early months after my children were through the stages I write about in this chapter. Would it have helped to know more? Definitely! I trusted and followed their feeding cues, so I get points for that. But I did not understand their sleep stages and that made matters worse with the boys. I regularly went to the rescue when they were sleeping lightly and not ready to get up. Kjerstin must have awakened herself in a more orderly fashion before she started to cry, so she saved me from that mistake, but even she alarmed me with all her snuffling, snorting, whimpering, and threshing about while she was in light sleep.

Having a greater understanding of my babies' personalities and temperaments would have helped me put away my agenda to get Lucas on a schedule. I finally gave up trying to turn him into the regular little baby his sister Kjerstin was, but I wish I had not done it at all. I could have made life easier for both of us by accepting his high activity and low consistency from birth. Curtis benefitted from his brother's influence, because I went along with his irregularity from the first. Actually, had I known about reading their sleep cycles, I think both my sons and I would have evolved a feeding routine a lot sooner.

FEED THE WAY YOUR BABY TELLS YOU

Central to the newborn challenge is getting on your baby's wavelength, learning to read the signs for how your baby feels and what they need. In fact, it is critical to know that your baby *has* signs and that you can read them. You get on their wavelength by by following the Satter Division of Responsibility in Feeding (sDOR):

You are responsible for *what* your baby is offered to eat and for following their lead with feeding. You work to calm them and feed in a smooth and continuous manner, paying attention to their feeding cues.

Your baby is responsible for *how much* they eat—and *everything else*: how often, how fast, how continuously, how skillfully.

What is your baby telling you?

We learn our methods from our babies: If it works, we keep doing it. If it doesn't work, we discard it. Many times, our trial-and-error sorting isn't even a conscious process. Parents who start out jiggling bottles, for instance, stop doing it within a couple of weeks because they unconsciously note that their baby only starts sucking again when they stop jiggling. Sleep cycles are less instinctive.

In one of my treasured oldie-but-goodie pieces of child-observation research, clinical psychologist Dr. Gail Price[1] video-captured feedings with mothers and their babies when the babies were under two weeks old. Afterward, she sat down with half of the mothers to watch their video and asked, "What is your baby telling you?" She did not coach in any way but only offered a calm and friendly presence. Mothers caught on quickly and could tell when what they were doing helped their baby calm down or eat better. One mother observed that her sleepy baby opened his eyes and sucked when she talked with him and when she touched his fingers, but not when she jiggled his body. Later that same mother observed, "I'm burping him so hard I look like I am killing him. Oh, you poor baby. Why didn't you tell me?" She was comfortable with her own criticism as long as she could apply a solution.

All of the mothers were interviewed when their babies were four to six weeks old. The half who had gone through the "What is your baby telling you?" exercise talked about paying attention to their babies' cues to guide feeding. They liked mothering because they felt effective and important to their babies. In contrast, mothers who saw the videos for the first time at four to six weeks were less aware of and knowledgeable about their babies' cues and not as likely to be on the same wavelength. They saw their babies as being set in their ways and didn't feel their own behavior affected their babies one way or the other.

The moral of the story is that your baby communicates with you, and that you can learn to read their language. Whether or not you use video to help you understand what your baby is telling you is up to you. Getting some distance might help you pick up on your baby's messages and your own behaviors that you miss when you are so involved with the situation at hand. It could help to have another person sit down with you, be a calming presence, and ask, "What is your baby telling you?" It doesn't get much better than that!

Pay attention to your baby's sleep cycles

For your baby to eat as well as possible and for feeding to be as routine as possible, time feeding for when your baby is hungry, calm, and awake but not overstimulated or exhausted from crying. Figure 7.1 addresses understanding and responding appropriately to your baby's sleep cycles. Wait until your baby is waking-up-and-drowsy before you pick them up. Hold, talk, and change diapers to bring your baby up to being wide awake and calm, or feed right away if they are already wide awake, calm, and show you they are hungry. Help your baby stay awake and calm by feeding in a smooth and continuous fashion until they show they have had enough to eat. Interrupt the feeding only to change breasts; burp only when they stop on their own. If your baby stops and seems comfortable, let them rest and look at you or talk a bit. The pauses in feeding are generally social times for babies. If you hold off and don't get too active, the pause can give a sweet little moment for you and your baby to enjoy each other before they go back to the business of eating.

FIGURE 7.1: UNDERSTAND AND RESPOND TO YOUR BABY'S SLEEP CYCLES

Let your baby sleep until they are waking-up-and-drowsy. Feed them when they become wide awake and calm. Help them stay awake and calm by gently cuddling, looking, talking, and stroking in a way they enjoy. Put your baby to bed when they are drowsy.	
YOUR BABY'S SLEEPING AND WAKING	**WHAT TO DO**
Deep sleep. Babies lie still, breathe deeply, and are not easily awakened.	Let your baby sleep.
Light sleep. Babies move around, make little noises, breathe fast.	Wait to see what happens. Your baby might wake up or go back to quiet sleep.
Waking-up-and-drowsy. Babies' eyes are open and they look sleepy. They might fuss a little.	Wait a bit. If your baby's eyes stay open or they keep fussing, get them up. Help them wake up by holding, talking, changing diapers.
Wide awake and calm. Babies' eyes are wide open and bright. They are relaxed.	Feed your baby. After feeding, enjoy holding, looking, talking, playing, or just being together.
Drowsy after eating and being together. Babies yawn and are sleepy and relaxed.	Put your baby to bed and let them go to sleep on their own. They may fuss a bit.
Upset and crying after being together. Babies are overstimulated, stiff, and look unhappy.	Soothe your baby by rocking, swaying, singing, shushing, and/or giving a pacifier.

Read your baby's feeding cues

Your baby knows how much to eat, and you can't guess or predict how much that is. Small or relatively thin babies do not eat less, and big and relatively fat babies do not eat more. In fact, it could be the opposite. Babies' food intake varies from day to day—sometimes by as much as 100 percent—and they still grow consistently.

Feed when your baby is hungry but not *too* hungry and stop when they are full but not *too* full. Figure 7.2 outlines what to look for in understanding your baby's hunger and fullness cues. The cues are just places to *start* in understanding what your baby is telling you. A baby is ready to eat when they look bright-eyed, curve their body toward you, curl their hands, suckle, and root for the nipple. They show positive body tension. A baby who is finished eating uncurls, relaxes their arms, legs, and hands, comes off the nipple, and might even push away. Their body tension is gone.

Your baby may want to continue suckling after they are full, and that's okay. You will get to the point where you can distinguish their self-soothing suckle from their eating suckle. Again, both are okay. You also get clues to understanding your baby's signs from reviewing the context—what has happened before? When has your baby previously eaten and slept?

Your baby's temperament and/or medical condition influence how easy or difficult they are to understand. The positive, relaxed, *easy-going* baby is more understandable than the *uptight* baby, who is erratic and difficult to read. A prematurely born baby might show hunger by becoming fussy and distractible and/or show they are full by coming off the nipple crying.

FIGURE 7.2: READ YOUR BABY'S FEEDING CUES

Feed when your baby is hungry but not *really* hungry. Stop feeding when they are full but not *really* full.	
I'm hungry or I want to talk Looks at your face Moves hands and arms toward you Raises head, turns toward you Smoothly moves arms and legs Eyes wide and face bright	**I'm really full** Pushes away Cries, fusses
I'm *really* hungry Makes loud feeding sounds Fusses Movements are jerky	**I need a break** Looks away Breathes fast, yawns Wrinkles forehead, frowns Face and eyes look dull
I'm full Stops nursing Relaxes Extends arms and legs Opens hands	**I *really* need a break** Arches back Pushes hand toward you Cries, fusses Falls asleep

It won't be long until you become expert with your own baby's cues, however unusual.

Accept your baby's eating attitudes and behaviors

Part of reading your baby's hunger and fullness signs is understanding and accepting your baby's eating attitudes and behaviors. Some babies love nursing and are content at feeding time. They nurse happily and kind of drift into getting enough, nursing more and more slowly and finally coming off with a contented little mouth-squeezing expression. Some want to eat often. Such babies might eat fast, can finish a nipple-feeding in no time at all, get full abruptly, and won't take another swallow. Other babies show combinations of the two. All are normal eating behaviors, and trying to modify them will cause no end of misery with your feeding relationship.

Some breast- or formula-feeding parents worry that their baby wants to eat more or more often than they think they should or more often than seems right. Not to worry. Trust your baby to know how often and how much they need to eat. How can a parent possibly know how much a baby needs to eat? Babies who want to eat more and more often are hungry and need more breastmilk or formula. They might need to nurse more often until their mother's breastmilk supply increases to meet their needs, or they might need a bigger bottle or even more than one bottle.

Understand control with feeding

Your baby wants to be understood, even at birth. They will do best with eating and last longer between feedings when you pay attention to them, trust what they tell you, and do what they want you to do. In other words, you let them be in control. Methods for keeping your baby in control are described in Figure 7.3. Because control is such a tricky concept, the second column might help more: what it looks like when you put *yourself* in control.

For your baby, your putting yourself in control makes feeding unpleasant. When feeding is unpleasant enough, often enough, long enough, babies develop lasting negative attitudes and behaviors around feeding and eating in general—and their time with you. On the other hand, newborns are flexible, and when you change your attitude and behavior with feeding, their attitudes and behaviors with eating change right along with yours.

FIGURE 7.3: KEEP YOUR BABY IN CONTROL OF FEEDING

You calm your baby and feed smoothly, paying attention to their cues to tell you how much, how fast, how often, how enthusiastically. Check yourself: Do you let your baby be in control of feeding?

You trust your baby and follow their cues	You put *yourself* in control
Feed your baby when they are awake and hungry.	Feed on a schedule.
Touch their cheek or lips and let them "open up."	Wake them up to eat.
Sit still and feed smoothly.	Make them wait.
Look, touch, talk, or sing in the way they like.	Push the nipple into their mouth.
Let them eat their way: much or little; fast or slowly.	Not pay attention to how they react.
Let them pause in eating to rest, "talk," or burp.	Move around, jiggle the bottle and/ or the baby.
	Try to get them to eat more after they show they are done.
	Stop feeding when they pause.

Teach your baby to go to sleep

Your baby can go to sleep on their own and, in fact, that is better in the long run than you rocking or walking them to sleep. By the long run, I mean you will thank yourself when your eight-month-old puts themselves to sleep and sleeps through the night and your older child is matter-of-fact about taking responsibility for their sleep. Those sleep patterns start right now.

Your baby's going to sleep on their own is part of their having achieved homeostasis. That grows out of the whole package we just discussed: understanding their sleep cycles, feeding according to their cues, and keeping them in control of feeding.

Put your baby to bed when they are calm and drowsy. They may yawn, rub their eyes, pull at their ears, or show Figure 7.2 "I need a break" signs. They might fuss when you put them down, but if all goes well, it will be a self-soothing kind of fussing. If at first they have more trouble going to sleep, you may choose to do a bit of low-key soothing as outlined in Figure 7.4. Whatever method you choose, do it slowly and calmly to give it time to work.

FIGURE 7.4: SUPPORT YOUR BABY IN GOING TO SLEEP

Your baby might go to sleep on their own or need a little help. Use trial and error with these methods. Give each about a minute, then wait five minutes to see if your baby calms down.

Put your baby to bed

- Put your baby down when they are drowsy after eating and being together. Consider swaddling them.
- Leave your baby alone to let them go to sleep on their own. They may fuss a little—or a lot.
- After a few minutes of active crying, show your face. Lean over and look at them. Hold your face about 10 inches away.
- Look, talk, sing, or shush in the way your baby prefers.
- Still looking, put your hand firmly on your baby's tummy and hold it there. Look, talk, sing, or shush gently.
- Still looking, talking or shushing, restrain one or both of your baby's hands firmly against their chest.

Take the next steps in soothing your fussy baby

- Pick your baby up and hold them snugly against your chest. Look and talk gently. Sing.
- Make a shushing sound.
- Swaddle your baby: Wrap them snugly in a blanket; look, gently talk, sing, or shush.
- Walk or rock, still swaddling, looking, talking, singing, or shushing.
- Put your finger or a pacifier in your baby's mouth. Swaddle, look, gently talk, sing, or shush.
- Go outside; go for a ride in the car; put your baby on the dryer, making sure they don't fall.

If you miss the early I-need-a-break messages, your baby will get more upset and stimulated and give you the I-*really*-need-a-break messages, arching, pushing away, fussing, and crying. Then you may have to do more soothing before you put them down: rocking, swaying, singing, shushing, and/or giving a pacifier. You don't need to soothe your baby to sleep. Put them down when they are calm and drowsy and ignore any further low-key fussing. You have done your bit by soothing them. See the later section "More about sleep."

GET ON YOUR BABY'S WAVELENGTH

Capturing your baby's attention without overwhelming them supports them in maintaining homeostasis. Some babies respond with calm and wakeful attention to talking, touching, movement, and having something to look at. Others are easily overwhelmed and fuss or go to sleep. An easily upset baby might prefer some ways of getting their attention over others. Over time, even easily upset babies can remain calm and alert with a variety of stimuli.

Talk in the voice your baby enjoys

Your newborn recognizes your voice and will turn toward you when you talk with them. Experiment with your speaking tone and tempo to see what your baby responds to best. You might find a sweet, soft voice works well, or a high-pitched, talking-with-baby voice. Experiment with making conversation. You might find that your regular talking voice is most interesting to your baby. At the same time as you experiment with what perks up and interests your baby, also be alert to what is overstimulating. That high-pitched baby voice—or your talking at all—may make them want to escape. Some babies get fussy when they are talked to while they eat, while others stay awake to eat only when you talk with them.

Hold and touch so your baby relaxes

Experiment with how snugly or loosely to hold your baby, how upright or flat. They will relax when they are in their preferred position but tense up or struggle when they are not. Hold firmly enough so your baby isn't afraid of falling, but loosely enough to give some room to maneuver. Your baby will be most relaxed when they are in a good feeding position: when their ear, shoulder, and hip are lined up. Keep their head straight or chin tipped up slightly while they eat.

Be mindful of how you touch, and do it slowly, smoothly, and firmly. Does your baby become calmer and more alert when you stroke their arms, hands, legs, back, or tummy or when you hold your hand firmly in place? Or does some or all of that touching upset them? Your baby is calm when they are relaxed and bright-eyed, overstimulated when they look away, breathe fast, yawn, frown, or lose that bright-eyed look. How does your baby react to tickling? I would guess, negatively. Keep in mind, it isn't *you* your baby is reacting to, but only what you are *doing*.

Move the way your baby likes

Experiment with movement. Is your baby's suckling more sustained and regular when you rock, or when you don't rock? Studies show that babies eat and grow less well when feeders jiggle the baby, jiggle the bottle, pull the nipple out of the baby's mouth and put it back in again, burp frequently, repeatedly check the level of milk in the bottle, continually arrange the blankets, and tickle the bottoms of the baby's feet.[2] Those methods for waking babies up and getting them to eat are so common that you may even have been taught them. Tradition is wrong on this one—these overactive methods absolutely do not work to make feeding pleasant for your baby. Babies don't enjoy eating and interacting when they are pestered and may fuss or go to sleep to make it go away.

Give them something to look at

Interested babies are wide awake and calm and do a better job with eating. They gaze longest toward faces or patterns of light and dark that resemble faces. Look at your baby while you feed and hold them a foot or less from your face. Your baby will periodically look directly at you but mostly seem to be looking at your ear or over your shoulder. At first, babies' peripheral vision is most developed—they see best out of the corners of their eyes or to the sides.

PLAY WITH YOUR BABY

Playing with your baby after feeding and while they are still calm and alert supports their homeostasis and helps them to eat well. Playing can introduce a slow-to-warm-up baby to enjoyment and coax an uptight baby to be more calm and sociable. It is just plain fun, and you certainly need some fun!

The imitation game

Babies love the imitation game. Put your baby in an infant seat and sit directly in front of them. Have a pleasant expression on your face, but don't smile, laugh, or gesture. Wait for your baby to take the lead. Sit quietly and look at your baby and let them look at you. Sooner or later, they will make a sound or gesture. Imitate what they say or do, but gently so as not to overwhelm them. Wait for another sound or gesture and imitate that. Keep waiting and copying until your baby looks away; then sit quietly and wait for your baby to look back and take the lead. You are telling your baby that you see them and hear them, but that you're not going to take over.

Play with language

Adding language to everyday tasks is fun and expands on the turn-taking that you have been doing all along with feeding. Babies love being able to anticipate what happens next and participate in the action. Brightly say "up you come" before you pick your baby up, then wait a bit. After a few repetitions, your baby will respond to your "up you come" by moving their arms and legs toward you in anticipation of being picked up. "Kiss your ear" can be a perfectly inspiring game. After a few times of your tipping them back and saying, "Kiss your ear," then tipping them forward to do it, your baby will curl forward for that kiss. Sing a little song, "Here we go to get some food" and look for signs of their pleasant anticipation of being fed.

Make up your own games

Patty-cake and peek-a-boo are repetitive games that parents have played forever, but the most fun games are the ones you make up as you go along. It's all just too captivating for words, and for your baby, your doing it makes it simply the best. However, keep in mind that such thrilling play can also be overwhelming for your baby, so periodically they will have to stop, look away, relax, and take time to settle down. Then they will return their attention to you and be ready to play again. Don't chase when they take one of those little time outs, and don't wander off. Wait your baby out, and soon they will return to the game.

ROUTINE YES, SCHEDULE NO

Letting a feeding routine develop is quite a different matter from imposing a schedule. Reading and responding to your baby's sleep cycles and hunger cues support evolving a routine. Their sleeping well and your following their feeding cues lets them eat well and that, in turn, lets them wait a bit longer before the next feeding. In fact, everything in the previous four figures supports working toward a routine. So does playing: It extends the time your baby is able to remain calm and awake.

- Figure 7.1: Your baby will eat as well as they possibly can when you allow them to cycle between deep and light sleep, wait to pick them up until they are waking-up-and-drowsy, and feed when they are awake and calm.
- Figure 7.2: Your baby eats most thoroughly when you feed when they are hungry and stop feeding when they are full.
- Figure 7.3: Letting your baby be in control calms them, lets them eat well, and lets them wait for the next feeding as long as is right for them.

- Figure 7.4: Supporting your baby in going to sleep on their own lets them cycle between deep and light sleep and only ask to be fed when they are waking-up-and-drowsy.

Differentiate frequent feeding from snacking

Some babies need to eat every two hours or even less. That is fine. Babies commonly cluster-feed, where they want to eat every hour or even more frequently, especially after a long feeding interval. That, too, is fine. But feeding at unnecessarily frequent intervals may or may not be fine, depending on what is going on.

Consider the snacking pattern. That is when a baby seemingly asks to eat, takes a few swallows, then loses interest or falls asleep. If your baby gets into a snacking pattern, be particularly careful to make each feeding as good as possible: properly interpret their sleep cycles, feed when they are wide awake, follow their feeding cues, and let them put themself to sleep when they are drowsy.

Consider the fussy, irregular baby whose feeding signals are difficult to interpret. Rather than making feeding the first solution, sort out what they want. Soothe them by holding, swaddling, talking, walking, or rocking. Be careful not to drift into being controlling: You are *not* using soothing techniques to feed them as a last resort or to stave off feeding. You are helping them to be calm and awake so they eat as well as possible.

MORE ABOUT SLEEP

This section repeats in detail what I summarized before. Understanding sleep is *that* important! Trusting your baby to guide the feeding process means feeding them when they are calm, awake, and hungry. That is easier said than done. You need to read your baby's sleep states and pick them up when they are awake but not *too* awake. Then you need to help your baby stay awake while they eat without having them get upset, enjoy them while they want to be enjoyed, and put them down when they have had enough. It is a process of trial and error that you will refine during the early months. Celebrate the moments when you and your baby are on the same wavelength and chalk the other moments up to experience. Your baby helps by becoming more and more settled and readable.

While it is important not to try to get your baby on a schedule, working toward a routine is another story. Reading and responding to your baby's sleep cycles and hunger cues will help move toward a feeding routine. Your baby will eat best and last longest between feedings when you pay attention to them and do what they want you to do with feeding.

Sleep cycles

Kari's mother explains:

> *Sometimes Kari sleeps quietly, but most of the time she snorts and sniffs and thrashes about. I used to jump with every sound, and when she was quiet, I kept checking to be sure she was still breathing! At first, I picked her up as soon as she made little noises and seemed to be waking up, but she was too sleepy to eat well or she got really fussy. It turns out she was in active sleep, and I was interrupting her sleep cycle. When she is ready to wake up, her eyes stay open, and she has a certain kind of cry. She quiets right down when I pick her up and by the time I change her diaper, she is wide awake and ready to eat. She eats well and doesn't get fussy. Afterwards, she stays awake a while, and when she gets drowsy, I put her down and she puts herself to sleep. She fusses a bit, but it seems more like she is singing herself to sleep than really crying.*

Deep and light sleep

Observations of sleeping newborns show that they go through two or three 60- to 90-minute deep/light sleep cycles. Babies are in deep sleep for about a third of the time, light sleep the rest.[3] Deep sleep is relatively easy to identify because your baby breathes regularly and doesn't move. Commotion generally doesn't disturb deep sleep, and if you try to wake up and feed a deeply sleeping baby, they remain drowsy and eat poorly. Until you learn to ignore it, light sleep can be nerve wracking. The lightly sleeping baby frowns, smiles, and grimaces, and their eyes move under their closed eyelids. They move around and appear to be waking up, but they actually will go back into deep sleep.

After a number of deep sleep/light sleep cycles, the baby enters the waking-up-and-drowsy stage. The waking-up stage looks a lot like light sleep, and sorting out the two can be challenging. The waking-up-and-drowsy baby's eyes stay open and they have the kind of glazed, heavy-eyed look that you and I have when we stumble out of bed in the morning. If you're not sure what you're seeing, give it some time. Your baby may go back to deep sleep, or they may be ready to wake up and will fuss to let you know. Fussing a bit is fine. Unless you let a baby cry a long time, you can easily soothe their waking-up fussing.

Becoming wide awake and calm

You can get on the same wavelength with feeding your baby when they are wide awake and calm. You quite naturally help a waking-up-and-drowsy baby become wide awake and calm by picking them up, talking, turning on the light, and/or changing their diaper. Soon your drowsy baby moves into the wide awake and calm state, becomes aware of their hunger, and announces it by looking at your face and showing "I'm hungry" signs: curling toward you, sucking. Be gently engaging but not exciting. Newborns are easily overstimulated, and then they are likely to tip over from wide awake and calm to upset and crying.

Your baby may need help managing their sleep cycle. Too-sleepy babies act ready to eat, then doze off before they seemingly have eaten much. A too-sleepy baby may not have enough wet or poopy diapers. Uptight babies have trouble being wide awake and calm. When you try to help them out of their drowsy state, they easily tip over into being flustered and start fussing and crying.

Easy does it. Look, touch, talk, and move your drowsy baby in gentle, low-key ways that let them open their eyes, brighten up, and remain calm. For both uptight and drowsy babies, maintain contact for a bit after feedings to help them gradually increase their calm and awake time. Play with them gently, in the way you have discovered that they like. Give them something to look at. Put them in their seat and take them with you as you move around the house. To know when enough is enough, be alert to messages that say, "I need a break." Their face and eyes may start to look dull and they may look away, breathe fast, yawn, frown, or hiccup. Then it is time to put them down for a nap.

Be consistent. The understandable error that parents of sleepy or unsettled babies often make is casting about, trying first one solution and then another: changing formulas, changing nipples, and changing soothing methods. All of that changing stimulates the baby more so they go into upset crying or go back to sleep to get away from it all. Pick a course and stick to it. It's hard without a feedback loop because you don't know what works and what doesn't. Keep being soothing, predictable, and gently engaging. Eventually, your baby's maturation and your tuned-in caretaking will pay off.

What sleep cycles are like for your baby

We can't think ourselves into your baby's skin, but let's try to understand what it might be like for them to have trouble waking up and staying awake to eat. Imagine yourself in a meeting right after lunch, fighting to stay awake. How tuned-in and effective will you be? Now imagine yourself having had too much caffeine or feeling so over-stressed that your nerves jangle. Just like your baby, it will be hard for you to get and stay focused so you can attend to the task at hand. Now imagine yourself in a state of flow, where you are calm, awake, tuned-in, and able to do what you need to do. Feeling that way is wonderful for you, and it is wonderful for your baby as well. Babies feel best, are most sociable, and are best able to eat well when they are calm and wide awake.

Sleep cycles vary

Right after birth, your baby may sleep for long stretches and sleep cycles may be somewhat mushy and ill-defined: sleeping and being awake for only short periods, eating often and irregularly. Crying tends to increase between the first and the sixth to eighth weeks of life. Babies generally cry about two hours per day early on, dropping to about 70 minutes per day by 10 to 12 weeks.[4] Most babies know the difference between night and day and sleep longer at night. Keeping the night feedings dimly lit, calm, uneventful, and as brief as possible helps babies further distinguish between night and day.

Beyond the basics, the variations are endless. One baby will come all the way up to a quiet alert state without any help; another baby will be drowsy for quite a while. A rare baby will sleep so long that they need you to intercept their drowsy periods to help them wake up to eat. That waking up strategy is only temporary. Helping your baby stay wide awake and calm during feeding and interested and relaxed for a while afterward helps them regulate their sleep cycles.

Be wary of interference

My young-mother friends tell me about current advice from health professionals and sleep blogs to wake a baby to eat every so many hours—often four—for the first two weeks. That interrupts their sleep cycle, and they don't eat as well. Along with that, parents are told not to let their baby nap for more than two hours in a stretch during the day so they sleep at night. Newborns don't need that. Even newborns know the difference between night and day and sleep for longer intervals at night.

As it says in the "Babies who require tube-feeding" section, prematurely born babies are particular targets for interference. While NICU feeding practice is changing toward cue-based feeding, many babies are still sent home with rigid feeding instructions: Feed every two hours and give a certain amount at every feeding. A young couple I met in Wyoming was saddled (no pun intended) with such a set of instructions, and it was making their lives miserable. They got special permission to attend my full-day feeding workshop for professionals and approached me during one of the breaks. They told me that they often had to wake their month-old baby up to feed him, and he was generally too sleepy to eat. Even if he happened to be awake at feeding time, he gave very hard-to-read signs, seemingly getting rigid and distracted when he was hungry and furiously coming off the nipple when he was full. The parents were relieved to get my encouragement to read and trust their baby's sleep cycles because that felt right to them. Understanding their baby's sleep cycles let them trust their observations that feeding him on a schedule made him too sleepy and/or irritable to eat. The same as other parents, they had good instincts.

Going back to sleep

Putting your baby to bed on his back decreases the risk of sudden infant death syndrome (SIDS).

At first your baby may go to sleep while they are eating. While it is *so* tempting to let them do it, they are likely to wake up sooner than if they finish eating while they are still awake. Going to sleep during the feeding can also keep your baby from getting enough to eat. Having the luxury of being an observer, I watched my granddaughter Marii dozing off during feedings and her mother moving her around and unwrapping her in unsuccessful attempts to wake her up. I suggested talking to her. So, my daughter started talking. She told Marii all about her day, the weather, dinner, and everything else she could think of. Amazingly, week-old Marii's eyes popped open, she looked bright, and she listened. It was as if Marii followed right along. And she ate while she listened.

Your baby's wakefulness after eating, however brief, gives you both a lovely time to cuddle, play, and socialize. This is a grand opening for the supporting parents of breastfed babies and has a function as well with respect to helping babies extend their times of being wide awake and calm. Babies who are held lots don't get spoiled. They actually cry less than babies who aren't held as much and, as I pointed out earlier, they are more cooperative as toddlers.[5] Give your baby something to look at or let them watch you and talk with them while you work.

After a while your baby will reach the I-need-a-break stage. They frown, yawn, squirm, hiccup, look away, or lose their bright-eyed look. It's best to put them down to go to sleep on their own rather than rocking or walking them to sleep. Use the methods in Figure 7.4 if they need a little help. An uptight baby who is not hungry—or any other baby—may need to cry a bit to get settled down. What could be more instinctive than going out and shutting the door when you are worn out from trying to get your baby to sleep?

Sleeping through the night

Being able go back to sleep on their own makes all the difference with your baby's sleeping through the night. Babies who can go to sleep on their own can cycle back into deep sleep from light sleep. As they get older and aren't as hungry at night, they put themselves back to deep sleep from light sleep. Babies who need to be rocked or walked to go to sleep will call for help when they are in light sleep. They need you to do what you did to put them to sleep in the first place. If it was rocking or walking, up you get. If it was letting your baby put themself to sleep, sweet dreams!

During the early months, your baby is hungry, needs to eat often, and wakes up at night to eat. The vast proportion of newborns are in no way nutritionally, emotionally, or developmentally ready to make it through the night without care and feeding. Most babies sleep for longer intervals at night. Being hungry arouses your baby from light sleep to waking-up-and-drowsy and, with your help, awake and calm and ready to eat.

Parents complain most often of sleep problems starting at age seven or eight months: They are tired of getting up at night to feed, rock, or walk their baby back to sleep. Parents long for the day when those intervals stretch enough so they can get a decent night's sleep. I must warn you that that particular problem started much earlier, with singing, rocking, or walking their baby to sleep rather than letting their drowsy baby put themselves to sleep. My friend and colleague Peggy commented that she made that mistake with her firstborn. By the time he was nine months old, he slept so poorly that they felt they had to do sleep training. The first night was awful when he cried for over half an hour. The second night he cried for a few minutes. The third night, both he and his parents slept through. She didn't make that mistake with her second-born. She put her down drowsy for naps and to sleep at night and her baby learned to self-soothe.

At some point, babies have the nutritional reserves to get through the night. Lightly sleeping, no-longer-hungry babies put themselves back to sleep, again, provided they put themselves to sleep in the first place. Michigan psychologist and infant sleep researcher C. Merie Johnson observed that when babies don't know how to put themselves back to sleep, they continue to signal their parents to do the singing, rocking, or walking that put them to sleep in the first place. The self-soothing infant who is no longer hungry at night goes back to sleep; the one who doesn't self-soothe calls for help. If you miss the early months, start during the day to teach your baby to self-calm and go to sleep. That self-calming might extend to night, or you might have to teach it at night as well. To address fussing and crying in general and when you put them down for a nap, in particular, review Figure 7.4, "Support your baby in going to sleep," page 189.

More about night sleeping

It is one of life's strange ironies that no matter how besotted we are with our babies, we are desperate for them to sleep. Johnson observed, based on parent surveys, that parents tried just about anything to get their children to sleep at night. They nursed them to sleep, eliminated naps, let them sleep in the same bed as parents, and even placed puppies in the crib.[6] Many times, feeding problems start when parents try to solve sleeping problems. Parents may start solid foods early or put cereal in the bottle in the mistaken belief that solid foods will get their child to sleep through the night. Some parents try to get their baby to eat more than they want at bedtime. None of the tactics work because they don't deal with the heart of the problem: babies who can't put themselves to sleep.

Because formula digests more slowly than human milk, formula-fed babies get over their night hunger earlier than breastfed infants. In fact, Johnson's studies showed that many breastfed infants continued waking up to be fed at night until they were weaned. Co-sleeping infants—the ones who sleep in the same beds with their parents—are two to three times more likely to awaken at night than those who sleep alone. Seventy percent of children with sleep problems had slept in the parents' bed all or part of the night in the month preceding the survey compared with 23 percent of the group without sleep problems.[6] But, which came first: the chicken or the egg? Are parents co-sleeping because their babies sleep poorly? It seems to me that it comes down to doing the best you can to read your baby's sleep and feeding signs, then doing what you have to do.

The American Academy of Pediatrics does not recommend co-sleeping, based on reports of infants who smothered or were injured falling out of bed when they were sleeping with their parents.

I hope I have made it obvious that I am not in favor of making *young* infants cry it out as a way of getting them to sleep through the night. Exhausted with getting up at night with one of my children, I was envious when a colleague boasted that all three of her babies slept through the night by age two weeks. My envy soon turned to horror: she let her newborns cry until they gave up.

MORE ABOUT CRYING

Of course, bedtime is not the only time your baby cries. Babies typically cry 2 to 4 hours a day in the first 6 weeks and then 1 to 2 hours a day at 8 to 10 weeks. Your baby's crying is a distress signal. Responding promptly is critical: Pick your baby up, cuddle them, talk, and move around. Then begin sorting out the problem. Until you know your baby well, you may not know the cause: tired, hungry, too cold, too hot, need to burp, poopy or wet pants, or too much stimulation. Do babies cry because they want company? Probably! Going-to-sleep strategies can do double duty with respect to helping your baby be relaxed and comfortable while they are awake.

Fussing is neither crying nor awake and content. Babies typically cry most during the late afternoon and evening.[7] Unfortunately, that is likely to be when their parents are most worn out!

Infant colic

According to research, 17 to 25 percent of infants have colic in the first 6 weeks, dropping to 11 percent by 8 to 9 weeks, and less than 1 percent by 10 to 12 weeks. With colic, the crying goes on and on and may be harsh sounding, it is unexplained, and despite your best efforts, you can't soothe your baby. Your baby's face may be red and frowny, fists clenched, abdomen tense, and knees drawn up. Such inconsolable crying can be a sign of a medical problem, and your doctor will evaluate your baby to be sure that is not the case.[7]

Among other issues, your doctor is likely to consider whether your baby has GERD—gastroesophageal reflux disease. Gastroesophageal reflux—spitting up—is common among young babies and is a cause for concern only if they have other symptoms such as choking, gagging, or refusal to eat. Projectile vomiting—vomiting with force—calls for medical attention.

Despite considerable exploration, no clear causes of infant colic have been identified, but the leading theory is newborn immaturity. The baby's nervous system and gastrointestinal tract, including gut bacteria, are not yet fully developed, and only time will address the problem. Sometimes it helps to get rid of allergens in your diet if you are breastfeeding or to try your baby on a hypoallergenic formula. Change formulas as a last resort as the change itself could be upsetting for your baby.

Parents may think their baby has colic when they actually do not. In one study, only 35 percent of infants who were perceived as colicky by their mothers were found to satisfy the three parts of the definition: starting in the early weeks, unexplained and inconsolable crying, and not associated with a medical condition.[7]

Consider your feelings

But does it really matter? Prolonged crying for any reason is hard on any parent. Parents who can't soothe their infant experience frustration, helplessness, fear, and loneliness and even have physical symptoms such as shortness of breath and headaches. Almost all parents have marital conflict related to their baby's crying and at times almost all resent their infant and have aggressive thoughts and fantasies.[8]

Feel your feelings and talk about them. Resentment and aggression are more likely to cause problems when you try to ignore them. Other parents share your feelings. According to folk-singer Rosalie Sorrels, many cultures have aggressive lullabies. I find that reassuring in a perverse sort of way, and I hope you do, too. Think about it:

Rockabye baby
in the tree top.
When the wind blows
the cradle will rock.
When the bough breaks
the cradle will fall.
Down will come baby
cradle and all.

Really? Down will come baby cradle and all? One origin story of the "Rockabye Baby" lyrics is that they were composed as a death wish directed at the infant son of King James II of England, hoping the baby would die and be replaced by a Protestant king. Maybe you don't need to know that. The point is that feeling aggression toward babies is common and expressing your aggression doesn't mean you will act on it. In fact, you are less likely to act on your negative feelings and darkest fantasies if you express them.

What to do about crying and/or colic

Once they have ruled out medical issues, parents say it helps most to have health professionals emphasize that there is no cure for the inconsolable crying. As with child temperament, you can relax and accept it. It also helps when others ask about how they, the parents, are doing rather than focusing only on the baby. My friend Patty felt immediate relief when her mother-in-law asked, "Don't you sometimes feel like throwing him out the window?" Feeling and doing are not the same!

Do the best you can to feed according to your baby's sleep rhythms and feeding cues. Go through the routine in Figure 7.4. Keep in mind that colicky babies are easily overstimulated, so be careful not to be so active that you contribute to the problem. Reassure yourself you are doing the right thing even if your baby can't respond right away. Let a routine evolve. Over the first six months, your baby will settle down, respond more to you, and become more understandable. Do the best you can with soothing, as long as you can, then put your baby to bed in a safe place, walk away, and let them cry it out. While it seems hard-hearted, the alternatives are worse: resenting your baby and being critical and hurtful with yourself and your spouse.

If you change your baby's formula, minimize the upset to your baby by doing it gradually. But first, consider whether your baby really *needs* a formula change. Despite the advertising, no bottle or nipple has been demonstrated to help with infant colic. In fact, changing could make matters worse. Changing nipples and bottles will upset your baby and can stimulate more crying.

MORE ABOUT DEVELOPMENT

Feeding is so much a part of your child's early years that feeding, loving, and development are inseparable. Being tuned-in, accepting, and savvy with feeding shows your baby you love them and supports them in emerging from the newborn period calm, connected, and ready to gradually engage in the world outside the two of you. Consider the first two stages: Homeostasis is getting settled down so your baby can sleep and eat well. Attachment is falling in love so feeding takes on even more of an emotional dimension. Each enhances the other. Being settled down and able to pay attention to others enhances a baby's ability to fall in love. Loving you and being loved back enhances a baby's ability to take an interest in what's happening and be more settled. Being calm and feeling securely loved support the toddler's risk-taking with independence and the preschooler's experimentation with how the world works. Figure 7.5 summarizes what your child accomplishes in each stage and how to feed them to support that accomplishment.

The stages and developmental tasks blend into each other, and a child continues working on one task when they pick up another. For instance, infants in general, disorganized babies in particular, and ill and neurodiverse children perhaps most of all continue to work on homeostasis throughout the first year and even longer. For another example, newborns can start to work from birth on separation/individuation—a toddler task—when you guide feeding based on information coming from them.

FIGURE 7.5: CHILD DEVELOPMENT AND FEEDING

Following sDOR supports your child's achieving their developmental tasks. Trying to get your child to eat certain amounts and/or types of food and/or grow in a certain way does not. The symbol (~) means ages vary for typical children. Ages vary even more for ill, vulnerable, and neurodiverse children.

STAGE	WHAT YOUR CHILD ACCOMPLISHES	HOW YOU HELP
Newborn ~ 0 to 3 months	Achieves homeostasis: becomes calm and understandable.	Feed smoothly based on their eating signs and sleep rhythms.
Infant ~ 2 to 6 months	Becomes attached: gives and receives love.	Feed based on their cues; smile and talk when they are ready.
Older baby ~ 5 to 9 months	Gets interested in things and people outside of the two of you.	Introduce solid food when they can sit up and open up. Give them things to look at and touch.
Almost-toddler ~ 7 to 5 months	Wants to do things themselves.	Let your child join you at family meals and eat with their fingers.
Toddler ~ 11 to 36 months	Finds out they are separate.	Follow sDOR; don't give food handouts; ignore pickiness.
Preschooler ~ 3 to 5 years	Experiments with the world. Imitates and tries to please.	Follow sDOR; avoid pressure, rewarding, shaming.

Sometimes children take developmental leaps, where they appear to suddenly move into the next stage. In reality, they have been working on getting there all along. As my colleague Pam Estes says, "Children don't do, don't do, don't do, and then they do." I talk more about separation/individuation in Chapter 10, Feeding Your Older Baby and Almost-Toddler, and Chapter 11, Feeding Your Toddler.

I have not heard this anywhere, but I observed with my own children that they became cranky when they were ready to take a developmental leap and hadn't yet gotten there. Consider that a hypothesis and check it out with your own child! Even if it isn't true, it helps with getting through some of the tough days.

Homeostasis

To eat well, your baby has to be able to maintain homeostasis: be wide awake and calm. You support homeostasis when you work to properly interpret their sleep states, feed in a smooth and continuous fashion, and pay attention to their messages to guide the feeding process. Babies are born with a longing to be understood and do best when you understand. Your baby feels understood when you do what they want you to do in taking care of them.

Your baby comes from a relatively quiet place into a busy world. To function in that noisy, colorful, smelly world, your baby, like all of us, has to learn to filter out distractions and attend only to the issue at hand. Think of having a conversation in the midst of a party or doing homework with the TV on. Homeostasis is being calm and focused in spite of outside stimulation. People who have attention deficit disorder have trouble filtering out stimulation.

In the midst of sights, sounds, and smells, a baby who has achieved homeostasis is organized. They can wake up, stay wide awake and calm enough to eat well, make the shift from waking to sleeping with little commotion, and remain comfortably asleep when asleep. It all flows from your waiting to pick your baby up until they are *truly* waking up and feeding according to their cues.

Your baby may have been born organized. Lucky you. A baby who has achieved homeostasis is easy to be with: They are not easily upset and when they are upset, they are relatively easy to read and calm. More to reassure you that it is not your fault than to scare you, not all babies are born organized. Some babies more than others have mellowing to do after they are born: They are erratic, hard to read, and difficult to settle. A baby's brain, nervous system, and GI tract continue to mature over the first several months and throughout the second year. In fact, the period of rapid brain growth extends over the first two years of your baby's life.

To extend the duration of your baby's remaining awake and calm, give them something to be interested in. Carry them while you go about your day, look and talk, hang a toy over the infant seat or crib. Babies and young children are easy to overwhelm, so respond quietly with less energy than theirs. Because your attention is pretty exciting, let your baby take breaks. They will look and seem interested for a time, then they will turn away. They turn away to calm down and keep from being overwhelmed by all the excitement of being with you. Wait it out, neither lose interest nor try to get your baby's attention. When they are ready, they will turn their attention back to you and the two of you can go back to looking and talking.

Attachment

The same as with homeostasis, your baby's ability to eat well depends on attachment. The same tuned-in and accepting feeding that supported homeostasis now supports attachment. A baby who feels understood, feels loved—and loving. Attachment is the falling-in-love stage where your baby watches, smiles, babbles, and reaches out to you to get your attention and keep you close. You naturally respond back by watching, smiling, babbling, and reaching. Your baby's feeding signs become signs of their attachment to you, and your responding says powerfully: I see and hear you, I care about you, and I want to give you what you need.

Going along with your baby's signs gives them the experience of being loved and lets them feel loving toward you. The same as earlier, talk and smile gently; don't be overstimulating or entertaining. When attachment goes well, the infant emerges with a sense of connection that prepares you both for the next stage of development: separation and individuation.

Attachment builds on homeostasis. To be ready for attachment, a baby has to be able to be calm and awake. For your baby to take pleasure in the outside world, some of the commotion within has to have subsided. Think of your jittery and overstimulated self. How sociable are you? Think of your tired and sleepy self. How much do you want to hang out and have a good time with other people? I rest my case.

Much is said about attachment parenting, a philosophy that promotes high levels of parental empathy and acceptance as well as continuous bodily closeness and touch. From the feeding dynamics perspective, while attachment is important, it is no more important than any other stage in development. Moreover, while empathy, acceptance, bodily closeness, and touch are important, your baby needs to balance such engagement with disengagement. The intermittent connections guided by your baby's sleep and feeding cues are part of the rhythms of your days with your baby.

Separation-individuation

Separation-individuation starts around age six months for a typically developing infant. This is the process by which your baby develops an awareness of their own self, separate from you. It is hard to imagine the opposite—the newborn experience of being continuous with you—but there it is. The first sign of your baby's awareness that you and they are *not* one and the same is their taking an interest in the world outside of just the two of you. Along with being able to sit up and open up for food, that social awareness is an indication for starting solid food. The older baby shows separation-individuation when they interrupt a nipple feeding to see who just walked into the room. The older baby starting on solid food—whom I call an *almost-toddler*—shows separation-individuation by refusing to let you feed them and insisting on feeding themself with their fingers.

Since we are concentrating on the first six months, we will talk more about separation-individuation later. For now, know that the toddler puts separateness to the test by struggling to manipulate and manage, by exploring, roaming out and coming back, and even defying. Having achieved homeostasis helps toddlers remain calm in the midst of the commotion of exploring and defying. Having achieved attachment lets toddlers take chances with roaming out and even being defiant: They have to love you and trust that you love them in return. Child development studies show that toddlers are more likely to be compliant with direction and limits when parents have sensitively responded to them when they were infants.[5]

Help can *really* help

Some parent-child combinations can complicate the developmental process to the point that getting some short-term help is in order. A child might be particularly disorganized and irritable or sleepy. Parents might be preoccupied, overstressed, depressed, or afraid of spoiling their baby. Achieving homeostasis can be challenging with a baby who was prematurely born, is ill, or is neurodivergent. Help can take the form of being a calming and supportive presence; asking how you are feeling; sitting down with you and your baby and asking the question, "What is your baby telling you?"; taking your baby for a walk while you catch a nap; or cleaning your house.

Be reassured that issues have to become extreme before they cause problems for the child. I once worked with an infant whose weight plunged off the growth curve during his attachment phase because his deeply depressed mother could not connect with him. Clearly, that family needed mental health counseling to address their issues. That was a lot different from new parents feeling overwhelmed and even depressed by all their responsibilities. Babies can cope with that!

CONSIDER PERSONALITY AND TEMPERAMENT

Your baby was born with certain personality characteristics, including activity level and regularity. It is both nature and nurture: these characteristics both persist and are modified by life experience.

Personality characteristics

In their famous and far-reaching studies of temperament, psychiatrists Alexander Thomas and Stella Chess observed that newborns differ in the nine personality characteristics outlined in Figure 7.6. These characteristics are the details that make up temperament (next figure). Knowing the details can help you understand and accept your baby.

FIGURE 7.6: PERSONALITY CHARACTERISTICS OF INFANTS AND YOUNG CHILDREN

Babies show both positive and negative characteristics: One who moans and wiggles with delight may also be offended if you do something not to their liking.	
Activity level. Kicks, moves, and squirms or sits or lies quietly; is likely to be more cuddly. **Rhythmicity**. Sleeps and eats at about the same times or rarely shows a pattern. **Approach-withdrawal**. Delights in anything new or gets upset. **Adaptability**. Adjusts readily to change or takes a while. **Intensity of reaction**. Moans in delight or objects strongly or reacts mildly or seemingly not at all.	**Threshold of responsiveness**. May react to every sight, sound, and touch at one extreme or tune out great commotion at the other. **Continuity of mood**. Is about the same day-to-day or has shifting moods. **Distractibility**. Can wait to eat if something else comes up or insists on being fed immediately. **Persistence and attention span**. Struggles to pick up food from a high chair tray or gives it a few tries and then waits to be fed.

Temperament

Temperament (Figure 7.7) is made up of combinations of personality traits. Thomas and Chess observed that about 40 percent of infants were "easy," 15 percent were "slow-to-warm-up," and 10 percent were "difficult." Thirty-five percent didn't fit into any of the categories. I appreciate the insights but not the terminology. The terms "easy" and "difficult" tell more about how grown-ups want babies to be than they do about the babies themselves. I prefer the descriptive terms *easy-going* to describe "easy" children and *uptight* to describe "difficult" babies. The term *slow-to-warm-up* is a fine descriptive term.

FIGURE 7.7: YOUR BABY'S TEMPERAMENT

You can be more patient and accepting when you understand your baby's nature. Your being accepting will let your slow-to-warm-up baby become easier to please and your uptight baby more flexible.

IF YOUR BABY IS:	WHAT YOU CAN DO TO HELP:
Easy-going: Relaxed, calm, and easy to please with clear signs. Eats and sleeps regularly.	Go by your baby's signs. Know that you can depend on your baby to show you what to do.
Slow-to-warm-up: Takes a while to get used to new experiences. Might not act pleased or happy, even when you get it right.	Respect your baby's sleep rhythms and eating cues even if it doesn't seem to help at first. Offer new experiences but don't get pushy. Stop when you see signs they want to stop.
Uptight: Wound up, touchy, and hard to figure out. Signs are not clear, except for being upset, and anything new is upsetting! You cannot predict when they will eat or sleep, be fussy or content.	Respect your baby's sleep rhythms and eating cues even if it doesn't work at first. Be sparing with new experiences and give time to adjust. Be as calm and consistent as you can. Get help if you need it.

The easy-going baby

The *easy-going* baby has regular sleeping and eating patterns, has a positive approach to new situations, adapts readily to change, and has an overall mild or moderate mood. It is easiest to be successful with *easy-going* babies. Their regular patterns and moderate responses make them easy to read, understand, and satisfy. Easy-going babies are born with homeostasis already in place.

The uptight baby

At the other extreme, *uptight* babies, through no fault of their own or anybody else, are negative, erratic, and difficult to read. They are likely to react negatively—and strongly—to new situations or new people. It is hard to know what uptight babies want. They cry a lot, cry loudly, are difficult to soothe, and have trouble falling asleep, staying asleep, and waking up enough to eat well. First, some encouragement: Bewitched parents of even the most challenging child are convinced their baby is perfect. Moreover, uptight babies who are parented with warmth and acceptance during the early months and years show the least behavior problems and greatest social skills of all children as first graders.[9] In the meantime, do the best you can.

Uptight babies have trouble establishing homeostasis, trouble that persists for at least the first year and probably longer. Study your child's sleep states and hunger cues and follow them as well as possible. Concentrate on the *quality* of feeding, not the *quantity* of food or the schedule. Brace yourself to be an advice magnet—and to ignore most of it. You will be told to stop breastfeeding (or scolded for not breastfeeding), encouraged to keep trying formulas or nipples until you find one that "works," advised to put your baby on a schedule, told that a schedule is the worst, or told to feed certain amounts. All of these strategies undermine a baby's homeostasis and make the problem worse, not better. Be skeptical of all input except "How are *you* feeling?" and "I can take him for a few hours." You know what is best for your baby, and with a bit of support, you will cope.

The slow-to-warm-up baby

The same as the *uptight* infant, the *slow-to-warm-up* infant is wary of new situations and new people but is more skeptical than downright rejecting. The *slow-to-warm-up* baby adapts slowly and has sleeping patterns that are somewhere between the two extremes: not as regulated as some, not so dysregulated as others. The *slow-to-warm-up* infant tends to be wary of new food experiences rather than offended by them.

The babies that don't fit in these three categories show other combinations of attributes. To read more about infant and child temperament, see the 1987 book *Know Your Child: An Authoritative Guide for Today's Parents* by Stella Chess and Alexander Thomas. It is an oldie-but-goody.

Help yourself with negative extremes

Keep a few points in mind about personality and temperament. First of all, you didn't cause it. For whatever reason, your baby came that way. Second, you absolutely have to stow your convictions about how you want things to go with your baby. The *uptight* baby is full of surprises, and you might as well relax and enjoy their surprises. Third, while your task early on is to help your baby be as calm and organized as possible, in the long run they need to learn to calm and organize themself.

Infants with a certain temperament won't necessarily be that way their whole life. Strongly reacting children can learn to calm themselves and deal with their own extreme responses rather than simply imposing them on other people. You moderate the uptight baby's extremes by being receptive to their messages as best you can rather than forcing them to become insistent in order to get your attention. You encourage the *slow-to-warm-up* child to become more adventurous by offering new experiences while being careful not to be abrupt or overwhelming. Both the *uptight* and *slow-to-warm-up* child push themselves along to learn and grow as long as we don't force them or rescue them. Then their negative tendencies are exacerbated.

VULNERABLE BABIES; CONTROLLING ADVICE

Parents of unusual or vulnerable babies are particular targets of controlling advice: advice that strays into the *yourself-in-control* column in Figure 7.3. Parents of the prematurely born are often told to feed their baby a certain amount, generally every two hours. The assumption is that such babies aren't capable of eating on demand. Parents of ill babies, babies with birth defects, and those who have medical, neurological, or physical limitations, or even relatively small babies are often given similar controlling feeding advice. Those taking-control methods spoil feeding. Trying to wake your baby before they are ready upsets them and makes them eat poorly. Trying to get your baby to eat a certain amount makes feeding miserable for both of you.

All of these vulnerable babies—or those *perceived* to be vulnerable—give hunger and fullness signs and they benefit from support with staying calm and awake during feeding. They give those signs even when they are tube-fed, and you can learn to read those signs in guiding when and how much to feed. There is more on this topic later in the section "Babies who require tube-feeding."

Exceptionally large or small babies

Trying to make babies eat more or less than they want ignores information coming from them and is profoundly disruptive of routine. It also distorts their attitude toward eating and ability to regulate their food intake. Even very young babies who are made to eat more than they want become revolted by food, upset during feeding, and prone to undereat when they get the chance. A few babies give in and eat the way their grown-ups want them to eat, eat more than they need, and their weight accelerates: it goes up faster than is right for them. Rather than achieving homeostasis, they become passive.

Even very young babies who aren't allowed to eat as much as they are hungry for become food-preoccupied and are prone to eat more than they need when they get the chance. Their weight is likely to accelerate:

to go up faster than is right for them. Rather than achieving homeostasis, they become chronically agitated.

Babies who don't eat "enough"

An infant who isn't eating enough is listless, falls off their growth curve, and appears dehydrated: dry skin, sunken eyes, few wet diapers. This is a medical emergency, and the child requires evaluation to identify the problem. Observing and evaluating feeding dynamics and correcting errors in feeding is an essential part of the solution. Even when the root cause is a medical one, the feeding relationship will be affected.

Given positive feeding dynamics, children who wear out before they seemingly get enough to eat might be helped by concentrating the formula. However, do it only with expert advice and supervision to guard against dehydration. Even then, babies are such good regulators that they can compensate by eating less of the concentrated formula. Such compensation is a sign that a child is regulating well and is growing at the rate that is right for them.

Prematurely born babies

Prematurely born babies in Newborn Intensive Care Nurseries (NICUs) are routinely tube-fed and must make the transition to oral feeding before they can be discharged. The trust approach is to cue-feed the orally fed babies; the control approach is to take over the *when* and *how much*. That is, it is assumed the babies don't have sleep cycles (Figure 7.1) or show feeding cues (Figure 7.2). Not true. A review of seven studies done in NICUs showed cue-fed babies took less time to achieve full oral feedings and had faster weight gains and shorter hospital stays.[10] The best part was that when they took their baby home, parents of cue-fed babies could feed them on demand based on sDOR: Parents knew their baby could be trusted to let them know when and how much they needed to eat.

In my view, a premature infant is ready to go home from the hospital when they are fed on demand. That is, their caretakers understand and support their sleep states, feed according to their feeding cues, and teach you to do the same. Demand feeding for NICU graduates is gaining ground, but it still may be unusual. Be prepared to receive—and resist—the all too common take-home advice to wake your baby to feed them a certain amount every two hours. Such methods are old-fashioned and sure to cause problems with feeding.

You can help teach your completely tube-fed baby to eat while they are in the NICU. Hold your baby close to you in feeding position while they are tube-fed and offer them the breast, a bottle, or a pacifier at the same time. That allows them to have nonverbal learning of what eating is all about: experiencing warmth and closeness and getting relief from hunger and fullness as they suckle. Feed your baby by nipple or by tube with their head elevated in the side-lying position or on their back. There is some evidence that premature babies eat more in side-lying position, although their oxygen saturation is about the same as when they eat on their backs.[11] I am not sure that eating *more* is desirable: The real issue is their eating as *much as they need*! If you have your baby lying on their side to eat, be sure their ear, shoulder, and hip are lined up, their head is higher, and that you hold the bottle straight in their mouth.

BABIES WHO REQUIRE TUBE-FEEDING

Babies need to be tube-fed when they can't eat as much as they need and their growth falters. A baby might have a chin, lip, palate, esophageal, or digestive system abnormality; neurodevelopmental issues such as difficulty coordinating sucking, swallowing, and breathing; low or high muscle tone; a serious heart condition; or developmental difficulties such as Down or Turner syndrome. In most cases, tube-feeding is supplemental rather than full, and it doesn't need to go on forever. Tube-feeding can be discontinued when a baby matures and their medical issues are resolved. But even with full tube-feeding, you can have a positive feeding relationship.

Don't be afraid of tube-feeding. It can help a great deal to preserve your feeding relationship and your quality of life overall. Also, don't be afraid of gastrostomy tube (G-tube) feeding through a surgical opening in your baby's stomach. It is minor surgery and may be preferable to a nasogastric tube—one that is threaded through your baby's nose and esophagus. The G-tube doesn't show and it doesn't interfere with suckling and swallowing. The G-tube can be removed when your baby gets strong and coordinated enough to eat on their own—and you are fully ready to trust them to do it.

Tube-fed children can still be *good eaters* as defined in Chapter 1. They can want to eat and enjoy being with their family at mealtime. Even if they can't eat enough on their own to support their needs, they can take an interest in food, sneak up on new food and learn to eat it (or at least ignore it), and to eat as much as they want.

Preserving the feeding relationship

I know this is asking a lot of you when you are coming to terms with your baby's condition and learning to manage it, but you can advocate for preserving your feeding relationship. Your doctors are understandably focused on your baby's survival. Their routine may call for your baby to be fully tube-fed rather than being allowed to eat orally to the best of their abilities and then supplemented by tube. The medical approach to tube-feeding is a control approach: certain number of ounces of breastmilk or formula per pound of your baby's body weight, fed every so many hours around the clock. Your baby may be over- or underfed, and they won't experience hunger and fullness.

In order to know what eating is emotionally and physically all about, your baby needs to suckle and be held close to you in feeding position at the same time as their hunger is satisfied via tube-feeding. Gaining such an instinctive sense of eating from the very first will let your child eat—or more-easily correct any gaps in learning to eat—when the medical procedures are resolved to the point that they are ready to eat normally. Suckling and being held close to you in feeding position also engages your baby's cephalic phase of digestion: It alerts their digestive system to prepare for the food that is coming and allows the system to work as smoothly as possible.

Consider trust-based tube-feeding

Some babies can eat enough to support their growth but feeding them can take hours and be exhausting for all concerned. In such cases, tube-feeding can help enormously. You can enjoy breast- or formula-feeding while you and your baby have the energy and enthusiasm. Then you can continue to hold and feed them from a soft medicine cup, syringe, or feeding tube while you go by their hunger and fullness cues. If your baby needs to be fully tube-fed, cuddle them while you feed and follow their sleep rhythms and feeding cues. If they are able, let them suck on your breast or a pacifier while you cuddle and tube-feed them.

Consider the insights of my ESI colleague Sarah Howe McKenna, RD, British Columbia nutrition support clinician. McKenna has helped many families make the hospital to home transition—from control to trust with oral- and tube-feeding. She says that at first it is daunting for parents to manage tube-feeding at the same time as they follow their baby's hunger and fullness cues. It takes a while to build trust, and tube-feeding may have to be adjusted to allow babies to experience hunger. The challenge is to feed on demand and let the baby eat orally to the best of their ability. Then supplement with tube-feeding, basing the amount on the baby's hunger and fullness cues. Babies' consistent growth indicates that feeding is going well, as does not showing any miserable "I'm too full" signs. Do seek help from a dietitian who is experienced with both sDOR and tube-feeding to help you balance your child's oral and tube-feed intake.

Trust your tube-fed baby's cues and growth

It is tempting to give too much by tube to get an exceptionally small baby to grow faster, but not wise on many levels. I cringe when I remember watching 18-month-old Nora being overfed by tube. She became more and more miserable, her face became more and more flushed, and she finally threw up. Nora had esophageal atresia: Her esophagus didn't go all the way through, and she had to be fed by tube until she was old enough to have it corrected surgically. Nora's weight had accelerated slowly over those 18 months, from the 10th to the 75th percentile.

I worked with Nora's parents after the surgery when she was ready to learn to eat. I encouraged them to follow Nora's hunger and fullness cues with tube-feeding and include Nora in family meals. Within a couple of weeks, she began finger-feeding herself bits of food, and she and her parents graduated from my care when she sat in my office chair and ate a Fig Newton! It helped that Nora knew what eating was all about. At first, she had had a surgical opening—a stoma—in her neck so she could eat from the nipple at the same time as the food dribbled out onto her neck. The stoma had to be removed after a few weeks, but that early experience still helped her.

WHAT COMES NEXT

The early relationship you establish with your baby forms the basis for everything that comes after with feeding and with parenting. One stage flows into the other. The infant becomes the toddler, then grows into the child who becomes the parent and then the elder. It is so good to be a part of all of this!

REFERENCES

1. Price GM. Influencing maternal care through discussion of videotapes of maternal-infant feeding interaction. *Infant behavior & development*. 1983;6:353–360.
2. Wright P. The development of differences in the feeding behaviour of bottle and breast fed human infants from birth to two months. *Behavioural Processes*. 1980;51:1–20.
3. Sander L. The regulation of exchange in infant caregiver systems. In: Lewis M, Rosenblum l, eds. *Interaction, Conversation, and the Development of Language (The Origins of behavior)*. Wiley; 1977.
4. Douglas P. Managing infants who cry excessively in the first few months of life. *BMJ*. 2011. doi:10.1136/bmj.d7772
5. Stayton DJ. Infant obedience and maternal behavior: the origins of socialization reconsidered. *Child Dev*. 1971;42:1057–1069.
6. Johnson CM. Infant and toddler sleep: a telephone survey of parents in one community. *Journal of Developmental and Behavioral Pediatrics*. 1991;12:108–114.

7. Zeevenhooven J. Infant colic: mechanisms and management. *Nature Reviews Gastroenterology & Hepatology*. 2018;15:479–496.
8. Levitzky S. Infant colic syndrome--maternal fantasies of aggression and infanticide. *Clin Pediatr (Phila)*. 2000;39:395–400.
9. McFarlane E. The importance of early parenting in at-risk families and children's social-emotional adaptation to school. *Acad Pediatr*. 2010;10:330–337.
10. Fry TJ. Systematic review of quality improvement initiatives related to cue-based feeding in preterm infants. *Nursing for Women's Health*. 2018;22:401–410.
11. Raczyńska A. The impact of positioning on bottle-feeding in preterm infants (≤ 34 GA). A comparative study of the semi-elevated and the side-lying position - a pilot study. *Dev Period Med*. 2019;23:117–124.

CHAPTER 8

Breastfeeding Your Baby

This chapter, the same as this book, is written for fathers as well as mothers. Within the context of breastfeeding, *mother* means the one who feeds the child. *Father* means one who takes equal responsibility for the child's care, love, nurture, guidance, and protection. With the exception of breastfeeding itself, fathers today play a lovely, creative, and active role in taking care of their infants and young children.

Adoptive mothers breastfeed, as do LGBTQ+ parents. You may prefer the gender-neutral term *chestfeeding*.[1] This chapter, and particularly the section, "Relactation and induced lactation," applies to chestfeeding as well as breastfeeding. I respect your preference, although I will continue to use the term *breastfeeding*.

IN THIS CHAPTER

This is a long chapter with lots of detail, so let's remind ourselves right up front: Breastfeeding is about love. Being successful with breastfeeding depends on your showing your love by getting on your baby's wavelength with sleeping and feeding.

At the end of the chapter, you will find Figure 8.5, "Many people contribute to successful breastfeeding," The list works well for a review of the topics in the chapter. It is a lot to take in at this point.

The discussion of *how to breastfeed* starts with "A tale of two babies," a feeding story that gives you an overview. Critical topics for you to understand are "Follow your baby's lead," "Develop a feeding routine," "Breastfeeding supply and demand," and "Knowing your baby is getting enough." "Breastfeeding anatomy and physiology" comes early in the how-to discussion because I think it supports breastfeeding to know how it works, but you might not agree. The rest of the chapter is about issues that may pop up: individual differences among babies, breast issues, and giving a bottle.

A word of encouragement: Veteran breastfeeders say this chapter gives you the information you will get from a book. They consider it to be accurate, informative, and supportive for anyone new to breastfeeding.

There is much to learn

Irrespective of terminology, biology, and gender, you have a lot to master. My goal in this chapter is to give you basic breastfeeding information as concisely as possible. Depend on your health professional to help you address special conditions and challenges. If you need it, track down this chapter's more in-depth references or seek out a breastfeeding specialist.

This chapter draws from much information in the rest of the book. Chapter 7 particularly, Understanding Your Newborn, outlines and elaborates on what you need to know to breastfeed your baby. Rather than giving page numbers when I refer to materials from Chapter 7, I depend on you to know where to find the information. Sections in other chapters are also important and for those I give page numbers. There are still a lot of them, and I beg your patience. I thought it was better to give page numbers than to make you dig around for the information.

You might also read parts of Chapter 9, Formula-Feeding Your Baby. I say the same there about the feeding relationship as I say here, but I say it in different ways and tell different stories. Particularly read Chapter 9 if you do any bottle-feeding, whether you choose expressed breastmilk or formula.

BEFORE BREASTFEEDING ISSUES

Chapter 6, Your Feeding Decision: Breastfeeding or Bottle-Feeding, emphasizes making the feeding decision that is right for you. While breastfeeding has unique nutritional qualities, breastfeed because you *want* to, not because you *have* to. Being comfortable with your feeding method and having a positive feeding relationship with your baby are more important than whether you breast- or formula-feed.

Whichever you choose, you are entitled to support from your health-care providers and help as you establish a positive feeding relationship with your baby.

Supportive obstetrical care

Discuss the delivery routine with your obstetrician. Breastfeeding goes better if you minimize sedation and anesthesia, and if you have access to your baby early and often. Understand how different forms of sedation affect breastfeeding. Make sure your baby can be with you in the delivery and recovery room.

Ask your obstetrician about hospital routines and ask about those routines when you tour the hospital. For specifics, see the section just below, "The breastfeeding-friendly hospital."

Your health conditions, medications, and drugs

Medications, including stimulants, caffeine and supplements, can pass from breastmilk to the baby. Do a web search for *drugs and other chemicals in human milk NIH* for a continually updated summary of what is safe—and what isn't—from the National Institute of Child Health and Human Development. When choosing your necessary medication, avoid the long-acting form (your baby has trouble detoxifying it), take medication right after you breastfeed, and watch your baby for unusual signs or symptoms such as changes in feeding or sleeping, increased fussiness, or rash. Birth control pills, especially the higherdosage ones, have been accused of (and defended against) decreasing breastmilk supply. Talk with your physician about using oral contraceptives and monitor your baby's growth if you decide to use them.

Certain antacids, anticoagulants, hormones, chemotherapy drugs for cancer treatment, anticonvulsants, laxatives, and illegal drugs are contraindicated for use while breastfeeding. Breastfeeding may or may not be contraindicated if you are HIV positive. Current studies show the risk of HIV transmission via breastmilk from an HIV-positive parent who is receiving antiretroviral treatment and is virally suppressed is less than one percent.[2]

Consider caffeine, alcohol, and smoking. Caffeine may interfere with relaxation, both for you and the baby. Alcohol in doses as small as a five-ounce glass of wine or a can of beer cuts down on oxytocin release and interferes with let-down. Smoking cuts down on prolactin release, and heavy smoking can reduce human milk production. Avoid exposing your baby to second-hand smoke.

Relactation and induced lactation

You may not have breastfed your baby right after birth because you or they were ill or you weren't with your baby. You can still breastfeed. Induced lactation and relactation are common historically and in other cultures. Stimulate your breasts ahead of time by massaging them and going through the motions of hand-expressing breastmilk. Nurse your baby early and often and continue to use manual stimulation. Babies less than three months old are generally more cooperative. Within two to three weeks, you are likely to be able to produce breastmilk; whether or not you produce enough to satisfy your baby's needs is another matter. You will be most successful as well as feel most rewarded if you put the emphasis on nurturing your baby and yourself with the feeding relationship, not on how much breastmilk you produce. You definitely need informed support. You may or may not be aided by taking medication: Discuss lactation-stimulating medications with your doctor.

With relactation and induced lactation you skip the colostrum phase, but other than that, the principles of supply and demand apply. Nurse your baby frequently, on demand, 8 to 12 times per 24 hours. Avoid baby-bottle nipples, pacifiers, and nipple shields. Give formula or donated human milk to provide for your baby's nutritional needs while you wait for your milk to come in. To avoid nipple confusion, consider using a supplemental nursing system that trickles formula from a reservoir through thin tubing onto your nipple as your baby nurses. As you produce more breastmilk, your baby's stools will become less formed and less smelly, and you can gradually slow the formula drip and then stop it altogether. Or not. You can have a lovely feeding relationship continuing to use a supplemental nursing system or even use it exclusively.

You may be able to relactate if your baby has been sick or premature and/or has spent days and weeks in the hospital. Premature infants can learn to breastfeed after initial bottle-feeding. Whether or not you are able to breastfeed fully, you can let your baby suck at your breast, with or without using a supplemental nursing system.

CONSIDER SUPPORT

You need to take care of yourself as you take care of your baby and learn to breastfeed. Give some thought to how you will do that.

Fathers as doulas

In cultures where breastfeeding is common and successful, new-parent doulas play an important role. You can learn to play that role. Feeding anthropologist Dana Raphael described the doula as the person who moves in with the new mother to give physical and emotional support, encourage confidence, and provide information. Surveys of success with breastfeeding parents found mothers assigned most importance to fathers' responsiveness. You are responsive when you find out and accept how your partner feels, even if those feelings are negative. Responsive fathers show and express their appreciation for and comfort with breastfeeding, run interference with other people, and pay attention to how their partner wants them to participate. Being responsive makes you a calming presence, which helps just by your being there and taking an interest. Doing household chores helps, but it is far down on the list.[3]

You both need support, so don't hesitate to let others know how you feel and ask for help if you need it. As a new father, you are likely to have negative feelings as well, and those feelings deserve airing and acceptance. Your responsibilities have increased tremendously, your life and schedule have become far more complicated, and if you are like most new fathers, you don't know what to expect or how to cope with a new baby. Many new fathers find babies only start to get interesting at around two to three months, when they interact more. At the same time, your partner is likely to be preoccupied with the baby, her moods may fluctuate, and she may be touchy, demoralized, and even depressed. Postpartum depression is real, and help is available.

Ask for help

Arrange for help ahead of time. You will both need it, and others want to help you. Tell your parents, or whoever parents you, that if they can squeeze out the time to be backup and support for you for a week or two, they will find it wonderfully rewarding and even healing. There is nothing quite like the satisfaction of helping a new young family get off on the right foot. Not only that, but they will likely find as I did that being with a newborn one step removed from their own babies was a wonderful way to put their own parenting in perspective.

Your new-baby helper can make sure there are regular meals, clean, do laundry, provide moral support, give encouragement, and add another set of eyes and ears as you try to understand what your baby is telling you. Most of all, they can be a calming presence while you get used to being parents. One of my colleagues wrote lovingly and fondly of her mother's help with new babies. One evening, her mother prepared a lovely dinner, lit the candles, and left her and her husband alone for a special and undisturbed time to themselves. What a wonderful gesture! The mother's giving her blessings to them as a couple was a powerful way of providing support to that young family!

At the very least, your helper can take an interest and *be there*. To understand why that helps, let us consider the early days of horse racing. Since highly bred racehorses are often jittery, especially in all the commotion before the race, trainers would put a goat in the pen with them. The placid, cud-chewing, unflappable goat would help calm the excitable racehorse. The saying, "get your goat" comes from competitor's stealing the goat, whereupon the horse would apparently get so upset it would lose the race. Don't forget where you heard it! It's a stretch, but the principle is the same. Many parents take turns with being the goat. When you are new parents, you both need a goat. A good goat is quiet, keeps advice to themselves, and is sensitive to parents' needs.

If you are particularly fortunate, you will have someone to sit down with you and observe feeding. They don't have to be a breastfeeding expert, just their presence can help you relax and observe and interpret your baby's messages. They can pick up on things you miss, and watching how they are with your baby can show you some different ways to engage.

If you can't arrange for help, at least cut yourself some slack. You don't have to know the answers, you don't need a clean house, and you can eat pizza. You do, however, have to share responsibility for observing, understanding, and making decisions about your baby—not just saying, "anything you want, dear." Inform yourself, think through the issues, and talk them over thoughtfully, like parents in the tale of two babies that I will soon tell you. Even if you have to leave to work or study, taking that responsibility will keep you an active participant in your baby's life.

The doula committee

Consider putting together a doula committee by drawing on your mothers, experienced friends, cooks, order-in sources, and cleaners. If you enjoy groups, get on the local breastfeeding grapevine or join an online chat group. The common thread for committee membership is comfort with breastfeeding. You will benefit from a knowledgeable, experienced, and supportive obstetrician, pediatrician, allied health professional, a hospital with breastfeeding-supportive routines, lactation counselors, and people who can provide ongoing situational and moral support.

Supportive obstetrical care

Discuss the delivery routine with your obstetrician. Breastfeeding goes better if you minimize sedation and anesthesia, and if you have access to your baby early and often. Understand how different forms of sedation affect breastfeeding. Make sure your baby can be with you in the delivery and recovery room.

The breastfeeding-friendly hospital

Hospital stays are short, but you are so receptive right after birth that the attitudes and behaviors you pick up there stay with you. Although pacifiers aren't recommended for breastfed babies, my hospital made pacifiers for babies with baby-bottle nipples, cotton, and tape. Months later, many parents still used those cobbled-together pacifiers! I am not recommending those nipples—store-bought ones are better. I am just pointing out how parents continue to practice what they see early on.

Find out about hospital routines and double-check what you are told. Talk to other parents who have delivered at the hospital, ask your pediatrician, and take a tour. Find out:

- If they encourage parents and babies to be together in the delivery room and right afterward.
- Whether they support rooming in and whether you want it.
- Whether they have a positive attitude about breastfeeding and give good instruction.
- Whether they have a certified lactation counselor.
- Whether they refrain from giving pacifiers, formula, or glucose water to breastfed babies.
- Whether they refrain from advising limits on nursing times.

Both of you need to hold your baby and spend time together during that important, exciting, and extremely receptive time right after birth. You will all be wide awake and seem to gaze into each other's souls. But don't take for granted that you will be given this time. I was surprised when my granddaughters, Adele and Marin, were judged "small" and immediately whisked away to be put into little warmers. They each weighed about six pounds, were in good shape, and their pediatrician pronounced them the healthiest twins he had known. Being twins and their small-but-normal size still set off the hospital routine. Not being able to get their hands on those babies was intensely frustrating for their parents.

Consider your own needs when you decide about rooming in. You may be tired or recovering after a cesarean section and need the rest. Also consider your need to have some early support as you get acquainted with your baby. Hospital staff can show you how to read your baby's sleep cycles, soothe and comfort them, and take care of their physical needs. They will tell you that all the racket they make while they sleep is just normal and not a sign they are waking up. You may need to learn diapering, holding, burping, and bathing. You will likely find one or two staff people who are a good fit for you.

Some hospitals still give glucose water before the milk comes in. This is not justified, even when a baby has jaundice. The main reason for avoiding glucose water is nipple confusion: The nipple on the bottle calls for a completely different nursing pattern than the breast.

The pediatric staff

Check the local breastfeeding grapevine to find a physician who is knowledgeable and supportive; not all are. A 2017 survey found that 65 to 76 percent of pediatricians recommend exclusive breastfeeding, 57 percent indicated that breastfeeding mothers can be successful, and 50 percent say the benefits outweigh the difficulties.[4] Despite American Academy of Pediatrics emphasis on breastfeeding,[5] the percentages I just cited have *decreased* since 1995. Reading between the lines, that decrease likely means that pediatricians have trouble helping when things get sticky. Up to a quarter of pediatricians indicated that they would recommend—erroneously—discontinuing breastfeeding for mastitis, nipple problems, seemingly inadequate milk supply, slow infant weight gain, poor health of the baby, and infant jaundice. To be clear, none of these issues means you have to stop breastfeeding.[4]

In their defense, pediatricians' hectic office schedules make it hard for them to find time to do breastfeeding counseling and problem-solving. However, pediatricians carry a lot of authority. Their positive attitude about breastfeeding and willingness to refer to someone who *does* have time and expertise can help enormously.

Increase your comfort and confidence by scheduling a predelivery visit with your pediatrician. Find out who at your doctor's office will be providing care. Since you may spend more office and telephone time with a nurse, nurse practitioner, or physician's assistant, you need to be comfortable with them as well. Don't hesitate to ask to speak and work with the person you want—not everyone is a good fit for everyone else. Gain an impression of your providers' ideas and attitudes about breastfeeding. Find out the frequency and scheduling of follow-up visits and how flexible they are about scheduling extra visits. Does someone in the office do breastfeeding follow-up? Do they call you or wait for you to call them? Keep in mind that after you deliver, you may not have much emotional or physical energy for seeking help.

The American Academy of Pediatrics recommends that both breast- and formula-fed babies be seen at three to five days with detailed, research-based guidelines for assessing you, your baby, and your breastfeeding relationship.[5] After that, the AAP recommends visits at one, two, four, six and nine months. If you are at all uncomfortable with how your baby is doing, ask for a two-week visit and more frequent visits after that.

Be wary of counterproductive advice

Pediatricians and other health workers love babies and want the best for them, but they are medical people and their primary concern is children's medical well-being. Your health worker might be experienced and responsive enough to say, "Follow your baby's cues, trust what your baby tells you," and even help you identify your baby's cues. The health worker who has the misfortune of being stuck in medical taking-control thinking might say, "Here's how much your baby should eat," "Don't feed him so often," or worst of all, "Get her to eat more—I don't care how you do it." There are a number of sections in this book about avoiding interference. The one that applies most to our current discussion is in Chapter 7, "Be wary of interference."

Interference is so much a part of feeding lore that health workers don't even know they do it. When you get counterproductive advice, discuss it with your care provider as tactfully as you can and tell them why it is not helpful. They are likely to be receptive because we all learn from our patients. You will be doing yourself the favor of recruiting support and helping other parents get better advice. You have my permission to copy this chapter for your health care provider.

EATING AND DRINKING WHILE BREASTFEEDING

You have to eat. You need strength, endurance, and emotional steadiness to be good parents. When you go without food, you will be worn-out, cranky, and discouraged. Be positive and reliable about taking care of yourself with food. If all goes well, you will be hungry, and your appetite will be good so you can eat as much as you want and need. If your appetite is poor at first, emphasize three meals a day and as many snacks as you need to feel comfortable and energetic. Your appetite will recover after a week or two, and eating can again be enjoyable.

Discover the joy of eating

Chapter 5 encourages you to use this time to discover the joy of being Eating Competent. You can only take another person, even an infant, as far as you have taken yourself. That means in order to trust your child, you have to trust yourself. To trust your baby to know how much to eat and, later on, to trust them to determine whether and how much to eat at family meals, you have to know about and trust those instinctive abilities in yourself. Moreover, you have to know it with your *body*, not your head. Take care of yourself and give yourself permission to eat food that appeals to you and eat as much as you want.

The Chapter 5 section, "The joy of eating during pregnancy," page 140, points out that pregnancy in general and eating during pregnancy in particular give you a priceless opportunity. You can use that time to gain respect for your body and for the miracle of giving birth. There is no better foundation for feeding your family than respecting your body, feeding yourself faithfully, and giving yourself permission to eat.

Forget about good-food/bad-food

During breastfeeding as well as during pregnancy and at other times, don't burden yourself with food prescriptions, portion sizes, and patterns. Instead, depend on being Eating Competent: Eat based on your body's wisdom. You don't have to worry about good-food/bad-food because as it says in the Chapter 1 section, "Eating Competence supports wellness," page 16: Competent eaters do better medically and nutritionally, have stable body weights, and feel good about their bodies. Competent Eaters are more active, sleep better, and have higher overall social and emotional functioning. Results with eat-this-don't-eat-that guidelines do not match that track record.

Being Eating Competent lets you choose food you enjoy and eat as much as you want at meals and at sit-down snacks as you need them. Being Eating Competent lets you include nutritious food, not because you *have* to but because you *enjoy* it. Use enough sugar, salt, and fat to make cooking and eating rewarding. For you to be faithful about feeding yourself, your food must be richly rewarding to plan, prepare, provide, and eat.

Drink as much as you need

Drink regularly throughout the day, but don't force yourself to drink more than you want. If you are truly dehydrated, your milk supply will decrease, but the idea that drinking more than you need will increase your breastmilk supply is simply wrong. Too much liquid intake can actually impair breastmilk production. You aren't supposed to consume any alcohol while you breastfeed, but you may be tempted to drink beer. It supposedly increases breastmilk production but, sadly, this isn't true. In fact, drinking more than a single can of beer or its equivalent can hinder let-down because the alcohol inhibits oxytocin release.[6] In addition, a certain amount of alcohol gets into the breastmilk, so consume any alcohol right after you nurse.

Just for curiosity: the numbers

Eating regularly and paying attention to your hunger and appetite and your baby's growth are the best guides to how much to eat while you breastfeed. Many variables affect energy requirement for breastfeeding, including your need, your baby's need, how much weight you gained during pregnancy, and your metabolism. Trust your hunger and appetite.

But, just for fun, let's look at the numbers. A newborn who eats a lot can take as much as 30 ounces of human milk a day. Closer to six months, some fully breastfed babies can eat 45 ounces or more. An ounce of human milk contains 20 calories, the same as an ounce of formula. While it is hard to say just how much extra food you need to support breastfeeding, a good guess is that 100 calories of your food convert into 90 calories of human milk. Using those numbers, you could begin by needing about 450 more calories a day to make enough breastmilk for your baby and about 1,000 calories a day toward the end of 12 months of breastfeeding. Maybe. Babies vary from one another in their calorie requirements by as much as 50 percent, and they frequently eat twice as much one day as another.

Since you can't go by the numbers to know how much to eat while you breastfeed, depend on being Eating Competent: Feed yourself faithfully and give yourself permission to eat. Eating regularly based on your hunger and appetite will give you as much as you need and is more than likely to give you enough protein, as well. You need only 12 to 15 grams more protein a day to support breastfeeding. An egg or a one ounce serving of meat, poultry, fish, or cheese offers 8 grams of protein. So do 8 ounces of milk or 4 ounces of cooked dried beans. An extra egg and glass of milk will provide for your additional protein needs. If your diet is low in protein, protein for breastmilk production is taken from your body's muscles and organs.

When to monitor weight

Your hunger and appetite will guide you in eating the amount you need to provide breastmilk for your baby. However, in some situations it can help to keep track of your weight. With respect to breastfeeding, monitoring weight is not to get your weight down but to make sure you aren't losing too much or too fast. If you lose no more than ½ pound per week, you are likely eating enough to support breastmilk production. If you gained less than the average of 25 pounds during pregnancy, particularly if you were slim to start with, follow your hunger cues to eat eat enough so you don't lose weight at all.

Enjoy regular and appealing meals that include fat for both nutritional value and pleasure. Since our current culture is so food-avoidant, fat-avoidant, and slimness-obsessed, I will belabor the point. A number of studies of lactation failure have identified part of the problem to be extremely poor food intake by the mother. Check yourself. Do any of these patterns describe yours?

- Low weight gain during pregnancy for whatever reason.
- Dieting to lose weight, both during pregnancy and lactation.
- Poor eating habits in general; too busy to eat.
- Very tired and seemingly experiencing some loss of appetite due to fatigue.
- Careful to avoid eating fat.
- Have a list of foods to avoid: fat, sugar, red meat, you name it.
- Not enough money to buy food.

If all has gone well, you have given up weight-reduction dieting during pregnancy. If not, now is the time to do that. Entice yourself to take time for meals and to eat enough by having food you enjoy. Emphasizing enjoyment lets you eat a greater variety of food which, in turn, supports nutritional excellence. Be as brave as you can about your weight and consider whether this is the time to develop a true appreciation for your body rather than thinking in terms of what you weigh and how you look. Consider what your body did for you and your baby during pregnancy! Consider what your body is doing for you and your baby during these early months!

Food money

If you worry about having enough money to buy food, get in touch with WIC: The Special Supplemental Nutrition Program for Women, Infants, and Children. Also consider applying for the Supplemental Nutrition Assistance Program (SNAP). Make use of food pantries. The nutrition programs may advise you to emphasize "healthy" low-calorie foods such as fresh fruits and vegetables and skim milk, but doing that doesn't make a lot of sense. Your and anybody else's first need is for calories. Emphasize strategies for getting enough calories when you shop and cook: Use higher-calorie versions of foods such as whole milk and canned fruit in heavy syrup. Have meals: They are the first line of defense in managing the food budget. Cook with fat, and include butter, regular salad dressing, and sauces at mealtime. Eat as much as you want to satisfy your hunger. For more, see the Chapter 5 section, "Address food insecurity," page 142.

Vitamins and minerals

"You lose a tooth with every child," the grandmothers used to say. Well, true—but not true. If need be, calcium will be taken from your teeth and bones for breastmilk production. You can protect your teeth and bones somewhat by drinking milk. Women who breastfeed past six months do break down bony tissue even if they are well-nourished. After weaning that bony tissue is built back up again, so the breakdown only becomes a problem when another pregnancy follows right after weaning.[7]

Your intake of manganese and iodine, vitamin A, vitamin C, and the B vitamins with the exception of folic acid is reflected in your breastmilk. Manganese is found in whole grains and nuts. Iodine is in iodized salt and is also present in ample quantities as a byproduct of the production of milk and commercially baked bread. Vitamin A comes from whole and fortified milk and from dark-green and deep-yellow fruits and vegetables. The only vitamins that are likely to present a problem, and only if you are vegan (eat no animal protein), are B6 and B12, so talk with your doctor about a supplement. In fact, get a consult with a dietitian, because eating successfully while vegan is challenging, especially during pregnancy and lactation.

The bottom line is that you can get what you need by being Eating Competent and therefore eating a variety of food.[8] If you feel more comfortable about your nutrition when you take a supplement, choose a broad spectrum (lots of different) vitamin-mineral supplement with generally no more than 100 percent of the Daily Value (DV) of any nutrient. Don't try to piece together a supplement package by taking a little of this and a little of that—or worse, a lot of this or that. Taking too much of any one nutrient can rob you of another nutrient or even be toxic. You don't need your prenatal vitamin when you are breastfeeding. On the other hand, if you have lost blood during delivery, you may need iron supplements. Ask your doctor.

Activity during breastfeeding

Trust your body to guide you in being active in ways that are right for you. If you are active for enjoyment and to take care of yourself, activity has the same physical, emotional, and social benefits now as at any other time. However, exercising primarily to lower weight can be demoralizing. Studies show that active mothers breastfeed just as well as mothers who are not active. Being more active means you need more calories and need to eat more, which you will do automatically by eating in accordance with your sensations of hunger and fullness. While generally active women who breastfeed have lower body fat than generally sedentary women, increasing activity during breastfeeding increases fitness but doesn't necessarily decrease body weight.

EARLY BREASTFEEDING ISSUES

Now we turn to issues that become important right after your baby is born.

Cesarean section

I hope you don't need this section, but if you do, you need it *right now.* When the placenta leaves the womb during delivery, high levels of pregnancy hormones (estrogen and progesterone) drop, which allows prolactin levels to increase and stimulates human milk production. Having the baby move through the birth canal isn't necessary to stimulate this change. Breastfeeding after surgical birth is the same as breastfeeding after vaginal birth except you are sore in a different place and sore for longer. Your stomach may be so tender when you hold your baby that for a time you may want to nurse lying on your side or using the football or Australian hold. Women who have cesareans may produce somewhat less breastmilk at first than those who have vaginal births.[9] But this doesn't have to stand in your way. Respect your baby's hungry days, be willing to feed frequently, and keep an eye on your baby's growth.

Skin-to-skin contact

After generations of whisking babies away right after birth to warming devices and medical procedures, the medical profession has acknowledged how stressful that is for both parents and babies. The American Academy of Pediatrics now endorses skin-to-skin contact for newborns and mothers for an hour after birth and as much skin-to-skin contact as you wish in the days following. AAP says such contact supports bonding, stabilizes babies and mothers medically, decreases infant stress overall, and particularly helps babies during necessary medical procedures such as blood draws.

Fathers and babies benefit from skin-to-skin contact as well and these same guidelines apply to fathers. Adoptive parents and babies benefit too, even if the baby is a bit older. AAP's warnings about safe skin-to-skin contact are obvious but important: Make sure your baby faces you, head straight up and turned to one side, legs bent, face away from your skin and out of the covers so they can breathe. Put your baby to bed when you are ready to go to sleep.[10]

Kangaroo care involves holding or wrapping your baby skin to skin inside your shirt. It is good for all babies but is particularly recommended for full-term infants who are neurologically, metabolically, or medically impaired. It can stabilize temperature, breathing, and heart rate, and calm your baby overall.

Baby's jaundice

Jaundiced babies have yellow skin, perhaps yellowing in the whites of their eyes, and their blood tests show high levels of bilirubin. Managing jaundice calls for your baby's getting enough to eat, and therefore to drink, and their passing stools.[11] Jaundice is more frequent with breastfed babies, particularly when they are premature. That is not because there is anything in human milk that causes it, but because milk production and therefore bowel function can be delayed. Formula-fed babies who don't eat much get jaundiced, as well. Normal full-term infants get jaundiced because they are born with a high red blood cell count that allows them to use the low amount of oxygen delivered to them across the placenta. After birth they don't need so many blood cells, so their bodies break down some of them. Bilirubin is the end product of that breakdown.

Excessive and prolonged jaundice can harm your baby, and your doctor will evaluate your breastfeeding routine and your apparent milk supply. If your breastmilk is relatively slow to come in, they may recommend temporary formula-feeding. They may also recommend treatment: Discuss it with your doctor. According to physician and breastfeeding experts Ruth and Robert Lawrence, to help prevent and address jaundice, nurse early and often. Avoid water and glucose water. Avoid formula supplements during the first few days as long as breastfeeding is going well. If bilirubin levels are particularly high or those high levels persist for several days, supplement with formula while continuing to nurse.[12]

Sleeping arrangements

To reduce the risk of sudden infant death syndrome, the American Academy of Pediatrics recommends "back to sleep": placing infants under age one year only on their back to sleep—not the side, not the tummy. Research on SIDS supports AAP's emphasis on having a firm sleep surface, room-sharing without bed-sharing, and taking care to keep covers off the baby's face. Additional recommendations for guarding against SIDS include breastfeeding, routine immunization, use of a pacifier (wait until breastfeeding is well established), and avoiding exposure to smoke, alcohol, and illicit drugs.

By the time you read this, there may be safety standards for bedside sleepers—the sort that can be easily accessed from your bed. Until then, AAP doesn't endorse them. AAP recommends against sleeping with your baby in your bed, even if you have a snuggle nest. If you choose to keep your baby in your bed, observe precautions: your little one is healthy; you remain awake and fully aware of what's going on around you; and there are no hazardous objects, pillows, or blankets to entrap a baby.

Your baby's head needs to be straight on their neck and shoulders—not tipped to the side or back—for them to breathe properly. Because of the difficulty of keeping your baby's head straight, don't let them regularly sleep in a car seat, stroller, swing, infant carrier, or infant sling. Don't sleep with your baby on a couch or in an armchair: The accident rate is high because babies can so easily fall down among the cushions.[10]

Enough background. Now let's get to the fun part: breastfeeding your baby. Let's begin with a story.

A TALE OF TWO BABIES

Meet Janet and David, Emily's parents, and Martha and Robert, Ryan's parents. All were first time parents. Both mothers had healthy and uneventful pregnancies, carried their babies to term, and had vaginal deliveries at breastfeeding-supportive hospitals. Both mothers were surprised at how awkward and selfconscious they felt as they were shown how to position the baby and help them latch on. Janet appreciated being helped to nurse while lying down, but Martha preferred sitting up. At each feeding, the hospital staff was careful to start the babies on alternate breasts and even suggested keeping track with a safety pin on the bra cup. While that seemed to be a silly suggestion at first, both mothers found they had difficulty remembering.

Getting started with nursing

All the parents were surprised to see that when their baby's cheek was stroked they turned toward the nipple, mouth open, searching for the nipple. Martha was startled when Ryan latched on: It was remarkable to see so much of her nipple and areola disappear into that tiny mouth. He put so much pressure on her areola that it almost hurt—in fact, it *did* hurt when he first latched on.

Emily took just the very end of Janet's nipple in her mouth and when she clamped down it hurt a lot! The nurse showed Janet the C-hold: flattening her nipple and areola between her thumb and forefinger and pressing in toward her chest wall to make it stick out before she placed it in Emily's mouth. It also helped to position Emily so her neck was extended and head tipped back a bit. That made Emily's mouth open farther so she could latch on better. Emily did better on one breast than the other, and the lactation counselor showed Janet and David how to get Emily's suck going on her less-preferred side by putting her finger, nail down, in Emily's mouth, and gently rubbing the roof of her mouth. When Emily actively started to suck, Janet quickly placed her on her breast and Emily took in the nipple and areola and suckled well. To understand proper latch-on, see the section, "Check for proper attachment," page 239.

Each couple was surprised at their baby's willingness to nurse to get the small amount of clear to yellowish colostrum that was available at first, and they had heard that colostrum had important immunity factors. They all still worried that the breastmilk didn't come before hospital discharge, and the sample formula kits looked appealing. They were reassured to know that babies generally don't get hungry until a few days after birth, and the 50 to 100 calories a day they get in colostrum generally satisfies them.

The first clinic visit

Both sets of parents had clinic visits about five days after their hospital release. By that time, both mothers' breastmilk had come in, and all were interested to see that, as they had been told, the "fore" milk at the beginning of feeding was thin and bluishlooking and the "hind" milk toward the end of feeding was creamier and more opaque. Janet said her breasts were full and she was aware of let-down—she could feel a tingling and prickling in her breasts. Martha said her breasts were soft and she couldn't feel any let-down, although she could tell by Ryan's slower, longer sucks that she had let down and he started getting milk.

David wanted to know what they were checking Emily for. "Jaundice, hydration, weight that hasn't gone down too far, and general signs that your baby is healthy," the doctor answered. "We also check whether the breastmilk has come in and how feeding is going. By now we like to see about six or eight wet diapers a day and that many of those diapers have at least a little poopy yellow stain." Both babies passed muster, both babies' weights were satisfactory, and Emily had gained back to her birth weight. Both sets of parents were advised to schedule a second visit in a month's time. Robert wasn't comfortable with waiting that long, especially since Ryan hadn't gained back to his birth weight, so he asked whether they could return sooner. The pediatrician reassured him that all was well, but Robert persisted, and they scheduled a visit two weeks later.

Emily was active and aggressive

After that early visit, our stories diverge. Emily kept Janet and David hopping. She was active, demanding, and dissatisfied, slept irregularly, and woke up crying and seemingly starved. She wanted to nurse at least every two hours all day and at least twice at night, although there was really no pattern. She nursed eagerly and had a powerful suck. She came off an empty breast crying and only stopped fussing when she got the second breast. She emptied that, as well, and seemed to look around for more.

David helped all he could by being encouraging and bringing Emily to Janet for the night feedings and by diapering, soothing, and dressing Emily. Janet was getting worn out, and David worried out loud that Emily's eating so often and seeming so unsatisfied meant that she wasn't getting enough to eat. Then, in the same breath, he announced to himself that he surely was changing a lot of wet, poopy diapers and that was supposed to mean things were fine. They kept track of Emily's pees and poops for a few days, making hatch marks on a piece of paper, feeling embarrassed for being so anal, so to speak. But it turned out to be reassuring, because Emily's output was just what they had been told it ought to be.

It didn't help when a visitor was critical of how often Emily ate and even suggested that Janet's milk disagreed with her and that Janet should give Emily a bottle so she would get on a schedule. Janet and David knew their visitor's ideas were simply wrong, but the whole episode upset Janet anyway. She was so tired she couldn't take much at that point. David told the visitor politely but firmly that Emily was doing just fine, and they wouldn't be using bottles any time soon. Janet was upset enough that she and David put in a call to the lactation counselor they had liked in the hospital. After asking a few questions about—what else, pees and poops—and how Janet was feeling, the counselor reassured them that they were doing well. That helped a lot, but they still worried and had to reassure each other all over again that they were on the right track.

Janet and David felt exhausted, harassed, and insecure when they presented Emily for her onemonth checkup. To her parents' astonishment, Emily had gained almost three pounds in that short time. Emily's eating pattern, although it seemed hectic and pressured, was just right for her and was apparently helping her thrive. Knowing that, her parents were able to relax and stop feeling like they were doing something wrong. Emily's eating schedule didn't get any less frequent for another month or so, but knowing all was well made it less wearing.

Ryan was sleepy and placid

Martha and Robert seemed to be having an easier time of it. Martha's mother came to stay with them for a couple of weeks, and that helped them calm down. Ryan seemed to be an easy baby because he slept three to four hours at a stretch. But when he woke up, he was still sleepy and during nursing, he did a lot of starting and stopping. He often drifted off to sleep before he had made much headway on the second breast, and they couldn't tell if he had gotten enough. Martha's mother wondered if that was all right, but she only voiced her concern when Ryan had two dry diapers in a row. She told Martha and Robert that she thought Ryan was too sleepy for his own good and they needed to give him some help staying awake to eat.

They weren't sure how to do that, and they found that the standard waking-up tactics didn't help: jiggling, tickling his feet, burping, unwrapping him and sitting him up. Then Martha's mother suggested talking with him. Martha started by talking in a gentle, soothing, commenting sort of voice, and when that didn't do much, she experimented with what tone of voice interested him. He perked up when Martha made conversation with him, so she chatted away while she fed him, telling him all about what was going on. Ryan's eyes opened wide and he looked at a spot above his mother's right ear. He ate steadily and was awake at the end of the feeding.

Between feedings, Robert helped Ryan get better at staying awake by holding him close to his face and talking with him. Ryan stayed awake and calm for a few minutes, then when he started to squirm and lose interest, Robert put him down for another nap. Within a day of Robert and Emily's helping Ryan be awake and calm for feeding and for a while afterwards, Ryan's sleep cycles improved. He started to wake himself up more thoroughly and stay awake while he ate. After another day or two, his pee and poop output reassured them they could trust him to eat. Read more in the Chapter 7 section, "More about sleep."

It was good that Robert had insisted on the two-week checkup because they needed reassurance. Ryan had gained back to his birth weight and seemed to be doing just fine. They told the nurse practitioner about Ryan's being so sleepy and she advised them that from now on they should wake him up every two hours to eat by unwrapping him, sitting him up, moving him around, sitting him up and bending him back and forth over his lap, and talking with him briskly. They protested that similar tactics hadn't helped to wake him up, but she pointed out that they had to work with him for 10 or 15 minutes.

It didn't seem right, but it was pretty hard to go against this seemingly expert advice. They tried doing the recommended gymnastics with Ryan every two hours, but it was a disaster. Ryan couldn't wake up when he wasn't ready, and he didn't eat well. They went back to following his lead with sleeping and eating at the same time as they kept a close eye on his nursing behavior, pees, and poops. He did fine. He kept himself for the most part on an irregular two- to three-hour schedule. When he woke up, he woke up thoroughly, ate well, and even stayed awake for a few minutes after he ate. Once in a while, he cluster-fed—he ate every hour for two or three feedings. When they went back for their one-month checkup they found he had continued to do well.

The experiences of these new parents represent more or less the normal extremes of newborn nursing behavior. Emily and Ryan challenged their parents in different ways, and both sets of parents did well with respect to reading the signs and evaluating what was going on with breastfeeding. That is not to say that it was easy. The parents were anxious and unsure of themselves, and only felt more comfortable after the breastfeeding and parenting began to feel more familiar to them. It helped even more when they got some outside confirmation that their infants truly were getting enough to eat and growing well.

BREASTFEEDING ANATOMY AND PHYSIOLOGY

Understanding how breastfeeding works will help you get your head in the game. Take a look at the breast cross-section in Figure 8.1. Lobules are the milk factories. The milk ducts carry the milk through the lactiferous sinuses just beneath the areola (the colored area around the nipple) to openings in the nipple. Your baby removes milk from your breast by squeezing the lactiferous sinuses between their jaw and tongue.

During pregnancy, breastmilk-producing anatomy and physiology grow and develop, and, by somewhere in the second trimester, you become capable of producing milk. Suckling and pumping without being pregnant does the same. Within three to five days after you have your baby, your breast lobules step up breastmilk production. That is an automatic process for all but a minority of mothers. Your breastmilk is "coming in" when your breasts feel fuller and heavier, and you may have some leaking. Only some of that fullness and heaviness is milk; most of it is increased blood and lymph circulation to your breasts. You make some breastmilk between feedings and store it in the lobules and ducts, but you make most of it when your baby starts to nurse.

Delivering breastmilk

When your baby suckles, the breast tissue matures further, you produce more prolactin, and you produce more breastmilk. When your breasts

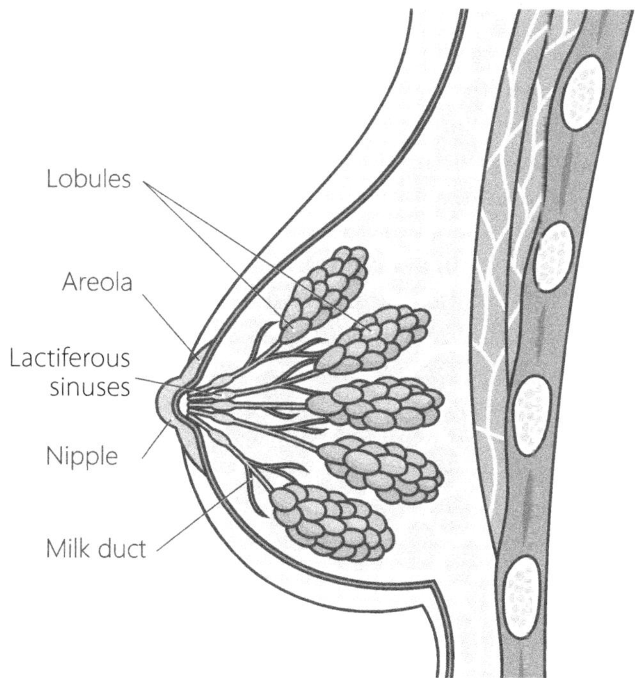

FIGURE 8.1: CROSS-SECTION OF A LACTATING BREAST

"empty" it is because the immediate supply of ingredients—components for making breastmilk—decreases. That supply is rapidly replenished. Between feedings you make some breastmilk, and your breasts may seem to fill up, but for the most part you are restocking prolactin for producing more breastmilk the next time your baby eats.

Squeezing on the lactiferous sinuses under the areola expresses breastmilk in a fine mist through nipple pores and into the baby's mouth. Rather than sucking, the process of breastfeeding is more accurately called *suckling*. Your baby sucks to make your nipple longer and to draw it and much of your areola into their mouth and keep it in place against the roof of their mouth. They squeeze the areola between their tongue and jaw to expel breastmilk, and their tongue moves back and forth as they swallow. Suction doesn't remove the milk but only holds the nipple in place in the baby's mouth. That's why the baby with severe cleft palate can't breastfeed: the opening in the palate interferes with suction.

To start with, Ryan got the lactiferous sinuses in his mouth; Emily clamped down on nipple. Ryan's latch-on felt like pressure and was a bit painful at first; Emily's *hurt*.

Let-down

Your breast simultaneously makes milk and delivers it to your baby during nursing. Milk is delivered from the lobules to the lactiferous sinuses by the let-down process. During let-down, oxytocin, a hormone produced by the pituitary gland, stimulates tiny muscles around the alveoli to contract and push the milk out of the ductules and ducts and into the lactiferous sinuses. Let-down delivers about half of the milk to the sinuses within the first two minutes of nursing, about 80 to 90 percent within the first four minutes. It takes longer than that for the baby to get it out, but the milk is available. In the early feedings after birth, it may take three minutes or more of nursing for let-down to begin. After a few days, your hormone production picks up and you can let down more readily. You may find yourself letting down when you hear a baby cry or when you experience strong emotions. Some mothers find let-down stimulates their need to urinate or have a bowel movement.

You may experience let-down as a tingling sensation, a feeling of pins and needles beginning right after starting to nurse and then going away gradually. Or you may feel nothing. You may feel contractions in your uterus, ranging from mild to painful, or feel intensely thirsty. As you nurse, milk may drip or spurt from the opposite breast. Even if you don't feel or see anything, you can tell during nursing that you are letting down because your baby's suckling pattern changes from short, choppy jaw movements to a long, rhythmic suck and swallow.

If you worry about let-down, consider the conditioning tactics in Figure 8.2.

FIGURE 8.2: HELP YOURSELF WITH LET-DOWN

Let-down is a conditioned reflex. To encourage let-down, focus your attention and set up associations.

- Slow down and pay attention to your baby and the feeding process. Don't let yourself get rushed, overtired, or distracted from your baby.
- Set up a little routine: Go to your comfortable nursing chair, get your nursing pillow and stool, get a drink and a snack.
- Breathe and be mindful to help yourself relax. Take a couple of slow, deep breaths, or use the breathing pattern that you used during labor a nd delivery.

Holding your baby

Hold your baby firmly so they don't feel they will fall, but not so tight they can't wiggle. Hold them tummy to tummy, lining up their ear, shoulder, and hip (Figure 8.3). Don't let your baby lie on their back with their head twisted. Try swallowing facing directly ahead and with your neck twisted. It makes a difference, doesn't it?

FIGURE 8.3: POSITION YOUR BABY

Here is how to hold your baby so they can breastfeed well:

- Lay them on their side with their stomach touching yours.
- Support their head and hold it slightly higher than the rest of their body.
- Face them straight ahead; don't let their neck be twisted.
- Hold their ear, shoulders, and hip so they are in a straight line.
- Have their chin tucked in and tipped slightly down, not tipped back.

Check for proper attachment

Make sure your nipple and areola are drawn into your baby's mouth. To remove milk from your breast, your baby's jaw and tongue need to be over the lactiferous sinuses, which are under the areola, the darker area around the nipple. Once the milk lets down, the properly placed baby's suckling pattern changes to a longer, slower rhythm and you may hear a low drawing sound. Some mothers say their baby's ears wiggle, indicating they are using their jaw in an appropriate up-and-down motion. The temples near your baby's upper jaw will also move in and out. Figure 8.4 gives signs that your baby is suckling properly. A poorly placed baby will only take the end of the nipple in their mouth. Experiment with improper latch-on by sucking only on the tip of your thumb. Notice what your tongue does. Then experiment with proper latch-on by inserting most of your thumb in your mouth. Notice how your tongue wraps around your thumb.

Check whether your baby can extend their tongue over the lower gum line. Some babies are "tongue tied." That is, the frenulum, the attachment of the tongue to the floor of the mouth, is too short to allow the tongue to move freely and may interfere with nursing. I say "may" because the advisability of clipping the frenulum to free the tongue is hotly debated in breastfeeding and medical circles. Suffice it to say that if your baby has trouble nursing, you need to seek experienced medical help.

FIGURE 8.4: CHECK WHETHER YOUR BABY IS PROPERLY LATCHED ON

Here are some indicators that your baby's mouth is properly attached to your nipple.

- Your baby's suckling changes from a short, choppy pattern to a longer, slower rhythm.
- You may hear a low drawing sound. With improper positioning, you hear a clicking sound.
- Your baby's lower lip is out and not tucked in.
- Your baby's cheeks are rounded and firm, not drawn in or dimpled.
- You can see their tongue beneath the nipple when you draw their lips aside.
- Much or most of your areola is in their mouth, not just the end of the nipple.
- You can feel the pressure on your areola, but it doesn't pinch.
- You have to break the suction to comfortably remove your baby's mouth from your breast.

Hungry days

As your baby grows, they stimulate you to make more breastmilk by having hungry days and eating more often. Your baby is hungry, not because your breastmilk supply is failing, but because their needs for breastmilk have temporarily exceeded your ability to produce enough. Nursing frequently makes you release more prolactin, grow more milk-making alveoli, ductules, and ducts, and produce more breastmilk.

It's not about filling and emptying your breasts, and thinking in those terms can lead you astray. One young mother was told that nursing more often than every 45 minutes didn't help increase milk production because it took the breasts longer than that to fill up again. Others are told it takes two hours. The upshot of that bit of misinformation, of course, is that it seems hopeless to feed, nursing mothers wait for their breasts to fill up, and babies cry from hunger. Forget that bit of destructive advice. If your baby wants to eat after a half hour, feed. Your baby will get a little breastmilk, and your milk-making and delivery systems will be stimulated. After a couple of days, your breastmilk supply will catch up to your baby's needs.

FOLLOW YOUR BABY'S LEAD

To help you get on your baby's wavelength with feeding, review the Chapter 7 section, "Feed the way your baby tells you." Bookmark those pages—they are important. Your baby will eat best and feel best about you both as well as maintain your breastmilk supply when you follow the Satter Division of Responsibility in Feeding (sDOR):

You are responsible for what your baby is offered to eat.

Your baby is responsible for *how much* they eat—and *everything else*: how often, how fast, how continuously, how skillfully.

Read your baby's feeding signs

As it says in Chapter 7, pay attention to your baby's sleep cycles and wait to feed them until they are wide away and calm. Emily's sleep cycles were not a problem: Her parents were relieved to let her sleep as long as possible, and she made it clear with her yelling when she was ready to wake up. Ryan was another matter. He had difficulty waking up and he had trouble staying awake long enough to eat. His mother helped by waiting to pick him up until he was waking-up-and-drowsy, not just in light sleep, then finding ways that worked with him to hold and talk with him so he could be wide awake and calm while he ate.

Again, from Chapter 7, "Read your baby's feeding cues," feed when they are hungry and stop when they are full. Keep your baby in control. If your breastmilk flows too fast and they seem to be gagging, hand-express a little breastmilk to slow down your milk flow. Don't interrupt feeding to burp. Only burp if your baby squirms or looks preoccupied, like they are full of air. Let your baby pause with eating and then go back to it. This is your social time. Be interesting, not exciting or overstimulating. Wait for their hungry signs to offer the nipple again, but don't get pushy–you are only checking to be sure they have had enough to eat.

Your baby's calm awake times after eating will get longer as they get older. Let them keep you company while you work, then do your best to put them to bed when they get drowsy, before they get overtired. An overtired or over-stimulated baby can need help going to sleep. Figure 7.4, "Support your baby in going to sleep," can help.

Understand your baby's development

The Chapter 7 section, "More about development" outlines what you do with feeding to help your child achieve those tasks. Emily and Ryan were working on their first developmental task: homeostasis. Emily was able to wake herself up to be fed and stay awake while she ate, but she needed help staying calm. Ryan was calm, but he needed help waking up and staying awake.

Understand your baby's temperament and personality

The Chapter 7 section, "Consider personality and temperament" helps you understand and accept your child's personality, realizing you neither created it nor caused it! Emily was an uptight, touchy baby who was challenging to figure out. Her parents had to be persistent in following sDOR by reading her feeding signs as best they could and being careful to keep her in control with feeding. Babies like Emily are challenging because at first, even excellent feeding and parenting doesn't calm them and you have to keep doing it anyway.

Ryan, on the other hand, was easy-going. His activity was low, he was even-tempered, and he was regular in his eating habits. Some easy-going babies get enough to eat and grow well, even though they sleep peacefully, wake up periodically to eat, then go right back to sleep. But at first Ryan's easy-going nature didn't serve him well because he had trouble staying awake long enough to eat well. His parents discovered that having conversations with him while he ate solved the problem, or his sleepiness could have led to growth faltering.

DEVELOP A BREASTFEEDING ROUTINE

Going through the motions of getting ready to breastfeed conditions you: It sets up let-down as an automatic response.

Get ready to breastfeed

Wash your hands before you feed your baby, after you go to the bathroom or change diapers, before you handle food, and particularly after you handle any meat, fish, poultry, or fresh produce. Use the handwashing technique you learned during the COVID epidemic or check the web for current guidelines. The bacteria that are on your breasts are familiar to your baby, so you don't have to wash your nipples or sanitize your clothing. Your regular showers will do.

Get yourself a drink and a snack if you are hungry. Silence your phone. Put a "no soliciting" sign on the door. Make a mental note or use a safety pin on your bra to help you remember which breast to start on.

Get comfortable to breastfeed

You will be feeding during most of your early time with your baby, so get as physically comfortable as possible. Here is what you need:

A good chair that supports your back and arms, fits your body, and lets your feet touch the floor.

A nursing stool that props your feet up at a proper height and angle.

A breastfeeding pillow that wraps around your body and curves under your elbow to give your baby space to lie with their tummy touching yours, holds their head at the proper height for nursing, and lets the muscles in your arm and back relax.

Most mothers nurse sitting up most of the time with their baby across their lap lying on their side. Some mothers use a football hold, where you hold a baby, head forward, on their back under your arm as if they were a football. My daughter used a twin-nursing pillow that wrapped around her body and went under both elbows so she could use a football hold to feed both Marii and Adele at the same time. Janet did many of Emily's night feedings lying down. Janet dozed during feeding but David stayed awake so he could keep Emily safe and put her back into her own bed when she finished eating. Also consider the Australian hold, where you hold your baby sitting up facing you and straddling your thigh, with your hand supporting the back of their head. Be careful to hold lower, where the skull meets the neck. Holding higher, toward the crown of the head, could set off their arching reflex.

You may get sore and tender and be aware of some discomfort each time your baby starts nursing. It is common at first for nipples to crack and even bleed. Varying your nursing position helps change the pressure points on your areola, so you don't get so sore in any one spot. Sharp pains in your nipple area could indicate that your baby is latched on improperly. If your nipple soreness is extreme or persists beyond the first week or two, get in touch with your lactation counselor.

BREASTFEEDING SUPPLY AND DEMAND

For the first few hours, your newborn is likely to be wide awake, and the next one or two days sleepy and not too interested in eating. Newborns wake up to eat, get a small volume of colostrum, and go right back to sleep. Most babies don't get too hungry until breastmilk comes in anywhere from day two to day five. Then your baby will wake up more often to nurse.

Your supply will match your baby's demand

Making enough breastmilk for your baby depends on supply and demand. At first your production is likely to be in balance with your baby's needs or maybe a little ahead. Your breasts will tone down production if your baby doesn't eat all that is available, although you may not be aware of it. After being in balance for a few weeks, your baby will get bigger and hungrier, need more, and demand to nurse more often.

Your breasts respond to your baby's more frequent suckling first by generating more breastmilk-making anatomy, later by making more breastmilk. After a couple of days of frequent nursing you and your baby are back in balance—for a while.

You will make more when your baby needs more

Even if your baby eats a lot, your breastmilk supply will match their needs. Twins can be successfully breastfed, as can triplets: the main deterrent is time, not breastmilk supply. In seventeenth century France, wet nurses were allowed to nurse up to six infants at one time, and foundling homes provided wet nurses for every three to six infants![12] Your baby may have hungry days at fairly predictable times, such as at seven to ten days of age, five to six weeks, and three months. Or not. Some babies have a hungry day every week and others seem to press for more food all the time. Emily was one of those pressing-all-the-time babies who gave her mother plenty of stimulation. Ryan was not so hungry, at least at first, so he wasn't as helpful to his mother in keeping up her breastmilk supply. It was good his grandmother identified his early too-sleepy patterns. If Martha's breasts had been under-stimulated much longer her production might not have recovered.

Hungry days

Hungry days are likely to be tough, tiring days. Your baby will be wakeful, hungry, and dissatisfied and you will seemingly do nothing but nurse. You may even ask yourself why you don't just give a bottle! Those hungry days have a developmental as well as a nutritional function. Often after hungry days, parents say their babies have increased their calm awake times. It helps to get through those tough days by making nursing, eating, and resting your main focus. Pretend you are snowed in and have to cancel your appointments.

Giving a formula bottle is tempting but it doesn't help with breastfeeding because your satisfied baby won't stimulate your breasts. Your milk supply will fall behind, and you will be stuck with giving a bottle. The next time your baby has hungry days, you will add more bottles. Some people with cooperative babies successfully supplement breastfeeding with formula feeding. For others, it is a miserable pattern because you feed and doubt, feed and doubt. If routinely supplementing with bottle-feeding goes on too long, a baby can start preferring the bottle and breastfeeding will be over. It doesn't have to happen that way, but you do have to know what you are doing and hang in there on those hungry days. Or not. You will be braver if you give yourself an out.

You do not *have to* breastfeed. Reread Chapter 6, Your Feeding Decision: Breastfeeding or Formula-Feeding, and decide again.

Relief bottles

On the other hand, a relief bottle or two can be helpful if you get too worn out or too far behind your baby's needs. It's a balance: A baby needs to be hungry enough to nurse well, but if they are too hungry, it can make them more sleepy and not as energetic about nursing. In general, properly using relief bottles requires phasing them out as soon as possible. Oral rehydration fluids, glucose water, or sterile water are not good substitutes for formula because they don't give enough calories.

Pumping—artificially removing milk from your breasts with your fingers or a machine—only helps with hungry days if the issue is your baby's inability to suckle. For such a baby, pumping your breastmilk and giving it to them via soft medicine cup, bottle, or feeding tube will preserve your breastmilk supply. However, pumping won't help if the issue is that your baby's hunger has gotten ahead of your breastmilk supply. Your baby's suckling is far more efficient at removing milk from your breasts and stimulating you to make more. Pumping in addition to frequent nursing may stimulate you to make more milk than your baby needs or it may not. The amount produced varies from person to person. Studies show that infants regulate the amount they eat based on how much they need, even if their mothers produce more because of pumping.[11]

You may need more or less breast stimulation than another woman, and your baby may be hungrier or not as hungry as another baby. My boys often had hungry days, grew like little weeds, and I hung in there despite entertaining fantasies of how life would be easier if I formula-fed them. For months, I carried my eager-eating boys around in a backpack as I went about my day. Charlotte Wright, a Scottish professor of medicine who does wonderful studies of children's eating and growth, helped me understand my experience. Dr. Wright found that mothers of taller, heavier, enthusiastically eating babies tended to stop breastfeeding earlier. Way too many people who don't understand normal child growth warn that such babies will be "obese" as adults. Dr. Wright isn't one of them. Her study found that those eager-eating babies were taller and heavier but not fatter than slower-growing, moderately eating babies.[13]

Depending on both breast- and bottle-feeding

Once you get past the early period when you are establishing your breastfeeding, you may find that you and your baby have more flexibility with respect to bottle-feeding. Some babies willingly nurse from both breast and bottle and happily eat either expressed breastmilk or formula. Using both breast- and bottle-feeding is more likely to be successful when bottle-feeding is done at predictable times, say at night or during the workday. The pattern to avoid is routinely giving the bottle after feedings because you doubt whether you produce enough breastmilk. In that case, it is better to use a supplemental nursing system.

Some fathers do the night feedings and take care of the bottles. You will come up with your own ways of working together to feed your baby.

A feeding pattern or snacking?

Feeding frequency is a highly individual matter that can only be determined by mother and baby. Breastfeeding babies typically eat about every two hours, but don't count on it. Ryan was naturally regular in his habits, and he and his parents fell into a fairly predictable and frequent feeding and sleeping pattern. But even Ryan could be unpredictable. He caught up in the morning after his longer night sleeping stretches by cluster-feeding. He ate twice or even three times in as many hours, then he went a longer stretch before he ate again. Emily's pattern was also typical, even if it was harder to live with. She was irregular, demanding, and dissatisfied, and in the early weeks she needed to nurse 12 or more times a day. That is tiring, especially when you combine it with all the other new-baby care. I once calculated that, on the smoother days, the feeding, changing, washing, cleaning, caring, and adoring of a new baby takes about six hours.

While frequent feeding is just fine, you may not want to let your baby get into a snacking pattern. That is when they seemingly ask to eat, take a few swallows, then fall asleep or lose interest. Or you may have been advised to "switch nurse," switch back and forth between breasts at each feeding, presumably to build your milk supply. Not a good strategy. Nursing briefly, your baby gets only the rapidly digested low-fat fore milk and not the more lasting, higher-fat hind milk and will soon want to eat again. Consistently getting too little fat and too much protein and milk sugar can also cause diarrhea and growth faltering.

Avoid a snacking pattern by reading and understanding your baby's sleep cycles and feeding when they are wide awake and calm. Review the Chapter 7 section, "Pay attention to your baby's sleep cycles." Martha and Robert kept their nerve and resisted bad advice by letting Ryan flail around during light sleep and waiting to get him up until he was truly ready to wake up. Then they gently moved him around and talked with him to help him stay calm and awake while he ate.

On the other hand, with respect to snacking, Mother Nature may be ahead of us. In cultures where mothers keep their babies with them constantly and use a frequent feeding pattern with short intervals between feedings, it appears that breastmilk has consistently higher fat concentrations.[14] The bottom line? It is up to you and your baby whether an around-the-clock frequent-eating pattern works for you.

Consider the length of feedings

Nurse long enough to empty your breast, but not so long that it wears you out. A newborn feeding can take an hour by the time you feed, burp, change, and play. Most of that has to do with inexperience and need for contact with your baby rather than with your baby's need for nursing. A hungry, vigorously sucking baby can get much of what the breast has to offer at any one time in four to five minutes, most of it in seven to ten. After that, it's just a trickle. Most babies will stop eating at that point, others will keep going.

Letting your baby actively nurse for 15 minutes on each side is more than long enough, although if you like letting your baby suckle longer, that's fine. If you don't enjoy prolonged suckling, and if your baby continues to have a strong sucking need, it is okay to use a pacifier. Wait until your baby is about six weeks old when your breastfeeding is well-established, then offer the pacifier but don't insist on it. Don't put honey on the pacifier because it could give your baby botulism, a type of food poisoning. Studies in Brazil, where the pacifier is standard equipment for every baby, indicate that pacifiers interfere with breastfeeding only when babies are pressured strongly to take them.[15]

To hold down on feeding times, don't overdo the ritual that goes along with feeding. Elaborate hand and nipple washing can wear you out. At night, consider using overnight diapers to cut down on the amount of fussing that goes along with feeding time. The less commotion that goes along with night feedings, the more likely your baby will go sweetly right back to sleep—and you, as well. By the way, keeping track of your baby's pees is more difficult with the highly absorbent overnight diapers.

By the time your baby is around six months old, feeding length will have decreased considerably and intervals between feedings increase. Older babies nurse fast and get on with what they were doing. They come off the breast to investigate any distraction, or, worse yet, try to look around without letting go! Because older babies can empty a breast in five minutes or less, their mothers worry that they are not getting enough to eat. Mothers also miss the long, quiet, intimate feedings. But those older babies maintain and even increase milk supply on fewer feedings and benefit from even brief intimacy.

KNOWING YOUR BABY IS GETTING ENOUGH

Rely on indirect evidence to know that your baby is getting enough to eat. That would be pees, poops, and growth.

Keep track of pees and poops

You won't always be so tuned-in to your baby's pees and poops! Expect every diaper to be wet and even contain a little poop. Once breastmilk comes in, a newly breastfed baby will likely have a bowel movement—a small amount of yellowish stain—in almost every diaper. Stools may be entirely liquid or soft, curdled, or seedy, like yellow cottage cheese. Early poops are the dark brown or greenish-black, sticky meconium that was in your baby's intestine before they were born. Colostrum appears to have a laxative effect, which helps the intestine start to work and expel the meconium. At times stools are an alarming green color that is of no consequence. Yellow or green, your baby's stools will have a sweet or cheesy odor.

Until you are comfortable that breastfeeding is on track, look for six to eight or more wet diapers a day. Remaining properly hydrated is particularly important for a newborn. Human milk composition is exactly right for your baby—it has the right amount of water, protein, sodium, and potassium. As a consequence, your breastfed baby's urine won't be very yellow.

Your baby may pass stools with no apparent effort, or may become preoccupied, stiffen, and turn red in the face. They may stop eating to fuss and grunt and not be able to continue until the job is done or even until their diaper is changed. Some babies don't like messy pants and will fuss and seem uncomfortable; others don't seem to notice. Breastfed babies usually don't get sore in the diaper area, particularly if you change a messy diaper promptly and clean your baby's bottom thoroughly. Cover any reddened areas with an ointment that stays on. My favorite is zinc oxide.

Evaluate your baby's growth

Your baby's weight pattern also indicates whether all is well. Review the Chapter 4 discussion, "Weight for age charts," page 104. Your baby knows how much to eat and how to grow. Fullterm, breastfed babies generally lose about five to seven percent of their body weight within two to four days after birth, and most regain to their birth weight by nine days of age. Formula-fed babies don't lose as much and regain faster.[16]

After that, your breastfed baby is growing well when their weight plots consistently on a particular percentile curve. For the first three months, breastfed babies grow at about the same rate or somewhat faster than formula-fed babies. After age three months, breastfed babies grow in length at about the same rate as formula-fed babies but gain weight at a somewhat slower rate. They drop by as much as one percentile grid line (say from the 50th to the 25th percentile) between 3 and 12 months.[17] That decrease in percentile is okay as long as it is smooth and slow.

Accept consistent growth

Guard against unconsciously trying to get your big baby to eat less or your small baby to eat more—and encouragement from others to do it. Some babies are very small and plot consistently at the lower end of the percentile curves. Your baby is doing well if they are alert, bright, developing normally, and have six or eight wet diapers a day, many of them with poops. On the other hand, contact your doctor and do problem-solving if your slowly growing baby has few wet diapers, their urine smells strong, and they don't have many poops. A too-slowly growing baby is apathetic, cries weakly, and has poor muscle tone.

Babies who are unusually large and plot at the upper end of the percentile curves are growing normally as long as they plot consistently on their growth percentile. Ignore health-policy-based judgments that a child growing at the 85th or 95th percentile weight-for-height is "overweight" or "obese." Read the Chapter 4 section, "Avoid applying BMI cutoffs," page 103. As preschoolers, 15 percent of relatively large babies reach BMIs at or above the 85th percentile,[18] which is to be expected statistically. Those who have an exaggerated concern about child "obesity" consider large babies staying large to be a serious problem. I consider it to be normal growth. Children come in a variety of sizes and shapes, and those sizes and shapes change as they get older. Remember Charlotte Wright's work: Big, fast-growing babies grow up to be taller and heavier but not fatter children.[13]

Do problem-solving with rapidly diverging weight

Whether a baby plots high or low on the weight percentiles, their weight can slowly and smoothly diverge up from their usual curve. That is more than likely to be a normal shift. However, flattening growth or rapidly abruptly and rapidly falling-off or climbing-up weight is a cause for concern that you need to address with your health professional. Do problem-solving with breastfeeding by taking particular care to follow sDOR. Understand your baby's sleep cycles (Figure 7.1), read their feeding cues (Figure 7.2), keep them in control of feeding (Figure 7.3), and support them in going to sleep (Figure 7.4). Keep records of your baby's pees and poops. Record a video and observe yourself: You may be interfering without realizing it. Ask an experienced person to observe a breastfeeding, looking for whether your baby is calm and wide awake, properly attached and suckling well, and shows sounds and signs of drawing in milk. Do not under any circumstances try to get your baby to eat more or less. Your baby will eat and grow well when your feeding relationship is good.

ALLOW FOR INDIVIDUAL DIFFERENCES

Much of individual difference in feeding has to do with the infant personality characteristics discussed in the Chapter 7 section, "Consider personality and temperament." Feeding an active baby with inconsistent eating and sleeping patterns is quite different from feeding a placid baby who is regular in their habits. Your baby's temperament determines whether they are relaxed and easy to understand and please or touchy and difficult to figure out. With an uptight baby, be persistent in following sDOR with all that entails as discussed in the Chapter 7 section, "Feed the way your baby tells you." It is difficult to persist with tuned-in and accepting feeding when your baby doesn't respond to your good care, but eventually what you are doing will work. Casting about for other solutions, trying this and that, will make matters worse.

Your baby may enjoy eating, eat fast or slowly, get full abruptly, or slowly drift off from nursing. The Chapter 3 section, "It's okay to love to eat," page 76, points out that these are normal variations in eating attitudes and behaviors and that those variations are entertaining and lovely. The problem is parents' and health professionals' entirely understandable tendency to react to children's extremes by trying to tone them down. Such toning down throws away trust in the baby to do their part with eating. The same thing can happen with the exceptionally large or small child or the one who eats an exceptionally large or small amount. Be aware of that tendency in yourself, resist it, and devote yourself to following your baby's lead with feeding. Interfering will make both you and your baby miserable and create the very issues you are trying to prevent.

The I-want-to-eat-all-the-time baby

It is hard to sort out what a fussy, irregular baby's signals mean. Do they want to eat? Do they want to be held and comforted? Are they overstimulated—having trouble being calm and alert? Do they want to go back to bed? Sort it out as best you can. If you aren't sure, it doesn't hurt to feed: Your baby will let you know soon enough that they aren't interested. The pattern to avoid is feeding to fix everything. Help your baby sort themself out by feeding when they are wide awake and calm. Pay attention to their sleep cycles (Figure 4.3) so they are truly waking-up-and-drowsy when you pick them up, then handle them slowly and quietly. Don't try to feed them when they are in deep or light sleep: It will make them eat poorly and be fussy. During feeding, follow feeding cues as best you can.

The too-sleepy baby

Too-sleepy babies sleep relatively long stretches, have trouble staying awake during feedings, and may show too few pees and poops. Not all babies who sleep a lot are too-sleepy babies. Relaxed babies with regular habits may sleep for three hours or more at a stretch and then wake up to eat well. The tactics for helping always-hungry and colicky babies be calm and wide awake also help the too-sleepy baby. When they fuss a bit and/or keep their eyes open, pick your baby up, talk, and move around. Vary your tone of voice and your speed of talking to find out what your baby responds to by being calm and wide awake. Change diapers and give your baby something to look at.

Don't overstimulate your baby by talking loudly, tickling, or jiggling. You are trying to help your baby take an interest, not upset them. Feed promptly when your baby shows "I'm hungry" signs. During feeding, experiment with talking, holding, and stroking in ways your baby responds to by staying awake and being relaxed. After feeding, maintain contact to gently support your too-sleepy baby's awake-and-calm time. Keep your baby with you in your arms, in a sling, or in an infant seat as you move around the house. Talk, look at stuff together. Put your baby down for a nap when they get drowsy.

The colicky baby

Babies cry a lot. The Chapter 7 section, "More about crying" tells you more than I hope you will need to know. Colic is the newborn pattern of unexplained inconsolable crying, fussing, and appearing to be in pain for part or in some cases much of waking time. Colic afflicts up to 25 percent of babies under age three months. Colicky babies apparently have nothing medically wrong with them, but they are not to be comforted, seemingly no matter what you do. The best guess is that colic is the result of a newborn's immature nervous or digestive system, and most babies outgrow the pattern by the time they are 3 to 4 months old. You do, however, need help from your doctor to diagnose your child's condition if your baby forcefully vomits rather than just spitting up, regularly seems to be in pain after eating, or if their growth falters.

Of course, you will try to soothe your baby, and good for you. Do the best you can as long as you can. Follow the advice in Chapter 7, "Feed the way your baby tells you." Pay attention to your baby's sleep cycles and feed when they are calm and wide awake. Read your baby's feeding cues; feed when they are hungry and stop when they are full. Keep your baby in control of feeding by calming them, feeding smoothly and continuously, and following their feeding cues. Support your baby in going to sleep by reading their drowsy cues and giving them a little help if they need it. Keep in mind that the overstimulated infant can act like they have colic, so be careful not to be so active that you contribute to the problem.

All your best efforts may not help at first and may not help for quite a while. After you have done all you can, put your baby to bed in a safe place, walk away, and let them cry it out. While it seems hard-hearted, the alternatives are worse: resenting your baby and being hurtful and critical with yourself and your spouse. Be reassured: This won't go on forever.

The baby with a cold or the flu

Infants with common diseases such as fever, upper respiratory infection, colds, diarrhea, or even chicken pox do best with continued breastfeeding. Babies with breathing problems seem to do better with breastfeeding than nursing from a bottle; they certainly do not do worse. Human milk isn't as concentrated in protein and electrolytes (sodium and potassium) so it isn't as dehydrating as formula. In fact, diarrhea and intestinal tract disease are less common in breastfed infants than in bottle-fed infants. Avoid abrupt weaning from the breast as that adds the trauma of weaning to the trauma of illness. Abrupt weaning could make your baby so listless they eat poorly, and you won't be able to tell whether the cause is the illness or the loss of breastfeeding.[12]

The baby who reacts to what you eat

Traces of what you eat show up in your breastmilk, although at levels too low to trigger allergic reactions in most babies.[19] Your breastmilk might taste like onion or garlic and your baby likely won't mind. In fact, breastfed babies appear to be more willing to accept solid foods when the time comes to introduce them, presumably because they already are familiar with flavors. Do, however, be careful not to eat too many prunes, plums, or other laxative fruits, as those could have the same effect on your baby.

Some unusual babies seem to get fussy, have symptoms of food sensitivity, or even seem to have allergic reactions when their mothers eat certain foods. It is hard to sort out a true reaction from coincidence, since all babies are at times fussy, spit up, are congested, or appear colicky. Generally, time is the only cure, but if you have a markedly fussy or colicky baby, it is worth a try to see if your food could be causing it. Your baby could have an immature or a particularly sensitive gastrointestinal tract and might do better if you kept your diet a little less challenging. Try removing the suspected food from your diet for a few days and see if symptoms disappear.

Mild to moderate reactions are quite different from those of a small percentage of exclusively breastfed infants who show frank allergy symptoms. Babies with allergies eat and grow poorly, develop eczema, or have stomach and intestinal symptoms such as vomiting with force (as opposed to spitting up), diarrhea, or have difficulty passing stools. The abdomen can be bloated and hard. Not surprisingly, they sleep poorly, are lethargic (you would be worn out too if you were hungry, itchy, and had a stomachache) and grow slowly. They can have crying episodes that last for hours.[20] Those symptoms can be a sign of a medical problem, and your doctor will evaluate your baby to be sure that is not the case as well as help you address your baby's allergies. Since your child's food allergies is likely to be an ongoing feeding issue, start now to establish a relationship with an sDOR-committed dietitian specializing in food allergies.

To continue breastfeeding, mothers of these highly allergic infants have to follow restricted diets. Whether or not it is necessary to wean such a highly allergic infant from the breast to a hypoallergenic formula depends on whether the mother can meet her own nutritional needs on that restricted diet.[20] For a discussion of hypoallergenic formulas, see the Chapter 9 section, "Specialized formulas," page 285. Talk with your pediatrician or dietitian about choosing a formula.

The vulnerable baby

The Chapter 7 sections, "Vulnerable babies; controlling advice," and "Babies who require tube-feeding," discuss feeding challenges on a whole different level. Vulnerable babies are capable of eating as much as they need; babies with certain medical conditions are almost always able to eat, but not as much as they need and may need help from being tube-fed, either with breastmilk or formula. Babies in both groups give feeding signs and, the same as with all other babies, it's about trusting your baby to eat to the best of their ability. Growing out of that trust, do what you do with other babies. Observe their sleep states and feed when they are calm and awake. Guide feeding based on information coming from them, being careful not to be controlling.

BREAST ISSUES

I hope you don't encounter any of these issues, but you need to know what to do to keep them from becoming problems. For instance, catching a plugged duct early and knowing what to do about it can prevent a breast infection. Breast issues are not a sign that breastfeeding is going poorly, but rather a common part of the process that you can hope to more or less take in stride as you work out your system.

Flat or inverted nipples

Adhesions in the breast tissue can make your nipple lay flat or dimple in when it is squeezed or stimulated rather than becoming erect. One or both nipples may be flat or inverted. Pregnancy or a baby with a strong suck can bring nipples out. These strategies might also help.

- Let your baby nurse promptly after birth.
- Flatten your areola between your thumb and forefinger, pressing in against your chest wall to help your nipple protrude.
- Hand-express a little milk just before you start to nurse to soften your breasts and make it easier for your baby to latch on.
- Use a breast pump just before you nurse—the suction will pull out your nipples and soften your breasts so your baby can latch on.
- Do a web search for a device to make nipples protrude. One of these gadgets might help.
- If your baby hasn't latched on by the time your milk comes in, begin bottle-feeding using expressed milk.
- Continue to offer your baby the breast when they are calm and your breasts are soft.

Being persistent in addressing flat or inverted nipples can be frustrating, time-consuming, and difficult, so seek help and support. One day your baby may suddenly latch on.

Engorgement

When your milk comes in, your breasts will get larger and fuller and may feel firmer. Engorgement goes beyond that. Engorged breasts can last for two to three days after your milk comes and are hot, heavy, hard, and painful. Nursing often helps to prevent engorgement. Let your baby nurse 20 minutes or more on the first breast and finish off with the second breast; use a breast pump if you are uncomfortable. Be sure to nurse at night even if the nursing staff offers to let you sleep, keep track of which breast you start on, and alternate breasts. Don't use a pacifier.

Use cold packs on your breasts between feedings and avoid putting heat on your breasts. Your nipples will be stretched flat by the engorgement, so help your baby latch on by hand-expressing some milk to soften your breast just before you feed, then compress the areola between your thumb and forefinger.

Some people swear by cabbage leaves. We are crossing into the realm of folk medicine, but if you are engorged, you will be happy to have something to try. Get a large head of cabbage, discard the dry, roughed-up outer leaves and remove two large inner leaves. Wash, pat dry, remove the center vein (for comfort) and crush slightly. Put a leaf inside each bra cup covering each breast. Reportedly, you will feel immediate relief. Keep changing the leaves every hour or so when they (the leaves) become limp and wilted. As soon as your breast softens and your milk begins to drip, breastfeed or pump. Although your breasts may still feel full, if your milk is flowing and your baby can latch on, you will be cured. Stop the cabbage—continual use is also a folk remedy for drying up the breasts.

If you don't get relief from self-help, get in touch with a lactation counselor.

Leaking breasts

Some breasts leak more than others, and some mothers are more annoyed and embarrassed by it than others. Firm pressure against your nipples may stop leaking. Fold your arms across your breasts and press firmly toward the chest wall or press with your thumbs and forefingers directly on the nipple. Protect your clothing by using absorbent pads or plastic bra liners. Absorbent pads keep your breasts drier, but either can hold moisture on your skin and cause irritation.

Sore nipples

Your baby puts most stress on your nipple at the corners of their mouth and where they stroke with their tongue. Be sure your baby is properly latched on. Shift the stress points by changing your nursing position—sit, lie down, use the football or Australian hold. For chafed or cracked nipples, use cool compresses after nursing and leave your bra and shirt open to expose your nipples to the air. Use your own milk as a lubricant.

Narrowed ducts

Narrowed ducts make breastmilk flow less freely. You experience the condition as a hard and tender area in your breast. Address it with heat and massage. With water from a hot shower flowing over your breast, massage from well behind the tender area toward the nipple. Try to time your shower so your baby will be hungry soon after. Massage the affected area while nursing. Hot compresses with nursing or pumping may also help.

Breast infection

A breast infection—mastitis—begins with a narrowed duct and is reddened as well as hard and tender. You feel like you have the flu: elevated temperature, aching all over, and worn out. See your gynecologist. They may or may not prescribe antibiotics. You can take acetaminophen or ibuprofen, but not aspirin. Rest as much as you can—your body needs help to fight off the infection.

You don't have to wean. Even if you are taking antibiotics, your baby won't get that much. The infection will go away faster if you keep the milk moving and keep emptying your breast. The trend is to avoid antibiotics and use the same strategy for a breast infection as for a narrowed duct. If you choose this approach, keep in touch with your doctor and expect to be better within 24 hours. You don't want to develop a breast abscess.

About 30 percent of breastfeeders get an infection during the first six weeks of nursing.[5] Causes seem to be not emptying breasts regularly, too-tight clothing, and too much fatigue and stress. Or nothing at all. I once got a breast infection that probably started with a narrowed duct, but since I was new to breastfeeding, I didn't notice it. My doctor advised me not to nurse while I was on antibiotics, but I found other advice I liked better (not always a wise idea) and continued nursing. It wasn't easy to go my own way because I worried about hurting my baby, but I'm glad I did.

Breast abscess

An untreated breast infection, especially if the breast isn't being emptied, may turn into a breast abscess. This is unusual but serious. It is a pronounced infection in a local area of the breast, accompanied by flu-like symptoms and a small, clearly defined, red, hot, painful area. Treatment is surgical drainage, similar to opening a boil. You can continue to breastfeed as long as your baby's mouth doesn't come in contact with drainage from the abscess.[5]

SUPPLEMENTS FOR BABIES

At birth, babies are at risk of bleeding because they have very little vitamin K in their bodies. As a consequence, it is critical for them to get vitamin K1 by injection soon after they are born. Your pediatrician will attend to that.

If you eat well, or even if you don't, your breastmilk will have ample vitamins and minerals, with the exception of vitamin D. Current trends for covering up with sunscreen or clothing keep children and grown-ups from making vitamin D with their skin. The American Academy of Pediatrics recommends supplements for all babies, children, and adolescents of 400 IU per day. An alternative strategy is to supplement the mother with 6,400 IU of vitamin D per day.[5] The increase from the previous recommendation of 200 IU per day is based on claims that high levels of vitamin D maintain innate immunity and prevent diseases such as diabetes and cancer. Those claims have not held up under further study. Don't give your baby or child more than 400 IU per day. Too much vitamin D can be toxic.

Iron is a debated-about supplemental nutrient. Regardless of maternal iron status, term newborns need little dietary iron because they get it from breaking down the extra red blood cells they were born with. Prematurely born babies, however, don't have the iron from extra blood cells and need to be supplemented from age two months. Although iron is in low concentrations, human milk provides protection against iron deficiency anemia for term babies during the first six months. Iron in human milk is about 70 percent absorbed, which is a relatively high rate. Furthermore, human-milk iron is carried in the form of *lactoferrin*, which prevents the growth of undesirable intestinal bacteria. Breastfed babies owe their sweet-smelling stools and likely resistance to intestinal upsets to a predominance of *lactobacillus bifidus*. Supplemental iron, on the other hand, nourishes undesirable intestinal bacteria as well as changes the type of intestinal bacteria. With greater access to iron, intestinal *Escherichia coli* grow more, make stools smelly, and increase babies' vulnerability to intestinal infections.

Fluoride supplementation is delayed for all infants until after six months of age. While fluoride is critical for dental health, too much can cause fluorosis, white mottling of the tooth enamel—or even colored mottling in extreme cases. Exclusively mixing infant formula with fluoridated water for a fully formula-fed baby can cause mild fluorosis.

GIVING YOUR BABY A BOTTLE

Whether you put breastmilk or formula into a bottle, attend to the feeding relationship as carefully as you do with breastfeeding. Human milk does not compensate for errors in feeding. Bottle-feeding lends itself to being controlling so you have to be particularly careful to follow your baby's feeding cues and avoid trying to get your baby to empty a bottle or eat certain amounts. Difficult as it is, be prepared to waste breastmilk. The Chapter 3 section, "Get comfortable with not knowing," page 79, addresses just that: You can't know how much your child *should* eat, and if you try, you are being controlling.

If you choose to use formula for a relief bottle, read the Chapter 9 section, "Infant formula," page 274.

Breastfeeding in your absence

Once your breastmilk is well established, you can continue to breastfeed fully or partially if your life takes you away from your baby for longer intervals. Your baby may have other ideas. Take a wait-and-see attitude, be prepared to adjust, and be honest with yourself: Is your approach to breastfeeding during your absences rewarding for you? Is it decreasing your stress level—or increasing it? Whatever happens, the pleasure, rewards, and contributions your breastfeeding has made until now remain.

Pumping every two or three hours or at the same intervals as you ordinarily breastfeed will keep up your breastmilk supply so you can breastfeed on days when you are with your baby. Even if you pump and have your child care provider give bottles during the day, you more than likely will have one or two night feedings. In fact, your older baby could have such a preference for nursing from the breast that they refuse bottles during the day and wait to eat until you get home. You may welcome night feedings as a way of squeezing in time with your baby—or you may not. Make night feedings easier by keeping them quiet and dimly lit and putting both of you back to bed drowsy. Some babies get by on solid foods during the day, but don't rush your baby into solid foods to prolong your breastfeeding.

Here is a little-known factoid: There is some evidence that breastmilk produced at night helps babies sleep and that breastmilk produced during the day helps them stay awake. If that is indeed the case, it could be good to keep the two separate and feed day breastmilk during the day, night breastmilk at night.[21] On the other hand, that may just be too complicated!

Teaching your baby to take a bottle

By the time your baby is four to six weeks old, it is safe to teach them to take a bottle, if you wish. Breastmilk supply and let-down will be well established, and your baby will be good at suckling. Fathers are likely to be most successful with the bottle project. Your baby knows their mother and expects to be breastfed; doing otherwise could be upsetting for them.

Bottle-feeding may be successful in the breastfeeding position, with your baby close to your face and their head, neck, shoulders straight. Or not. A colleague said that the breastfeeding position upset his sons, presumably because what he had to offer did not meet their expectations! He and each of his boys had better success when he propped them up in the crook of his thigh and he fed looking straight at them. Whatever works, do the feeding yourself. Except for rare occasions, don't pass your baby around to others to be bottle-fed. Your baby is most comfortable with you—you know them best and you can read their signals.

A baby's whole world is focused on their mouth. Changing from breast- to bottle-feeding is huge for them, especially if the bottle contains formula, which tastes different from human milk. Practice when your baby is a little hungry but not famished. Being too hungry will make them desperate to eat and not willing to experiment. Stow any ideas about how you want your baby to eat and take it slowly and gently. Your baby needs time and repeated unpressured exposure to gradually get used to the feeling of the silicone or rubber nipple in their mouth, learn to suck and swallow in a different way, and catch on to the fact that the stuff coming out of the nipple is food.

Break it down into simple steps. Brush your baby's lips and wait for them to open up before you put the nipple in their mouth. Follow their lead: At first, they will spit the nipple out; later, they will leave it there. After a number of repeats, your baby will comfortably accept the nipple and let it be in their mouth. Plan on a few more sessions for them to figure out how to suckle and take a bit of breastmilk or formula: Putting drops of formula or breastmilk on the nipple helps. Plan to have still more sessions before they take enough to constitute a feeding. Trying to make this process go faster will make it go slower. Eventually your baby will get so they can take a bottle, even if they don't enjoy it as much as breastfeeding.

Some people swear by one type of nipple, others another. Some brands claim to mimic the shape of the extended nipple and areola. More importantly, pick out a nipple and stick with it. If you use formula, choose one and stick with it. Changing nipples or formula makes the process all new to your baby and they have to learn all over again.

Pumping breastmilk

Breast pumps remove milk from your breast with suction. Start experimenting with equipment and learning to express and store breastmilk several weeks before you need it. You may be comfortable with expressing breastmilk, or you may not. You may be able to get a significant amount of breastmilk when you express, or you may not. Some mothers can get eight ounces of breastmilk at a time, most express a couple of ounces. Some mothers use wearable breastmilk collectors. Some pump for the occasional relief bottle. Some pump exclusively and bottle-feed their baby expressed breastmilk. Most are somewhere in between. To pump exclusively, keep up your breastmilk supply by pumping as often as your baby normally breastfeeds, more often during their hungry days.

With respect to equipment, practices are changing so rapidly that it is best to check with a lactation counselor or support group. Here are some issues to consider. Some people purchase breast pumps, others rent and purchase their own fittings (the hoses and valves, flanges that go on the breasts and bottles for catching the milk). You may need to be measured for the correct flange fitting. Also consider purchasing multiple sets of flanges to help with washing up. For occasional use, you can experiment with a smaller mechanical breast pump, try the hand-operated piston, or remove milk from your breasts with hand expression. For any method, start with breast massage. Wash your hands, then stroke from the outside edge of the breast toward the nipple, applying gentle but firm pressure with the palms of your hands. Alternate your hands as you work around your breast, stroking from the shoulder down, the side in, the waist up, and the breastbone in. Massage around each breast several times before you start pumping.

At first plan to express three to five minutes on each breast. Later you can work up to ten to fifteen minutes. Your milk will first come out in small spurts, may flow freely, or may come out in starts and stops. Don't worry if nothing comes out the first few times you try. You may find that briefly repeating the massage helps to work the milk down. You may also find it helpful to switch from one breast to another because the second breast will let down milk in response to stimulus to the first.

Using water or a few drops of breastmilk, moisten the funnelshaped flange of the breast pump and place it over your breast. Let your nipple slide along the inside of the top part of the flange until it lines up with the opening in the center if the flange. Sliding helps stimulate the let-down reflex; moistening lets the flange make a better seal with your breast. Hold the flange just tightly enough against your breast to make a good seal, but not so tightly that it digs into your breast and pinches off the milk flow. Stop pumping one minute after the milk has slowed and break the seal by pressing your finger between your breast and the flange. After each use, thoroughly wash all parts of the collecting apparatus that comes in contact with the milk. Rinse thoroughly and allow to air dry.

To hand express, lean over a sterile container for catching the milk, place your thumb and index finger on your areola about an inch back from your nipple, right over the lactiferous sinuses. As you press inward toward your chest wall, squeeze your thumb and forefinger gently together. The repeated motion is to push back and squeeze, push back and squeeze. Keep your thumb and finger in the same position until no more milk comes out, then rotate to another position and repeat.

Storing breastmilk

Human milk spoils easily and must be promptly packaged and stored. Do a web search for *CDC breastmilk storage*. Microwaving is not recommended but if you do, follow the directions in Figure 9.1, "Safe microwaving," page 274. Discard any unused breastmilk after the feeding.

I feel more comfortable with prompter and shorter storage times than those recommended by CDC. For recommendations on safe milk handling, I talked with Robert Bradley, PhD, at the University of Wisconsin Food Science department. Based on considerable research on freezing milks of all kinds, Bradley recommends keeping unfrozen human milk in the refrigerator for no more than 24 hours and frozen human milk at 0 degrees Fahrenheit or lower for no longer than 45 days. Freeze human milk for storage right after you collect it. Dr. Bradley says you can freeze small amounts as you go along and combine them in the same container, as long as the quantity you add (the justcollected, liquid milk) isn't greater than the amount that is already frozen. Putting too much liquid milk in with the frozen milk thaws it, impairs the quality, and even lets bacteria grow.

Human milk is raw milk and contains many active enzymes that function even at freezer temperatures. The fat in human milk may separate and even cling to the side of the container, but when the milk is warmed and swirled about it mixes in. Protein clumps with freezing and may plug the nipple, although the human milk is as nutritious as ever for your baby.

CHECKLIST FOR SUCCESSFUL BREASTFEEDING

Here, as promised, is Figure 8.5.

FIGURE 8.5: MANY PEOPLE CONTRIBUTE TO SUCCESSFUL BREASTFEEDING

As you review the list below, you may be surprised at how many people support you and your baby. That is positive for us all. We all benefit from helping to raise children.	
Mother Is healthy; has nipples baby can suckle Eats well enough and gets pretty good rest Is as relaxed and positive as possible Maintains sDOR Understands supply and demand Accepts help and support Minimizes alcohol and smoking Avoids street drugs	**Baby** Neurological and medical conditions allow breastfeeding Can wake up and stay awake to eat Can suckle
Extended family Emotional support: listening, encouraging Social support: accepting, encouraging Situational support: housekeeping, running errands Parenting support: observing baby, feedings Providing a calming presence	**Workplace** Allows leave time Gives breaks for breastfeeding or expressing Provides privacy for breastfeeding or expressing Provides cold storage for expressed breastmilk Provides close-in parking places for new parents
Child care Follows sDOR Has procedures that support breastfeeding Has a private place for nursing	

Health care providers	
Before the baby comes	**At the hospital/birthing center**
Discusses particular concerns about breastfeeding Addresses breastfeeding pros and cons Physically assesses breasts and nipples Teaches sDOR	Appropriately manages anesthesia during labor Has breastfeeding-friendly policies and procedures Has knowledgeable and skillful staff
Following discharge	
Recommends follow-up visit early after discharge Provides support for problem-solving	

ENJOY YOUR ADVENTURE

Maintain a positive and flexible attitude. Keep in mind that any amount of breastfeeding is a success. It is all a grand experiment. Do your thinking, planning, and providing to set yourself up as well as you can to breastfeed. Then let go of it. You can't control the outcome. Given your particular physiology, circumstances, and baby, you may or may not be able to fully breastfeed your baby. The bottom line is feeding your baby in a way that you both enjoy and that supports your baby's growth and development. Achieving your breastfeeding goals need not contradict that, but if it does, your baby's growth and development comes first. However long or however much you breastfeed your baby, sooner or later you have to stop. That stopping is one of those necessary losses that you will encounter throughout your child's growing-up years. No matter what happens, you are special to your baby, and that won't change.

This has been a long chapter, with lots of detail. Here is a summary of the basic points:

- Enjoy your baby.
- Take care of yourself: eat well, drink enough, rest enough, and avoid getting physically over- stressed.
- Follow sDOR: Go by your baby's cues to feed them when they are hungry, awake, and calm, and let them eat how much, how fast, and how enthusiastically they want.

- Make yourself comfortable to breastfeed and cuddle your baby: Look at them and hold them in good position, talk and touch gently in a way that lets them relax.
- Be sure your baby is properly latched on to your nipple and areola. Know your baby is getting milk from their longer, slower suck-swallow motions and a drawing sound.
- Keep the feeding smooth and steady. Only stop when your baby pauses and rests, then wait and let them go back to eating if they want to.
- Wait to feed until they are fully awake and help them stay awake by looking and talking while they eat. Work toward having your baby stay awake through the whole feeding.
- Enjoy your baby.

REFERENCES

1. Rosen-Carole C. Chestfeeding and lactation care for LGBTQ+ families lesbian gay bisexual transgender queer plus. In: Lawrence RA, Lawrence RM, eds. *Breastfeeding (Ninth Edition)*. Elsevier; 2022:646–650.
2. Abuogi L. Infant feeding for persons living with and at risk for HIV in the United States: clinical report. *Pediatrics*. 2024. doi:10.1542/peds.2024-066843
3. Rempel LA. Relationships between types of father breastfeeding support and breastfeeding outcomes. *Maternal & Child Nutrition*. 2017. doi:*https://doi.org/10.1111/mcn.12337*
4. Feldman-Winter L. National trends in pediatricians' practices and attitudes about breastfeeding: 1995 to 2014. *Pediatrics*. 2017;140. doi:10.1542/peds.2017-1229
5. Meek JY. Policy Statement: breastfeeding and the use of human milk. *Pediatrics*. 2022. doi:10.1542/peds.2022-057988
6. Food & Nutrition Board. *Nutrition During Lactation*. Institute of Nutrition, National Academy Press; 1991.
7. Worthington-Roberts BS. Lactation: Basic considerations. In: Worthington-Roberts BS, Williams SR, eds. *Nutrition in Pregnancy and Lactation*. WCB McGraw-Hill; 1997:316–346.
8. Satter Eating Competence Model (ecSatter): Evidence-based research. *https://www.needscenter.org/resources/satter-eating-competence-model-ecsatter/*
9. Feldman-Winter L. Evidence-based updates on the first week of exclusive breastfeeding among infants ≥35 weeks. *Pediatrics*. 2020;145. doi:10.1542/peds.2018-3696
10. Task Force on Sudden Infant Death Syndrome. SIDS and other sleep-related infant deaths: updated 2016 recommendations for a safe infant sleeping environment. *Pediatrics*. 2016. doi:10.1542/peds.2016-2938
11. Lawrence RM. Normal growth, growth faltering, and obesity in breastfed infants. In: Lawrence RA, Lawrence RM, eds. *Breastfeeding (Ninth Edition)*. Elsevier; 2022:298–325.
12. Lawrence RA. Breastfeeding infants with problems. In: Lawrence RA, Lawrence RM, eds. *Breastfeeding (Ninth Edition)*. Elsevier; 2022:474–514.
13. Wright CM. How does infant behaviour relate to weight gain and adiposity? *Proc Nutr Soc*. 2011;70:485–493.

14. Dettwyler KA. Infant feeding practices and growth. *Annual Review of Anthropology*. 1992;21:171–204.
15. Victoria CG. Pacifier use and short breastfeeding duration: cause, consequence, or coincidence? *Pediatrics*. 1997;99:445–453.
16. P. D. Macdonald PD. Neonatal weight loss in breast and formula fed infants. *Archives of Disease in Childhood - Fetal and Neonatal Edition*. 2003. doi:10.1136/fn.88.6.F472
17. Kramer MS. Feeding effects on growth during infancy. *The Journal of Pediatrics*. 2004;145:600–605.
18. Berkowitz RI. Growth of children at high risk of obesity during the first 6 y of life: implications for prevention. *Am J Clin Nutr*. 2005;81:140–146.
19. Gamirova A. Food proteins in human breast milk and probability of IgE-mediated allergic reaction in children during breastfeeding: a systematic review. *J Allergy Clin Immunol Pract*. 2022;10:1312–1324.e8.
20. Rajani PS. Presentation and management of food allergy in breastfed infants and risks of maternal elimination diets. *J Allergy Clin Immunol Pract*. 2020;8:52–67.
21. Hahn-Holbrook J. Human milk as "chrononutrition": implications for child health and development. *Pediatr Res*. 2019;85:936–942.

CHAPTER 9

Formula-Feeding Your Baby

As I have said before, when I talk about "you" and "your baby," I am thinking of parents of either gender. One of you will likely take primary responsibility for your child, and the other play a supportive role, but not necessarily. However you work it out, you both have a role to play, and you both are responsible for understanding and making decisions about parenting in general and feeding in particular. Formula- or human-milk feeding with a bottle gives you both the opportunity to be mainstays in feeding. You know your baby best, and your baby eats best when you feed them. A person who regularly takes care of your baby makes a good substitute, and once in a while it is okay to let someone else do a feeding. But for the most part, keep feeding to yourselves. Your baby feels most secure and eats most capably with you. You are best at tuning in on what your baby wants and needs.

I wish I had a magic wand to resolve any negative feelings you have about formula-feeding. It is all so unnecessary! Bottle-feeding can be as much about love as breastfeeding. Being successful with bottle-feeding depends on your getting on your baby's wavelength with feeding, sleeping, and crying. Instead of beating yourself up for your feeding choice, get to know and understand your baby and know that—absolutely—you and your bottle-fed baby can have a splendid feeding relationship.

I hope your health care professionals are accepting of your choice as well. The same as you, they want to take good and loving care of your baby, and your formula-feeding with a bottle is part of that good and loving care. Understand where they are coming form: Standards of practice say health professionals have to encourage breastfeeding and they are subjected to a *lot* of breastfeeding promotion.[1]

THE FEEDING RELATIONSHIP

The bottom line is having a good feeding relationship with your baby, and you have chosen the feeding method that will best allow you to have that relationship. Feeding is about loving and respecting, about knowing your baby, doing what is right for them, and being successful with them. Because you and your baby spend most of your early months together with feeding, feeding provides your best opportunity to get to know your baby. Feeding gives your baby powerful messages: I see you; I value you; I respect you; I am willing to go to some trouble to work things out with you. Feeding well satisfies your needs, as well. You need to know you can give your baby what they need to make them happy.

At the same time as I support you in choosing to formula-feed, I trust you to take it the rest of the way to having a positive feeding relationship with your baby. Be forewarned that bottle-feeding lends itself to being controlling—to trying to get your baby to eat certain amounts and/or in a certain way. To guard against being controlling, wait for your baby to open their mouth before you put the nipple in. Feed when your baby wants to eat, not on a schedule; feed as fast or as slowly as your baby wants to eat; feed as much or as little as your baby wants to eat, not to empty the bottle. Sit quietly and feed smoothly: Bottle-feeding parents tend to interrupt the feeding to check the level of formula in the bottle, wipe the baby's mouth, arrange the baby's clothes, and burp the baby.[2] Hold your baby so they relax and seem comfortable. Don't prop the bottle or put your baby down to sleep with a bottle. Don't feed them in an infant seat, even if you hold the bottle for them. Only burp them if they seem full of air. As outlined in the Chapter 7 section, "Routine yes, schedule no," let a routine evolve. Don't try to force a schedule.

This chapter draws from much information in the rest of the book. Pay particular attention to Chapter 7, Understanding Your Newborn, which outlines and elaborates on what you need to know to bottle-feed your baby. The section, "Feed the way your baby tells you" and the figures below are particularly important:

- Figure 7.1: Understand and respond to your baby's sleep cycles.
- Figure 7.2: Read your baby's feeding cues.
- Figure 7.3: Keep your baby in control of feeding.
- Figure 7.4: Support your baby in going to sleep.

Rather than giving page numbers when I refer to materials from Chapter 7, there are so many that I have omitted them in this chapter.

Sections in other chapters are also important and for those I give page numbers. You might also read parts of Chapter 8, Breastfeeding Your Baby. I say the same there about the feeding relationship as I say here, but I say it in different ways and tell different stories.

IN THIS CHAPTER

This is a long chapter, so let me tell you what's here so you can whittle it down to size. The first 20 pages are about getting your ducks in a row before your baby is born. You can think now about taking care of yourself and making ahead-of-time equipment decisions: water, nipples, bottles, bottle warmers. This section helps get you started thinking about choosing infant formulas. I hope you can skip the sections on specialized and emergency formulas, but they are there if you need them.

Then, we get to what I consider the fun part: parenting with feeding. Follow your baby's lead, know how not to get derailed, let your baby determine how much and how often, don't worry about spoiling your baby. You might want to skip ahead and read that section first. It will keep you going while you take care of business with the other information.

Toward the end we discuss challenging babies and babies with diarrhea.

TAKE CARE OF YOURSELF

To take care of your baby, you need to take care of yourself. Feed yourself well, attend to your physical comfort, and address your emotional needs.

Get the meal habit

If all goes well, you will use your getting ready to be a parent to become Eating Competent: To discover the joy of eating, as outlined in Chapter 5. Your eating has everything to do with the way you feed your baby. To trust your baby to know how much to eat and, later on, to trust them to determine what to eat from family meals, you have to trust your own instinctive abilities with eating. Chapter 5 will help you with that.

Get into the meal habit now, so it is well established by the time your baby is born. You will need your strength, endurance, and emotional steadiness in order to be good parents. When you are hungry or go without food, you will be worn-out, cranky, and discouraged. Be positive and reliable about taking care of yourself with food. Eat enough and manage your time so you can have three meals a day and as many snacks as you need to feel comfortable and energetic. Drink enough but not too much. Quench your thirst, but don't force yourself to drink more than you want.

Arrange for your feeding comfort

In the first few months you will spend most of your time with your baby feeding them, so arrange to be physically comfortable and protect your back. Sitting comfortably will help you sit still and not fidget with the bottle.

Sit so you don't strain your back and legs. Get a good chair that supports your back and arms and fits your body. Support your feet well on the floor or get a footstool that holds your feet at the proper height and angle. Consider getting a feeding or nursing pillow. That big, C-shaped pillow gives your baby space to lie comfortably in front of you and curves under your arms to support your elbow so you can support them. Do NOT confuse the feeding pillow with the baby *self-feeding* pillow, an appalling contraption that lets you prop your baby's bottle. Propping your baby's bottle is not good *at all*. Your baby needs you to hold them while they eat, both for nurturing and for safety, and you need it, too.

Take care of your needs

Read the Chapter 8 section, "Consider support," page 220. Both bottle-feeding and breastfeeding parents need support when they are first learning to be parents. Accept support from your family and other loved ones when it is offered. Recruit an experienced teacher and support person. Have regular and frequent office visits with your pediatrician.

You will likely play the doula role for each other: give physical and emotional support, encourage confidence, and provide information. Again, we can learn from breastfeeding parents: Breastfeeding mothers say information is least important; responsiveness is most important. You are responsive when you find out and accept how your partner feels, even if those feelings are negative. Responsive parents show and express their appreciation for and comfort with formula-feeding, run interference with other people, and pay attention to how their partner wants them to participate. Responsiveness makes you a calming presence, which helps just by your being there and taking an interest. Doing household chores helps, but it is far down on the list.[3]

As a new father, you are likely to have negative feelings as well, and those feelings deserve airing and acceptance. Your responsibilities have increased tremendously, your life and schedule have become far more complicated, and if you are like most new fathers, you don't know what to expect or how to cope with a new baby. Many new fathers find babies only start to get interesting at around two to three months when they interact more. At the same time, your partner is likely to be preoccupied with the baby, her moods may fluctuate, and she may be touchy, demoralized, and even depressed. Postpartum depression is real, and help is available.

BEFORE-BIRTH FORMULA-FEEDING ISSUES

Do your best ahead of time to ensure that you have a safe water source and choose nipples, bottles, and formula. Infant formula has a separate section starting after this one.

The water supply

The water you use to reconstitute concentrated or powdered baby formula has to be clean and low in lead, nitrate, sodium, and pesticides. It may be fluoridated. If you have your own well, have your water tested at least once a year by the state laboratory of hygiene for cleanliness, nitrate, arsenic, and pesticide levels. If you have any doubt concerning the safety of your well water, purchase bottled water for your baby. City water supplies as well as commercially bottled water are required by law to be periodically tested to be safe. Don't use softened water, as the softening process adds sodium. You do not have to boil water unless you have a vulnerable baby or have reason to believe your water is contaminated with bacteria or parasites. Boiling doesn't get rid of lead, nitrate, sodium, and pesticides: It actually concentrates them. For more issues about water, do a web search for *Environmental Protection Agency (EPA) Safe Drinking Water Information.*

Test for nitrate

Nitrates occur naturally in soil, plants, and water. Infants under age six months can't properly metabolize nitrate: They chemically change ingested nitrate to *nitrite,* which displaces oxygen in red blood cells. Babies who consume too much nitrate develop a condition, methemoglobinemia, or blue baby, that interferes with the oxygencarrying capacity of the blood and can make them very ill. City drinking water is continually tested to be sure the nitrate level is within the safe range of less than 10 parts per million (ppm). Well water might contain more than that. With rising population density and more and more people moving into agricultural areas, nitrate in well water is an increasing problem. Be particularly careful to test after heavy rains, flooding, irrigation, or fertilizer application near your well. Again, boiling the water doesn't help: It only concentrates the nitrates.

Home water purification units

Carafe filters and counter-top units remove bad tastes, odors, chlorine, and organic chemicals, but do not remove lead, nitrate, sodium, or pathogens. Some filters remove only sediment. Only filters that have been rated as 1 micron absolute or smaller will get rid of *Giardia* and *Cryptosporidium*, parasites that are common causes of waterborne disease outbreaks. Home water purification systems that use a process called reverse osmosis remove *Giardia* and *Cryptosporidium*. The process also removes fluoride, an advantage for reconstituting baby formula, a disadvantage for other older family members. If you have a reverse osmosis unit, you will know it. The units are expensive, require a large storage tank and have a separate faucet. Check when you shop to find out what is removed by your water purification unit.

Nipples

Marketing plays on any guilt you may have about formula-feeding, so know this: Despite advertising to the contrary, no nipple, bottle, or nursing system totally mimics the breast. Baby-bottle nipples feel different in the baby's mouth.

It's hard to know ahead of time which nipple will work for your baby. Consider getting a nipple flight: a selection of nipples to try out. Do a web search for *baby bottle nipple variety*; you might get lucky. You are looking for a baby-bottle nipple that fits the size and shape of your baby's mouth and is stiff enough not to collapse when your baby suckles. A baby with a strong suckle needs a stiffer nipple that flows more slowly. A baby with a weaker suckle or who tires easily needs a softer nipple that flows more rapidly. The hospital nursing staff can tell you if your baby has a stronger or weaker suckle. Standard, non-latex nipples are softer and easier for babies to squeeze than silicone nipples, which tend to be firmer. Once you choose a nipple, try to stick with it. Babies generally prefer the nipple you started with and are upset by switching from one nipple to another. You have to put up with the disposable nipple-bottle assemblies in the hospital but make the switch to your own as soon as you get home.

The nipple determines the rate at which your baby gets the formula. The flow rate is good when your baby is able to nurse smoothly, steadily, and continuously. You can get an idea about flow—what your baby gets via suckling—by holding the bottle upside down. The formula needs to come out in steady drops that follow each other closely, but not in a constant flow. A too-slow nipple can frustrate and wear out your baby; a too-fast nipple can gag and frighten them. If you are forced to change formulas, again check the nipple flow. Some formulas are thicker than others and flow differently.

Baby bottles

It seems to me that glass or stainless-steel baby bottles are best because they don't give off particles or chemicals. Glass and stainless-steel bottles are easy to clean. They have enough weight to stay put in the dishwasher and stay hot so they dry fast. Glass and stainless steel in a heated bottle stay warm longer while you feed your baby and stay cold longer in a diaper bag. Stainless steel has the added advantage of being opaque, which may help you to go by your baby's feeding cues rather than by how much formula is left in the bottle.

Silicone is better than plastic because it gives off fewer chemicals and no microplastics. Silicone doesn't break, although it does scratch, but it is difficult to break a glass bottle. Avoid cute bottle designs or bottles shaped to make them easy for a baby to hold. A child who is old enough to enjoy an animal-shaped bottle or hold it themself is ready to be weaned from the bottle.

Plan to warm—or not warm—the bottle

Babies don't seem to mind whether their bottle is warmed or straight out of the refrigerator, as long as it is the same from one feeding to the next. It might feel more nurturing to you to give your baby a warmed bottle, and your breastfed baby might accept a warmed bottle more readily. However, there is much to recommend cold bottles: You can feed immediately, there is no waiting if your baby takes more than one bottle, and cold bottles are easier to manage when you are away from home.

If you warm your baby's bottle, do it right before feeding. Don't let bottles stand out of the refrigerator to come to room temperature between feedings. You might want to invest in a baby-bottle warmer, and some of the stainless-steel bottles have warming gadgets built in. Otherwise, set the bottle in a container of hot tap water or hold it under hot running tap water. Test a few drops on the inside of your wrist. If it's the right temperature, you won't be able to feel either warm or cold because it will be the same as your body temperature.

Although microwaving formula bottles is not recommended, half of parents heat bottles in a microwave.[4] As a consequence, Maternal & Child Health Nutrition Specialist Madeleine Sigman-Grant developed guidelines for doing it safely. Follow the Figure 9.1 directions. Be sure to shake the bottle after microwaving and do the wrist test. Dr. Sigman-Grant found no nutrient loss with microwaving formula.[5]

FIGURE 9.1: SAFE MICROWAVING

A microwaved bottle that feels lukewarm on the outside may contain pockets of scalding liquid. To avoid burning your baby, carefully follow these procedures. These procedures for safe microwaving were carefully developed.[1] Share them with anyone who cares for your baby.

- Microwave the bottle without a nipple or cap (so it doesn't explode).
- Heat a four-ounce bottle no more than 30 seconds; an eight-ounce bottle no more than 45 seconds (on full power).
- After microwaving, replace the nipple assembly and mix the contents of the bottle by turning it upside down, then right side up, 10 or more times.
- Check the temperature by placing a few drops of liquid on your wrist. It is the right temperature when it feels neither warm nor cold.
- If it's too hot, wait. If it's too cool, remove the cap and heat a bit more.

Sigman-Grant M. Microwave heating of infant formula: A dilemma resolved. Pediatrics. 1992;90:412–415.

INFANT FORMULA

Since your baby can only cuddle, root, and suckle, they must be held and fed by nipple, and you must use infant formula. Give your baby infant formula until they are well-established on table food, which for typical babies is toward the end of the first year, later for babies with issues. Infants are nutritionally vulnerable, and what they eat has to be uncompromisingly appropriate. Infant formula must be easy to digest, must supply all babies' nutritional needs, and must not disrupt babies' fragile body chemistry. Human milk and standard commercial formulas adequately fill these specifications. Specialized formulas address other needs as well and are reviewed later in this section. Those include partially predigested formulas, hypoallergenic formulas, formulas for infants born prematurely, and formulas that correct for inborn errors of metabolism.

Choosing formula

Formulas come ready-to-use, as concentrated liquid, or in powder form. Most parents start their baby on whatever formula their hospital uses and continue to use that brand as long as they need formula. Most hospitals let formula companies take turns supplying formulas, so there is no endorsement. Most WIC (Special Supplemental Nutrition Program for Women, Infants, and Children) programs hold competitive bidding to choose baby formula manufacturers. That means they tend to use formulas from major manufacturers, which may or may not be more expensive than less well-known formulas of equal quality, such as store-brand formulas. Babies get attached to their formulas, so it is best to switch to your chosen formula right after you get home. If you have a strong family history of allergies and are able to pay the extra cost, discuss with your doctor putting your baby on an extensively hydrolyzed formula.

Despite the availability of so-called "follow-on" formulas, you do not have to change formula as your baby gets older, even if you continue to give formula after age one year. Your older baby will continue to grow and do well on their infant formula.

Avoid formula switching

For most babies, any of the standard formulas work just fine. Once you start on a formula, keep using the same one if you possibly can. Studies show that parents make frequent formula changes based on their baby's spitting up, crying, and constipation.[4] Changing formula is unlikely to address those issues. Examine feeding if your baby fusses during or after feeding, spits up, pulls off the nipple, or doesn't seem to want to eat. Are you feeding when your baby is calm and alert? Are you going by your baby's feeding cues to let them eat the amount they want and need? Are you doing your jobs and letting your baby do theirs? All those issues are addressed in Chapter 7, Understanding Your Newborn.

Persistent feeding problems are likely due to your baby's physical, nervous, or digestive system immaturity. Discuss persistent problems with your baby's doctor. Changing formulas is likely to make the problem worse because your baby will have to cope with what, for them, is a huge change. Babies settle down with time.

You might have to change formulas if you and your health care professional determine that your baby needs a hypoallergenic formula. The WIC program might also change vendors. Change from one formula to another slowly and give your baby time to adjust. Mix the old gradually with the new until you make the shift. Your baby experiences their whole world through their mouth, and for them small differences in thickness or flavor can be extremely upsetting. Make sure the new formula works with the old nipples: Drops should follow each other closely but not be continuous when you hold the bottle upside down.

Avoid formula substitutes

Despite the ready availability of infant formulas, a sizeable number of people give their babies inappropriate food. Even before the 2022 infant formula shortage, over 25 percent of parents gave their under-six-month-old baby cow or goat milk, sometimes watered down, sometimes unpasteurized. That percentage increased to almost half during the shortage. Not a good idea. Babies can't properly digest even pasteurized cow and goat milk, and it doesn't help to add solid foods: The combination may or may not add up to nutritional adequacy. Around 10 percent of parents of young infants used toddler formulas, which are marginally okay for toddlers but too high in protein for infants. Some parents tried to fill their babies up with solid foods, and that does not work either. Trying to get a too-young baby to eat solid foods can spoil the feeding relationship.

Do not under any circumstances give your baby unpasteurized cow and goat milk: Unpasteurized milk carries a high risk of contamination that can make your baby sick. Even when cow and goat milk are pasteurized, unmodified milk doesn't give babies all the nutrients they need. Not only that, but pasteurized, unmodified milk sets up such a tough, cheese-like curd in the stomach that it is hard for babies to digest and is likely to give them a stomachache. Formulas are balanced and carefully tested to support babies' nutritional needs. Formulas are heated to above pasteurization levels during production so they set up a soft custardlike curd in the baby's stomach, and that is easy to digest. Unmodified cow and goat milk are too high in protein, and the excess protein can stress babies' kidneys. For some unknown reason, babies bleed from their intestines when they are given even pasteurized cow milk and that can cause anemia.

Common infant formulas

Seventy-five percent of formulas fed to U.S. infants are cow-milk based; 25 percent are soy-based. Enfamil, Similac, and Good Start are the most commonly available cow-milk-based formulas. They and their store-brand equivalents made by Up & Up, Signature Procare, Members Mark, Mama Bear Advantage, Parents Choice, Tippy Toes, and others are suitable for most babies.

Soy-based formulas include Isomil, ProSobee, Alsoy, and their store-brand equivalents. Babies might be put on a soy-based formula if they develop a cow milk sensitivity or allergy, although up to 10 percent of babies with cow-milk allergy also react to soy.[6] Your doctor may determine that your baby needs a soy-based formula in the unusual case that they become lactose- (milk sugar) intolerant following a bout of severe diarrhea. You can also get lactose-free, cow-milk-based formula: The label will say something like Lactofree, which can either be a brand name or a generic description.

Beyond the lactose intolerance or cow milk allergy experienced by far fewer than 25 percent of babies, why are so many babies being fed soy-based formula? Is it because soy is one of those currently favored plant foods, assumed to be somehow better than cow milk? If so, it's the wrong reason. Babies develop as many allergic reactions to soy-based formulas as they do to cow-milk-based ones. While soy can certainly contribute to a healthy diet, there is nothing inherently superior about it. In fact, soy-based formulas are relatively high in aluminum, which puts them out of the running for preemies, and they provide a level of phytoestrogen (a form of the female hormone estrogen) that is high enough to influence the menstrual cycle of humans.[7] The U.S. National Toxicology Program monograph on the safety of the use of soy formula states that the use of soy-based infant formula poses minimal concern, emphasizes a lack of data from human subjects, and points out that aluminum has not been demonstrated to be toxic for humans. My point of view: Why risk it if you don't have to?

Formula safety

The U.S. Food and Drug Administration sets and enforces strict regulations so the infant formulas you find in your grocery store, pharmacy, or discount store are safe. FDA specifies 30 nutrients in specific amounts that must be included in infant formulas. Any ingredient used in infant formula must be safe and suitable for such use.

It was FDA scrutiny that contributed to the 2022 formula shortage by discovering *chronobacter* contamination in the powdered baby formula of a major manufacturer and withdrawing it from the market. Babies were getting sick and even dying. During the formula shortage, imported formulas with unfamiliar brand names began to appear in U.S. retail markets; those are also subject to FDA scrutiny and are safe. Their formulations and instructions are a bit different: They may contain a bit less iron but still an adequate amount, and the instructions are in milliliters and grams. You can find conversion instructions on the web.

Here is a big *however*: Formula ordered directly from other countries bypasses FDA scrutiny and may or may not be safe.

Formula ingredients

If you have a particular interest, you can shop for what you consider important by reading labels and nutritional lists of ingredients. You may or may not find nutrition and ingredient information on the web, so you may need to spend some time in the store doing your research. Ignore label claims, which are there for marketing and don't give accurate information. Manufacturers promote qualities shared by all standard formulas, such as being pure, pesticide free, having 20 calories per ounce, having 30 basic ingredients including iron, being non-GMO, having no artificial flavors, sweeteners, or colors, and being gluten free (there *is* a possibility for cross-contamination, so look for *gluten free* on the label). Over half of infant formulas claim to be better for infant colic and gastrointestinal symptoms, claims that have no basis in fact.

Other ingredients vary among formulas. Manufacturers make unsubstantiated claims to sell their product. Here are a few of those claims: Added probiotics produce soft stools and support the immune system. Oligosaccharides protect against intestinal infection. Omega-3 fatty acids (DHA) support brain development. Lactoferrin (human-milk form of iron) protects against anemia. Lutein ensures eye health. Manufacturers may boast about avoiding palm oil or corn syrup solids, but both are perfectly nutritious for babies and suffer only from negative press.

Infant formulas are so tightly controlled that "organic" means little and may not be worth the considerable additional cost. You do not have to pay extra to get the qualities that organic formula manufacturers boast about. Standard formulas are pure, pesticide free, use non-GMO ingredients, and can claim being "closest to breastmilk." GMOs are barred from use in infant formula and baby food.

Some formula manufacturers make an issue of the whey/casein ratio. Whey protein predominates in human milk and is more digestible for human infants; casein predominates in cow milk and is less digestible for human infants. However, casein in formula is heat treated, which makes it digestible. As a result, most babies digest both high-whey and high-casein formulas well, although an occasional baby seems to do better on Good Start, which is the only baby formula that is 100 percent whey. Similac is 80 percent whey and 20 percent casein. Enfamil is 60 percent whey, 40 percent casein. Other formulas will state their whey/casein ratio on the label.

Expense

Infant formulas are expensive. You can get help purchasing formula if you qualify for the WIC program or the Supplemental Nutrition Assistance Program (SNAP), often called Food Stamps. Consider applying. Those programs are set up as a nutritional safety net for people who need a bit of help for a while. Do this for your baby.

Beyond getting help for purchasing formula, know that powdered and concentrated liquid formula tend to be the least expensive, ready-to-feed most expensive. Standard-brand formulas, Enfamil, Similac, and Good Start tend to be more expensive than store-brand formulas, which are just as good.

Hydrolyzed formulas contain casein that has been broken down (hydrolyzed) into smaller proteins, making it more easily digested. Both whey-based and hydrolyzed formulas might be marketed as "partially hydrolyzed," "easy-to-digest," "calm," or "gentle." Your baby might do better on a hydrolyzed formula, but research shows that only extensively hydrolyzed formulas help with allergies and occasionally with colic.

Some parents start infants early on solid foods as a way of cutting down on formula costs, but that isn't a good idea. It doesn't save much money and starting solids too early can cause nutritional and food-refusal problems. Your baby will be ready to start learning to eat solid foods when they can sit up, open their mouth when they see the spoon coming, close their lips over the spoon and transfer food from the front of their mouth to the back. About that time, they will be able to digest and absorb the nutrients in solid food.

Stools with formulas

Breastfeeding parents have the special treat of tracking their babies' pees and poops as a way of knowing they are getting enough to eat. No sense letting them have all the fun! You will know how much formula your baby eats, but pees especially—and poops to a certain extent—give you a second opinion that feeding is going well. Your formula-fed baby ought to have six or eight wet diapers a day and likely have two to three poops. Observations from the University of Connecticut Health Center found infants receiving Enfamil had two or three mushy or watery stools a day. Infants on Nutramigen (hydrolyzed formula) had twice as many stools as infants on Enfamil and stools tended to be watery. Infants receiving ProSobee (soy formula) had hard/firm stools about a third of the time and had two or three stools a day. Babies fed ProSobee more commonly strained with defecation. Babies had yellow, brown, and green stools, with green being most common with iron-fortified formulas (Enfamil, ProSobee, Nutramigen). Spitting, gassiness, and crying were common and the occurrence was about the same for all formula groups.[8] Hard, dry stools may indicate incorrect preparation of formula.

Formula for your older baby

Wait to feed your baby whole pasteurized milk, using a cup, along with meals and snacks until they are at least a year old *and* they are well-established on table food. You don't have to switch your baby to pasteurized milk. The same infant formula you have been using all along is right for your baby the whole first year and even longer. If your baby has been ill or gotten a slow start for whatever reason, you may want to give infant formula until you are confident that they are well on their way nutritionally. As long as you give formula from the cup, in fact, there is no need to be in a hurry about getting off it.

Leave your prematurely born baby on infant formula until 12 months corrected age and they are well-established on family food. That might take a while. Because of early medical procedures done to the mouth, your prematurely born baby is likely to be slow and cautious about new mouth experiences. A new nipple, new formula, or new method of eating are scarily unfamiliar, and they need time to get used to them. Take your time. Your baby will eat solid foods eventually and get there faster if you don't feel you have to hurry them up.

There is no need to use toddler formula or toddler milk, often labeled "follow-up," "growing up," or "transition formula." For the infant, toddler formula is nutritionally inferior to infant formula and, for the toddler, no better than whole pasteurized milk. Toddler formulas are typically billed as a safety net for picky eaters, which they are not. Pediasure by Abbot Labs markets to pediatricians as the solution for children's picky eating. Its packaging says, "Studied in children at risk for malnutrition" and uses marketing buzzwords like, "Gain and grow with immune support," "Non GMO," "Clinically proven to help kids grow." In reality, giving toddlers and older children formulas such as Pediasure interferes with and delays their learning to eat and, in the long run, impairs their nutritional status. As we will address in the following chapters, there are many ways to address picky eating, and giving a child a special formula isn't one of them.

Supplementary vitamins and minerals

Brand-name infant formulas are nutritionally complete and don't need to be supplemented with any other vitamins or minerals. Commercial-formula-fed babies get adequate amounts of all vitamins and minerals and don't need supplements. There is nothing to be gained by nutritional supplementation and something to be lost. Too much of any nutrient can give undesirable side effects and decrease absorption of other nutrients. The Chapter 10 section, "Nutrients and your older baby," page 343, discusses specific nutrients in more detail.

Intramuscular vitamin K1 is routinely administered to all infants on the first day of life to reduce the risk of vitamin K deficiency bleeding.

Fluoride

To protect against fluorosis—mottling of teeth—formulas are low in fluoride, and fluoride supplementation for infants is delayed until after six months of age.[9] The water you use for diluting your baby's formula is likely to contain fluoride. Check with your doctor. You may need to use bottled water but do check that it doesn't have fluoride in it. We will discuss fluoride further in Chapter 10.

Iron

The American Academy of Pediatrics recommends iron-fortified formula from birth for all bottle-fed babies. Iron in red blood cells carries oxygen to all parts of the body. When children don't get enough iron, they may become anemic: look pale, act cranky, and lack energy. For the term infant, the issue is prevention of the iron deficiency anemia that can appear after age six months and more often after a year of age. The newborn needs and uses very little dietary iron before age four to six months. Prematurely born babies don't have the iron stores and need to be supplemented by age two months.

You may have heard warnings that iron-fortified formula is constipating and upsets babies' stomachs. It does not. Double-blind studies—where neither researchers nor mothers knew whether the babies were taking iron fortified formulas—found that babies on both formulas had the same numbers of stomach and intestinal upsets and the same amount of constipation and diarrhea. If you are still unconvinced and you still want to use the non-iron formula, you must give your baby iron drops. See your health care provider about a recommendation for iron drops and about instructions for proper dosage.

PREPARE FORMULA EXACTLY RIGHT

Although modern formula-feeding is convenient and safe, it is important not to become casual about the mechanics of preparation. The water supply must be clean and safe and even boiled for some infants, the nursing equipment sanitary and comfortable for both feeder and baby, and the formula prepared precisely according to directions. Small errors in measurement can change the formula concentration, and that can have serious consequences for your baby. Too-concentrated formula (made up with too little water) can stress your baby's kidneys and digestive system and cause dehydration. Too-dilute formula (made up with too much water), can slow babies' growth.

Common errors in formula preparation

Modern formula preparation is deceptively simple—so simple, in fact, that it is easy to become lax and inattentive, and to make some serious errors. People not only make mistakes, sometimes they vary the concentration of infant formula on purpose. A 2009 survey of infant formula-feeding practices showed that mothers put in more or less water than recommended believing it would control constipation or diarrhea, slow the baby's growth, or get them to grow faster. Sometimes they acted on the advice of their doctors. At times they diluted formula to save money or make it last longer or adjusted water when package sizes did not come out even with the baby's bottle. Some mixed formula with warm tap water (which is likely to be softened and therefore contain sodium), and some added cereal to the bottles.[4]

Don't get it *close*—get it *right*

Follow instructions exactly when you prepare formula. Measure liquids with standard clear measuring cups that have the volume marked off. If you boil your water, measure it afterward because the evaporation from boiling will change the measurement. Get your eye down even with the level of water on the side of the measuring cup or rigid-sided bottle to measure liquid accurately. Don't measure in baby bottles that have disposable plastic inner liners—the markings are not accurate.

Ready-to-feed formula generally comes in quart containers that say *ready to feed*, and you can pour it directly into the bottle and feed it. Ready-to-feed formula also comes in disposable baby bottles. Liquid concentrated formula generally comes in 13- or 14-ounce containers and you dilute the concentrated formula 1:1 with water. If you make up one bottle at a time, be very sure your measuring equipment is accurate. To make up the whole container, use the container to measure an equal volume of water for diluting. Store the diluted formula in the refrigerator in a clean, covered container or in clean, covered, individual baby bottles.

Powdered formula comes with a little scoop for measuring and directions for how many ounces of water to use per scoop. Use the scoop provided in the formula container and throw it away when the container is empty. Use the scoop according to directions: exactly how to fill the scoop, whether to scrape it against the can or a straight edge, whether to shake or tap it. The way you fill, scrape, and tap affects the measurement. Use the new scoop that comes with each new can: It could be slightly different. If you change formulas, again study the directions.

Keep formula fresh and cold between feedings

An opened can of liquid formula or formula reconstituted from powder must be kept tightly covered, refrigerated immediately, and stored in the refrigerator for no more than 48 hours. Store an opened can of formula powder in a cool, dry place and use it within a month after you open it. Because even carefully handled powdered formula can contain a small number of undesirable bacteria, it wouldn't hurt to store the opened container in the refrigerator.

Keep your refrigerator temperature between 35 and 40 degrees Fahrenheit, a temperature that is as cool as possible without freezing. Formula that is between 40 and 140 degrees (optimum temperatures for bacterial growth) for two hours or more is contaminated and must be discarded. Discard any formula left in a bottle an hour after the feeding starts. Bacteria from your baby's mouth gets in the bottle during nursing, so once you have fed from a bottle, don't reuse it because the bacteria can multiply rapidly. Keep time and temperature in mind when you carry bottles in a diaper bag. Have the formula very cold when you pack it, and tuck in an ice pack.

Develop and maintain high standards of sanitation

There is no way of knowing how often babies get sick from contaminated formula. Be conscientious about cleanliness when you handle your baby's formula, bottles, and nipples, even when your baby gets older. Babies have low immunity to bacteria in the digestive tract and are more sensitive to irritating substances than older children or adults. The baby who has diarrhea or is vomiting from a food infection risks dehydration.

It is easy to make mistakes. Observations of infant formula-handling show that 55 percent of parents did not wash their hands with soap before preparing infant formula, 32 percent did not take the ring and nipple apart and scrub the crevices, and 6 percent did not discard formula left standing for more than 2 hours.[10]

Wash your hands before you feed your baby; before you handle food; after you go to the bathroom or change diapers; and after you handle any meat, fish, poultry or fresh produce. Use the handwashing technique you learned during the COVID epidemic. Change your hand towel daily or more often if it stays damp. Use regular hand soap. Anti-bacterial cleaners contain antibiotics, and routine use of antibiotics tends to produce antibiotic-resistant bacteria. For tough disinfecting jobs, use chlorine-type bleach.

Bacteria require three conditions to multiply: nutrients, heat, and moisture. Use a clean dishcloth and start with a clean sink or dishpan.

If you use a bottle brush, wash and rinse it carefully after each use and put it where it can quickly dry and stay dry. Anything left wet provides a medium for bacterial growth. Take the nipple out of the nipple ring and take apart any other baby-bottle components. Carefully scrub the bottles and nipples in hot, soapy water, force water through the holes of the nipple, then rinse in water as hot as your hands can stand. Be sure that you get all the suds off, as dried soap scum contains food particles and, again, provides a good medium for bacterial growth. Invert the bottles on a drying rack, put the nipples in a clean strainer, and let air dry. Keep your tools and work surfaces clean and dry.

You can depend on your dishwasher for washing equipment, bottles, and nipples as long as the drying cycle gets up to 180 degrees and the rinse cycle gets rid of the caustic dishwasher detergent. Take the nipple ring and nipple apart, pre-rinse the bottles and nipples to get the milk film out, and force water through the holes of the nipple. Consider getting a basket to contain the small pieces and keep them from floating around in the dishwasher.

Clean the exposed top of the formula can and other equipment you use in formula preparation. Let air dry. Promptly refrigerate opened formula.

Sterilize for more protection

The Centers for Disease Control and Prevention recommends sanitizing equipment in boiling water for infants under two months, prematurely born babies, and those with compromised immune systems due to illness (such as HIV) or medical treatment (such as chemotherapy for cancer). Do a web search for *How to Clean, Sanitize, and Store Infant Feeding Items.* Health departments in England and Australia, and likely other countries as well, recommend always boiling water and sanitizing equipment. The heated drying cycle in your dishwasher sanitizes your equipment. Lacking that, sterilize by boiling everything for five minutes before you make up the bottles: the water used in formula preparation, the bottles, the nipples and nipple covers, and the measuring and mixing equipment. Let the equipment air dry, and store it in a clean, dry place. You can also sterilize by following the directions for your microwave or purchase a commercial sanitizer.

Unless you have a vulnerable baby, after the first few months you still have to be careful about being clean, but you don't have to sterilize. In fact, today's thinking is that exposure to allergy-causing substances early on can cut down on allergies later on. The exception is exposing your baby to food pathogens, which can overwhelm their ability to maintain hydration and biochemical balance. With careful handling of formula and equipment, you keep the bacterial level down and let your baby gradually develop the ability to live with necessary germs.

Honey

Don't give your baby honey before age one year because it could cause botulism, a type of food poisoning. Don't put honey on the pacifier, and don't give your baby anything that is baked with honey. Baking doesn't destroy the botulinum spores that grow and cause the poisoning.

SPECIALIZED FORMULAS

Babies need special formulas when they have allergic reactions, have difficulty eating enough to satisfy their nutritional needs, or have particular health conditions that must be managed with careful nutritional manipulation. This discussion will get very deep, very fast so concentrate on what you need to know: Why your baby might need a specialized formula and what those formulas are. Figure 9.2 lists formulas commonly used for food intolerance, allergy, or digestive difficulty. These are the common brand names; you can find additional formulas with these characteristics on the web. Formulations are constantly changing and so are the names, but the categories—partially hydrolyzed, extensively hydrolyzed, amino acid—are likely to stay the same. Consider this to be background information. To make proper use of these formulas you need advice and support from your health care provider.

FIGURE 9.2: MODIFIED FORMULAS

For infants who have food intolerance, allergy, or digestive difficulty. Protein is modified. Fat and carbohydrate, indicated in parentheses, may also be modified.

Partially hydrolyzed protein.

- Gerber Good Start Gentle
- Abbot Similac Total Comfort

Extensively hydrolyzed protein. "Predigested," "hypoallergenic."

- Abbot Alimentum
- Enfamil Nutramigen (Corn syrup solids, modified cornstarch)
- Pregestimil (MCT oil, corn syrup solids, modified tapioca starch)

Amino acid, "elemental."

- Nutrica Neocate
- Abbott Elecare

Food allergy or intolerance

A true food allergy affects the immune system. For people with allergies, even small amounts of the offending food can trigger a range of symptoms, which can be severe or life-threatening. In contrast, food intolerance often affects only the digestive system and causes less serious symptoms. Babies can also react to certain foods when they are ill. Depend on your health professional to help you sort it out. Since your child's food allergies are likely to be an ongoing feeding issue, start now to establish a relationship with a sDOR-committed dietitian specializing in food allergies. It could save you a lot of misery in the form of feeding problems.

Symptoms of food allergy include itchy mouth and throat; rash or eczema; diarrhea, cramps, nausea, vomiting; swelling of the face or tongue; and trouble breathing. Babies can also show extreme irritability, either as a stand-alone symptom or as a result of the other symptoms. While a baby's food intolerance might be addressed with a partially hydrolyzed formula, addressing food allergy requires an extensively hydrolyzed formula. Formulas for food allergy hydrolyze (break down) the protein extensively or reduce it to its most elemental form: amino acids. Extensively hydrolyzed formulas can be labeled *hypoallergenic* if they have been tested to demonstrate that infants with defined symptoms do not react when they are given these formulas.[6]

Partially hydrolyzed infant formulas (Gerber Good Start Gentle and Abbot Similac Total Comfort) are not hypoallergenic. They may be recommended for preventing allergies, but they don't help.[11] Extensively hydrolyzed formulas (Gerber Extensive HA, Abbot Alimentum, Enfamil Nutramigen and Pregesimil) *do* help.[6] Amino acid formulas are hypoallergenic but have other intended uses.

Extensively hydrolyzed or amino acid formulas (Nutrica Neocate, Abbot Elecare) are generally used when children have gastrointestinal tract impairment: They have chronic diarrhea, malabsorption, short gut syndrome, Crohn's disease, or HIV/AIDS. Amino-acid-based formulas are the most hydrolyzed of all. About 10 percent of infants do not respond to extensively hydrolyzed formula and need to be put on amino-acid-based formula.[6]

With respect to colic, although the majority of infants with colic do not respond to extensively hydrolyzed or amino acid formula, those with severe colic may benefit from a one- to two-week trial.[12] However, abruptly switching formulas could agitate your baby and exacerbate their colicky symptoms. Extensively hydrolyzed formulas have pronounced bitter, sour, and savory tastes compared with standard formulas and human milk, which have milder flavors.[13] Switch by diluting your current formula with about 10 percent of the new formula (9 parts old formula and 1 part new formula) and gradually work up.

It may reassure you to know that babies who had been fed extensively hydrolyzed formulas had more tolerance for strong flavors than those on standard formulas. They ate significantly more savory-, bitter-, and sour-tasting and plain cereals than did the human-milk- or cow-milk-based-formula-fed infants.[13]

Digestive difficulties

The oil in the extensively hydrolyzed Pregestimil comes in the form of medium-chain triglycerides—MCT oil. Your doctor may recommend Pregestimil if your baby has had part of their intestine removed, has cystic fibrosis, or gets diarrhea from other dietary fats. Medium-chain triglycerides don't require the usual digestion before they can be absorbed. Do a web search for *infant formula with MCT oil* to find other brands.

The carbohydrates in Nutramigen and Pregestimil, both extensively hydrolyzed, come from corn syrup solids and modified food starch. Both carbohydrates can be digested by babies who have trouble digesting other sugars such as lactose (milk sugar) or sucrose (table sugar). Do a web search for *lactose-free infant formula* to find other brands.

Prematurity

Products for infants who were born prematurely such as Similac Neosure or Enfamil EnfaCare offer more calories and higher levels of protein and other nutrients per ounce, including calcium and phosphorus. These formulas support optimal growth and development so that catch-up growth started in the hospital can continue at home. Standard formulas have 20 calories per ounce; formulas for preterm babies have 22 or 24 calories per ounce. According to the American Academy of Pediatrics, until they reach 5.5 to 8 pounds, babies are generally recommended to have a 24-calorie-per-ounce formula (e.g. Enfamil®Premature 24 cal/fl oz). After that, they can go to a 22-calorie-per-ounce transition formula (Enfamil NeuroPro™ EnfaCare® 22 cal/fl oz) and stay on that until they are 9 months corrected age. After that, they can have standard 20-calorie-per-ounce formula or finish out the first year with the 22-calorie-per-ounce formula.

Do not concentrate regular formula to make it higher in calories. That concoction would be too high in protein and low in water and will not provide the proper level of all other nutrients for your nutritionally fragile infant.

Inborn errors of metabolism

Babies are tested at birth for inborn errors of metabolism (IEM). These are genetic disorders that impact the function of enzymes leading to the abnormal metabolism of protein, fat, or carbohydrate. Due to the lack of sufficient enzyme activity, one or more byproducts of the incomplete nutrient breakdown process accumulate to toxic levels within the individual, while other compounds may become deficient. The most common inborn errors of metabolism are cystic fibrosis, fructose intolerance, galactosemia, maple sugar urine disease (MSUD), and phenylketonuria (PKU). A baby with cystic fibrosis is likely to require supplemental enzymes and the others require a specialized infant formula. Your baby will be tested at birth for these and other disorders and, if diagnosed, referred to a specialty clinic for careful dietary management.

EMERGENCY FORMULA

We are going to be haunted by the 2022 infant formula shortage for a long time. Parents coped with lack of formula availability by increasing breastfeeding, increasing use of banked donor human milk, changing formula brands, and desperately scouring the shelves in grocery, pharmacy, and big-box stores. Nearly half of families used at least one feeding practice that was dangerous for babies, such as watering down formula or giving even pasteurized cow or goat milk.[14]

We hope it won't happen again, but just in case, here is an emergency fallback evaporated-milk formula that you can use with your healthy baby until commercial formula is available. This recipe was safely used for decades by formula-feeding parents. It is still used for cultural and economic reasons in parts of Canada among Aboriginal peoples, where they don't have the nutritional safety net of the US WIC and SNAP programs. Babies do well on this formula, provided they are supplemented with vitamin C.[15]

I debated long and hard about giving you this recipe, because the American Academy of Pediatrics does not approve of it, and the World Health Organization says it should be used only under direct health care provider supervision. I decided to give it to you on the grounds that it is far better than the dangerous alternatives parents were forced to use during the formula shortage. However, you must do your part by following these instructions absolutely *to the letter*. Simple as it is, the evaporated milk formula has been calculated very carefully to give it appropriate calorie and nutrient density and to provide the proper proportions of protein, fat, and carbohydrate.

Use ***evaporated*** milk, not pasteurized milk or condensed milk. Evaporated milk is a canned cow's milk product that has been concentrated by removing half the water. In contrast to raw or even pasteurized milk, the canning process heats evaporated milk to a high enough temperature to make it digestible: It sets up a soft curd in the baby's stomach. Evaporated milk also doesn't cause the intestinal bleeding that is a problem with pasteurized milk. Again, *evaporated* milk is not the same as *condensed* milk. *Condensed* milk has a lot of added sugar—more than the added sugar in the evaporated milk formula recipe—and is used for baking.

Making evaporated milk formula

The recipe is in Figure 9.3. Do not use versions of this recipe you find on the web. Some are inaccurate, such as one starting with a 13-ounce can of evaporated milk (cans have been 12 ounces for decades). Some are dangerous, such as the one recommending diluting evaporated milk 1 to 1 with water and not adding sugar or syrup.

FIGURE 9.3: EVAPORATED MILK FORMULA

Measure absolutely accurately when making this formula and store it carefully. While it has been used for decades to raise healthy babies, it is not recommended by AAP. Supplement with a good source of vitamin C.

- One 12 ounce can whole evaporated milk, fortified with vitamins A and D.
- 17.5 ounces tap water (525 grams).
- 1 ounce (2 tablespoons) sugar or corn syrup (30 grams). *Do NOT use honey.*

Mix well, portion into absolutely clean bottles using an absolutely clean funnel, cover, and refrigerate.

Clean all mixing utensils, bottles, nipples, and bottle covers scrupulously. Do not substitute other milks or change the proportions of evaporated milk, sugar, or water. The addition of sugar or syrup along with extra water is critically important because the carbohydrate content of the evaporated cow's milk is too low for your baby and the protein content too high. Do not use honey as a sugar source because honey is often contaminated with botulinum spores that babies cannot neutralize in their stomachs and will therefore make them sick. The standard proportions of milk, sugar or syrup, and water are appropriate from birth through age 12 months and even after, if you choose to continue formula after the first year.

PARENTING WITH FEEDING

Now let's turn to your relationship with your baby around feeding. We begin by discussing issues that are important right after birth.

Skin-to-skin contact

After generations of whisking babies away right after birth to warming devices and medical procedures, the medical profession has acknowledged how stressful that is for both parents and babies. The American Academy of Pediatrics now endorses skin-to-skin contact for newborns and mothers for an hour after birth and as much skin-to-skin contact as you wish in the days following. Let me do a friendly edit and include fathers in that guideline. The AAP says such contact supports bonding, stabilizes babies and mothers medically, decreases infant stress overall, and particularly helps babies during necessary medical procedures such as blood draws. The AAP's warnings about safe skin-to-skin contact are obvious but important: Have your baby facing you, head straight up and turned to one side, legs bent, head away from your skin and out of the covers so they can breathe. Put your baby to bed when you are ready to go to sleep.[16] Kangaroo care involves holding or wrapping your baby skin to skin inside your shirt. It is good for all babies but is particularly recommended for full-term infants who are neurologically or metabolically impaired. It can stabilize temperature, breathing, and heart rate, and be calming.

SIDS

To prevent sudden infant death syndrome, the AAP recommends "back to sleep:" placing infants under age one year wholly on their back to sleep—not the side, not the tummy. Research on SIDS supports AAP's emphasis on having a firm sleep surface, room-sharing without bed-sharing, and taking care to keep bed covers off the baby's face. Additional recommendations for guarding against SIDS include breastfeeding, routine immunization, use of a pacifier, and avoiding exposure to smoke, alcohol, and illicit drugs.

Safe sleeping

The AAP recommends against sleeping with your baby in your bed, even if you have a snuggle nest. By the time you read this, there may be safety standards for bedside sleepers but until then, the AAP doesn't endorse them. If you choose to keep your baby in your bed, observe precautions: Your little one is healthy, you are fully aware of what's going on around you, there are no hazardous objects, pillows, or blankets to entrap a baby.

Your baby's head needs to be straight for them to breathe properly—not tipped forward or to one side or the other. Because of the difficulty with keeping your baby's head straight, don't let your baby regularly sleep in a car seat, stroller, swing, infant carrier, or infant sling. Don't sleep with your baby on a couch or in an armchair: The accident rate is high because babies can so easily fall down among the cushions.[16]

Post-hospital followup

The AAP recommends an office visit at three to five days for both breast- and formula-fed babies with detailed, research-based guidelines for assessing you and your baby.[1] Fullterm, formula-fed babies generally lose about four percent of their body weight within two to four days after birth, and most regain to their birth weight by seven days of age.[17]

After that first early visit, AAP recommends first-year visits at one, two, four, six, nine, and twelve months. If you are at all uncomfortable with how your baby is doing, ask for a two-week visit and frequent visits after that.

FOLLOW YOUR BABY'S LEAD WITH FEEDING

Your baby will eat best when you follow their lead in feeding. In order to do well with feeding, get on your baby's wavelength and trust information coming from them. Your baby knows how much to eat to grow in the way that is right for them. Your baby will eat best and feel best about you and about themself when you follow the Satter Division of Responsibility in Feeding (sDOR):

- You are responsible for *what* your baby is offered to eat.
- Your baby is responsible for *how much* they eat—and *everything else*: how often, how fast, how continuously, how skillfully.

Your job with formula-feeding is straightforward: Keeping your baby's needs in mind, you get to choose the formula that goes in the bottle. After that, it is all up to your baby: when, how much, how often, at what level of skill, how long, how fast. Your job is responsive feeding. Feed promptly when your baby asks to be fed—when they are wide awake and not upset from crying. Help them to remain calm and wide awake by feeding in a smooth and continuous fashion, paying attention to their feeding cues. They want to eat when their eyes are wide open and their face looks bright. They want to stop eating when they relax and let go of the nipple. Respond to the I'm hungry and I'm full cues in Figure 7.2, not the *really* hungry *or really* full cues.

Check your baby's suck and swallow. Like breastfed babies, bottle-fed babies suckle: They suck the nipple to hold it in place and squeeze the "shoulders" of the nipple between their tongue, jaw, and palate to pump out the milk. If all goes well, your baby will feel relaxed in your arms, move their arms and legs easily, be able to eat from the bottle smoothly and steadily, and comfortably suckle and swallow. They will eat fast or slowly; a little or a lot; seem to enjoy it or be ho-hum about it. They will eat until they show signs they need a break or have had enough.

I hesitate to even suggest how long feeding will last, but you might appreciate some rough ideas. At first, a feeding can take up to an hour. After you and your baby become more familiar with the process, newborns can take 20 to 40 minutes to eat, 3- to 4-month-olds 15 to 30 minutes, babies over 6 months 10 to 20 minutes. Do troubleshooting if your baby doesn't seem to make much headway on their bottle in those *approximate* times. If they also snort, cough, choke, come off the nipple to cry, arch their back, or kick and squirm, something may be wrong. It might simply be that the bottle or the nipple isn't working properly—feeding too fast or too slowly—and you need to adjust it or get a stiffer or more-pliable nipple. It could be a vacuum in the bottle—adjust the nipple ring. It could be that you are having trouble reading and responding to your baby's feeding cues: Have someone you trust observe a feeding. It could be that your baby has trouble suckling or coordinating their suck, breathe, and swallow. Talk with your pediatrician. Ask them if you should see an occupational therapist.

Read your baby's sleep

Feeding when your baby is hungry, calm, and awake is easier said than done. See the Chapter 7 section, "More about sleep." As outlined in Figure 7.1, babies cycle two or three times during any sleep episode between deep sleep, when they lie still and are difficult to wake up, and light sleep, when they move around and make noises. Don't pick your baby up during light sleep: They need to go back to deep sleep. They won't wake up fully and won't eat well. Wait to pick up your baby until they are in the waking-up-and-drowsy stage.

It's not easy to tell waking-up-and-drowsy from light sleep, but you can do it with practice. Your baby's eyes will be sleepily open, and they may fuss a bit to get your attention. Pick them up, talk, change their diaper, move around a bit, and let them become wide awake. If they do, it's feeding time. If they don't, let them sleep on your chest or put them back to bed. Does your baby want to eat right after they get up, or do they take their time waking up? Socialize a bit if that is what your baby wants, but don't make your baby wait to eat until they are worked up or exhausted from crying.

Supporting your baby in going to sleep allows them to sleep as long and as well as possible and, over time, evolve a feeding routine. Put your baby to bed when they are calm and drowsy. They may yawn, rub their eyes, pull at their ears, or show Figure 7.2 "I need a break" signs. They might fuss when you put them down, but if all goes well it will be a self-soothing kind of fussing. If at first they have trouble going to sleep, you may choose to do a bit of low-key soothing as outlined in Figure 7.4. Whatever method you choose, do it slowly and calmly to give it time to work.

Understand control with feeding

Because bottle feeding lends itself to being controlling, you must take particular care to trust your baby, follow their cues, and avoid putting yourself in control. As outlined in Figure 7.3, sit still and feed smoothly. Let your baby eat fast or slowly, much or little. Be interesting, not exciting or stimulating. Let them pause to rest during feeding. This is your social time. Offer the bottle again without getting pushy—you are checking to be sure they have had enough to eat.

Keeping your baby in control of feeding is particularly important for irritable, difficult-to-understand, and colicky babies—and it is particularly challenging. Those babies, through no fault of their own or anybody else, are born unpredictable, easy to upset, and hard to interpret. Keeping such babies in control of feeding helps them get more calm and understandable, but it takes patiently doing the same tuned-in feeding over and over again. On the other hand, if you happen to have a compliant, placid child, you may be able put yourself in control and get away with it—at least for a while. But sooner or later your child will come to resent being overruled and you will have trouble. If it doesn't happen for the first few years, I promise you it will when they are a teenager.

Maintain good feeding position

Your baby can lie on their back or their side to eat as long as you are careful to present the bottle from straight on; keep their ear, shoulder, and hip lined up; and keep their head higher than the rest of their body. Supporting your arm on a feeding pillow and your baby's head on your arm holds their head higher than the rest of their body, which helps swallowing and keeps formula out of their inner ear. Throughout the feeding, hold the bottle at an angle that continuously fills the nipple, keeps it comfortable in your baby's mouth, and allows them to eat smoothly. Those who worry unnecessarily about overfeeding babies and making them too fat make an issue of the angle and recommend having it be just steep enough to fill the nipple with formula or flat enough for pacing. If your baby likes those angles, use them; if they don't, don't.

Emptying the bottle creates a vacuum that has to be released to avoid slowing the rate of flow and collapsing the nipple.[18] Your baby may come off the nipple to let in air, or you may have to adjust the nipple ring to continuously let air into the bottle.

Hold your baby so they can clearly see your face. Newborns can only focus on objects that are a foot or so away and they gaze longest at faces. Your baby will look toward your face or just over your ear and then look away. Looking away gives them a break from all the excitement of eating and connecting with you. Keep looking and wait. After they settle down, they will look back, and you don't want to miss it!

Be wary of interference

This book is longer than I had hoped because I am forced to address interference. It takes so many forms and so many of those forms are subtle. Trusting your child with feeding means ignoring the advice of those who don't. Let's take a look at some interfering advice.

Feeding by the clock seems never to go away and managing children's eating is always with us. "Paced bottle-feeding" is gaining popularity even among lactation counselors and in WIC clinics. Pacing is interrupting bottle-feeding every three to five swallows—20 to 30 seconds—by stopping the flow of milk. Paced feeding levels the bottle with the nipple still in the baby's mouth until the nipple empties and the baby has to stop eating. Presumably that gets babies to eat more slowly, take breaks, and "reduce the risk of overfeeding." All of those reasons belong in the Figure 7.3 column, "You put *yourself* in control." Babies can be trusted to eat slowly (if they *enjoy* eating slowly), take breaks, and not overfeed themselves. How would you like to be interrupted every 30 seconds when you were trying to eat?

Interfering advice is often clothed in the term "responsive feeding" and is paradigm straddling rather than trust paradigm. Because it has elements of positive feeding, tactics labeled "responsive feeding" are often difficult to detect. You may have been given soothe-sleep advice: essentially to feed as a last resort after swaddling, shushing, swinging, diaper-changing. That is quite different from observing your baby's sleep states and feeding when they are calm and awake. You may have been advised to stop feeding your baby at the first sign they are finished, even if they are pausing to rest or socialize. Babies eat less with both soothe-sleep techniques and stopping at the first sign of satiety, but *less* is not what you want. You want your baby to eat *as much as is right for them.*

By the time you read this there are likely to be other sneaky ways of being controlling, so it is up to you to detect them. Consider *intent*: Is it to enhance the feeding relationship and your baby's enjoyment of eating and your enjoyment of feeding? Or is it to control how much your baby consumes?

FEEDING CAN GET DERAILED

While bottle-feeding an infant seems straightforward, there are many ways it can get derailed. Contrasting those going-wrong ways with the going-right ways we just considered will give you a greater understanding. Let me tell you about a classic study by Mary Ainsworth, a well-known developmental psychologist and pioneer in attachment studies. Dr. Ainsworth observed 26 mothers and their babies in the feeding situation.[19] Of the 26 mothers, 7 did well with feeding.

As long as the mothers paid attention to the baby's signals and guided feeding by those signals, the feedings were positive. However, when the mothers ignored what their babies told them and put themselves in control of feeding, the infants ate poorly. Although she did not measure how much the babies ate or what they weighed, Ainsworth did note that the overfed babies were heavier, and the babies who were fed arbitrarily or impatiently were underweight.[19]

Demand feeding

Seven of Ainsworth's mothers were sensitive to their babies' signals and fed skillfully. They presented the nipple so the baby could take it easily, fed smoothly, and they and their baby enjoyed each other.

Three mothers tried to get their babies on a schedule and their tactics interfered with establishing a feeding routine. They delayed feeding their hungry babies until they became over-hungry and upset. Feedings were tense and unhappy. Because the over-hungry babies had trouble settling down, they did not eat well and were soon again hungry.

Feeding errors

Four mothers seemed so eager to be finished caring for their babies that they put them down whenever they paused or smiled or fussed during the feeding. Some mothers appeared to want to feed in a hurry. The nipple holes were so big the babies choked and gagged and paused in the feeding, whereupon the mothers assumed they were full and terminated the feedings.

Five of the mothers tried to get their baby to eat past the point they indicated they were finished so they would sleep longer. In the latter case, the babies spit out the nipple, struggled, and tried to turn their heads to get away. But the mothers persisted in pushing the nipple into the baby's mouth and holding it there until the baby gave in and suckled. Needless to say, the feedings were tense and anxious.

LET YOUR BABY DETERMINE HOW MUCH TO EAT

Some parents choose to formula-feed so they can be sure their baby gets enough. You can tell that your baby is *getting* formula, but going by *how much* doesn't tell you if they are getting *enough*. The only way you can know they're getting enough is if they are satisfied after eating and they grow well, the same as with breastfeeding. Only your baby knows how much is enough, and you must go by what they tell you.

Babies vary in how much they need to eat

You can't predict how much a baby needs to eat. As I discussed in the Chapter 3 section, "Get comfortable with not knowing" page 79, the amount they eat can vary a great deal feeding-to-feeding and day-to-day.

Ignore charts on the formula package or the web that tell you by age how many ounces your baby needs per feeding. At any one feeding, let your baby eat until they show they have had enough, even if it is half or twice as much as another feeding—or half or twice as much as another baby! Make another part of a bottle if they want it. Stop feeding after only part of a bottle when they show they aren't interested in eating any more. While you will have to throw away that partially eaten bottle, my ESI colleague Peggy Crum has a suggestion for when your baby wants more than one bottle: Make an extra bottle for each feeding. If you don't use it, refrigerate it and use it to start the next feeding.

Guard against being cued by the bottle

Watching the level of formula go down in your baby's bottle can make you unconsciously guide feeding based on their emptying the bottle rather than how much they want to eat. Human Development and Family Studies professor Allison Ventura observed what happened with feeding when she took away the bottle-emptying information. She observed mothers feeding one day from a clear bottle, another day from a weighted, opaque bottle. Some mothers were equally attentive and responsive to their baby's cues with either bottle. Other mothers were more attentive and responsive to their baby's cues with the weighted, opaque bottle and less attentive and responsive when they could see the level of formula in the bottle. Babies of less-responsive mothers ate more.[20]

The baby's eating more is not the problem—or the solution. The problem is their eating more than they *want* and losing track of their internal cues of hunger and fullness. Unless you correct your ways with feeding, the tendency to eat based on information coming from you can stay with your child throughout life and undermine their ability to eat the amount that is right for them. The moral of the story: Tune in to your baby! Being able to see how much your baby eats can make you controlling with feeding. To guard against that, keep your baby in control of feeding (Figure 7.3).

Respect the difference among babies

Your baby's food intake depends on their activity patterns, metabolism, growth rate, and body size and shape. Those, in turn, are predominantly determined by genetics. You can't tell by looking at them whether a baby will eat a little or a lot. Studies of young infants by Harvard nutritionist Jean Mayer showed that the fattest babies tended to eat the least and were the least active, the leanest babies ate the most and were the most active.[21] The point? These tendencies are constitutionally determined and can be changed only with extreme effort and at a high risk of being destructive.

As I point out in detail in Chapter 10, Feeding your Older Baby and Almost-Toddler, a bit of mistaken advice that simply does not go away is that babies need to be put on solid foods when they take 32 ounces or more of formula. Wrong! A 15-pound baby may be only three months old and eat that much, and that is too early to start solid foods.

Day-to-day intake varies

A Texas anthropologist who kept a daily record of a baby boy's food intake from age one week to nine months observed his formula intake at age two months to range from 9 to 15 ounces a day; at age four months it ranged from 10 to 35 ounces a day. His formula intake dropped off when he was started on solid foods. As he took more solid food, he took less formula, but his formula intake continued to fluctuate.

Although the little boy's food intake was highly variable, his growth was smooth and consistent. It was also interesting that while his growth was average—right at the 50th percentile—his average formula intake was relatively low.[22]

I worked with a mother of a baby who needed to gain weight so he could have surgery for a heart defect. She was tremendously reassured by learning about babies' fluctuating food intake. It helped her keep her spirits up when her baby had his natural small-eating days. It also helped her to resist being pressured by others into trying to get him to eat more than he took voluntarily.

LET YOUR BABY DETERMINE HOW OFTEN TO EAT

As with quantity, give your baby control of how *often* they eat. You may be asked about the number of times your baby eats in a day or even *told* how many times! Parents appear startled by the inquiry and will respond with something like, "Well, let me see, she wakes up in the morning and wants to be fed, that's one time, and then sometimes she wants to be fed again about 9:00, but sometimes she doesn't, and then. . . ." They simply don't know. Good for them! If you regularly wash a batch of nipples and bottles, you will have a general idea of the number but, beyond that, you may not know. It is as it needs to be.

Your baby will eat as often as they need to. As they get bigger, when their stomach holds more and they are able to digest more at any one time, they will eat less frequently. By the time they are 12 to 15 months old, they will probably eat about six times a day: three meals and three snacks.

Eating at night

Your baby wakes up at night because they are hungry and need to eat. If you don't struggle with it, it will be easier to get up! The more accepting and responsive you can be with your baby, the faster they will mature and the sooner they will get to the point where they can sleep through the night. By age six months, 60 percent of babies sleep for six-hour stretches at night, with girls and formula-fed babies sleeping longer.[23]

Don't give cereal to hasten sleeping through the night—it doesn't help and can create a host of problems. You can be most helpful to your baby with sleep issues by paying attention from the beginning to their sleep cycles and putting them to bed when they are drowsy but not asleep. While it is tempting and rewarding to rock or feed your baby to sleep, you will also be planting the seeds for later sleep problems. You are teaching them that they can't go to sleep without your help, and they will continue to demand that help as they get older. On the other hand, waiting to put your baby to bed until they are over-tired and over-stimulated can make it hard for them to go to sleep.

YOU WON'T SPOIL YOUR BABY

Parents often worry that being accepting and responsive to their baby's appeals will spoil them: They will ask all the more for attention. The opposite is true. Babies who regularly get their needs met demand less attention, not more.

Understand child development

Your baby emerges from the undefined world of the womb into one full of sights, sounds, and movement. To keep from being overwhelmed by all the commotion, the newborn has to establish homeostasis: screen out enough of the stimulation so they can remain calm. That allows them to avoid getting upset or going back to sleep to get away from it all. You help them with homeostasis by paying attention and doing what they need you to do. You let them sleep until they show signs of waking up. Then you help them be calm and wide awake for feeding by holding them securely with a little wiggle room, keeping their head higher than the rest of their body for feeding, and talking and stroking in ways they enjoy. Hold your baby's head at the base of their skull. Holding higher stimulates an arching reflex. Babies show they are calm and wide awake by relaxing, appearing bright-eyed, and more-or-less looking at you. Actually, they look past your ear.

After two or three months, your baby is ready for attachment and does best when they can connect with you. They smile and babble to get your attention and you smile and babble back. They reach and you reach back. Or you start the smiling, talking, and reaching and give them time to respond before you continue the "conversation." Following your baby's lead and feeding the way they want to be fed is the very best thing you can do to let your baby achieve homeostasis and attachment.

CHALLENGING BABIES

Ask any parent with two or more children: No two babies are alike. Babies vary in size, shape, temperament, the ability to remain calm in the midst of commotion, activity level, physical sturdiness, and efficiency of eating. I could go on. Each baby offers particular rewards. Each parent is more challenged by some temperaments than others. It will be sheer luck if you get a comfortable fit between your baby's personality characteristics and yours. If you are a mild-mannered person, an aggressive, active baby may challenge you considerably. Or vice versa. Help your baby do well with sleeping and eating, but don't try to change them. To appreciate and enjoy your baby, you may have to examine how you think and feel about how things *should* go with feeding and sleeping.

The Chapter 7 sections, "Vulnerable babies; controlling advice" and "Babies who require tube-feeding," discuss feeding challenges on a whole different level. Vulnerable babies are capable of eating as much as they need; babies with certain medical conditions are almost always able to eat, but not as much as they need, and may need to be tube-fed. For both groups, as with all other babies, it's about trusting your baby to eat to the best of their ability. So do what you do with other babies. Observe their sleep states and feed when they are calm and awake. Guide both bottle-feeding and tube-feeding based on information coming from them, being careful not to be controlling.

DIARRHEA

Frequent liquid stools can reflect a change in bowel habits or an illness. A change in bowel habits can be caused by teething, a dietary change, or who knows what else and is simply a nuisance. Disposable diapers help sop up the mess, but often time is the only solution. Despite their runny stools, children's appetites are generally unchanged.

Norovirus is another story. It can cause dehydration, especially if the child is also vomiting, has fever, or both. If dehydration goes too far, the child may have to be hospitalized and put on intravenous fluids. While this is serious, it is unusual for dehydration to get to the point of being a medical emergency. Norovirus is highly contagious, so consider washing your baby's hands after you have been out and about. They touch more than you realize: shopping carts, toys that get dropped, strangers' hands …

Norovirus is likely to spoil your baby's appetite, but if you keep calm and don't pressure them to eat, their appetite will recover nicely. Talk with your health care provider about taking care of your child when they have a stomach and intestinal virus. You are likely to be advised to offer a commercial oral rehydration therapy fluid (ORT) and feed as usual to the extent of your child's hunger and appetite. ORT brand names include Pedialyte, Infalyte, Nutramax and Rehydralyte. It is no longer recommended to stop feeding while your child is ill or substituting some other dietary concoction like the traditional BRAT diet (bananas, rice, applesauce, tea, and toast). If the BRAT diet is new to you, forget you ever heard it! It doesn't work and is nutritionally inferior to your baby's formula.

Don't substitute fruit juice or drink, sports drinks, Jell-O, soda or any other liquid for the ORT or the formula. Any of them can worsen diarrhea by allowing undigested sugar into the child's colon, which in turn attracts water and nourishes undesirable bacteria. The commonly used apple juice is particularly undesirable because it contains fructose, which is poorly digested, and sorbitol, which isn't digested at all. Both fructose and sorbitol attract fluids into the intestine and make stools more liquid.

ENJOY YOUR ADVENTURE

I hope you emerge from this long and detailed chapter feeling confident about your decision to formula-feed. I also hope that many if not most times you and your baby are on the same wavelength with feeding. If you have a challenging baby, those sweet times will be *moments*, but those moments will increase with your devoted attention. Through it all, remember that you are special to your baby. No one else can do it better.

Here is a summary of this chapter's basic points:

- Enjoy your baby.
- Take care of yourself: Eat well, drink enough, rest enough, and avoid getting physically over- stressed.
- Choose the nipples, bottles, and formula that are right for you and your baby. Avoid changes if you can.
- Make yourself comfortable as you cuddle and feed your baby. Look at them, hold them in a good position, and talk and touch gently in a way that lets them relax and stay awake.
- Follow sDOR: Go by your baby's cues to feed them when they are hungry and fully awake; let them eat how much, how fast, and how enthusiastically they want.
- Keep the feeding smooth and steady. Stop only when your baby pauses and rests, then socialize, wait, and let them go back to eating if they want to.
- Time feedings based on your baby's sleep rhythms. Wait to feed until they are fully awake; put them to bed when they are drowsy.
- Enjoy your baby.

REFERENCES

1. Meek JY. Policy Statement: breastfeeding and the use of human milk. *Pediatrics*. 2022. doi:10.1542/peds.2022-057988
2. Wright P. The development of differences in the feeding behaviour of bottle and breast fed human infants from birth to two months. *Behavioural Processes*. 1980;51:1–20.
3. Rempel LA. Relationships between types of father breastfeeding support and breastfeeding outcomes. *Maternal & Child Nutrition*. 2017. doi:doi.org/10.1111/mcn.12337
4. Lakshman R. Mothers' experiences of bottle-feeding: a systematic review of qualitative and quantitative studies. *Archives of Disease in Childhood*. 2009;94:596–601.
5. Sigman-Grant M. Microwave heating of infant formula: a dilemma resolved. *Pediatrics*. 1992;90:412–415.
6. American Academy of Pediatrics Committee on Nutrition. Hypoallergenic infant formulas. *Pediatrics*. 2000;106:346–349.
7. Suen AA. Developmental exposure to phytoestrogens found in soy: new findings and clinical implications. *Biochemical Pharmacology*. 2022. doi:doi.org/10.1016/j.bcp.2021.114848
8. Hyams JS. Effect of infant formula on stool characteristics of young infants. *Pediatrics*. 1995;95:50–54.
9. Clark MB. Fluoride use in caries prevention in the primary care setting. *Pediatrics*. 2020. doi:10.1542/peds.2020-034637
10. Labiner-Wolfe J. Infant formula-handling education and safety. *Pediatrics*. 2008;122:S85–590.
11. Davisse-Paturet C. Use of partially hydrolysed formula in infancy and incidence of eczema, respiratory symptoms or food allergies in toddlers from the ELFE cohort. *Pediatric Allergy and Immunology*. 2019;30:614–623.
12. Lucassen PL. Effectiveness of treatments for infantile colic: systematic review. *BMJ*. 1998;316:1563–1569.
13. Mennella JA. Early milk feeding influences taste acceptance and liking during infancy. *Am J Clin Nutr*. Sep 2009;90:780s–788s.
14. Cerniogl o K. Infant feeding practices and parental perceptions during the 2022 United States infant formula shortage crisis. *BMC Pediatrics*. 2023. doi:10.1186/s12887-023-04132-9
15. Friel JK. Eighteen-month follow-up of infants fed evaporated milk formula. *Can J Public Health*. 1999;90:240–243.
16. Task Force on Sudden Infant Death Syndrome. SIDS and other sleep-related infant deaths: updated 2016 recommendations for a safe infant sleeping environment. *Pediatrics*. 2016. doi:10.1542/peds.2016-2938
17. Lawrence RM. Normal growth, growth faltering, and obesity in breastfed infants. In: Lawrence RA, Lawrence RM, eds. *Breastfeeding (Ninth Edition)*. Elsevier; 2022:298–325.
18. Ross E. Supporting oral feeding skills through bottle selection. *Perspectives on Swallowing and Swallowing Disorders (Dysphagia)*. 2015;24:50–57.
19. Ainsworth MDS. Some contemporary patterns of mother-infant interaction in the feeding situation. In: Ambrose A, ed. *Stimulation in Early Infancy*. Academic Press; 1969:133–170.
20. Ventura AK. A pilot study comparing opaque, weighted bottles with conventional, clear bottles for infant feeding. *Appetite*. 2015;85:178–184.
21. Rose HE. Activity, calorie intake, fat storage, and the energy balance of infants. *Pediatrics*. 1968;41:18–29.
22. Adair LS. The infant's ability to self-regulate caloric intake: a case study. *J Am Diet Assoc*. 1984;84:543–546.
23. Pennestri M-H. Uninterrupted infant sleep, development, and maternal mood. *Pediatrics*. 2018. doi:10.1542/peds.2017-4330

CHAPTER 10

Feeding Your Older Baby and Almost-Toddler

Parents can have misgivings about starting solid foods with their baby. Is it because they feel responsible for getting their child to eat "healthy food?" Is it because they have heard stories about picky eaters and worry that solid food refusal—or less-than enthusiastic acceptance—is the beginning of the end with enjoyable feeding? The many books promoting the one-size-fits-all approach of "baby-led weaning" tacitly build on those fears by promising problem-free feeding throughout life. It is an empty promise: This stage will not make or break you with feeding. Problem-free feeding depends on following Satter Division of Responsibility in Feeding (sDOR) throughout the growing-up years.

It's too bad that parents find this transition stage in feeding so worrisome, because it can be a lot of fun. I am captivated by watching babies eat, and my audiences are charmed by videos of babies being spoon-fed. It seems that when they are in the driver's seat parents get worried. Relax. You've got this.

IN THIS CHAPTER

This chapter has a lot of detail, so let's cut to the chase. Well, two chases. First, introducing solid foods is about leadership and acceptance. You show your baby what they have to learn with food and eating and accept their reaction while they learn it. They may be enthusiastic, offended, or bored; they may eat or not eat. To be entertained as well as informed, skip ahead to the feeding stories in the section "Be prepared for adventure," page 326. Trust that when you provide your baby with continued opportunities to learn, they will get around to eating. In adhering to the giving-autonomy part of sDOR you are demonstrating love. Earlier, you showed your love by feeding on demand. Now you show your love by supporting your baby's sense of *agency*—their feeling of being able to determine whether, how, and how much they eat.

The second chase is about the mechanics of choosing feeding methods and food that are in concert with your child's developmental readiness. At first their oral-motor ability lets them eat smooth and soft food. As their ability to control their mouth and fingers matures, you follow their lead to offer soft, then thicker and lumpier food, then small-to-gradually larger pieces of soft family food. When they can eat with their fingers, you let them join in with family meals and eat soft family food.

The third section of the chapter starting with "Choosing food," page 333, addresses food and supplemental nutrients. All of it is intended to reassure you: What you eat is okay for your baby; you just need to modify the texture to match their oral-motor ability.

THE GOAL IS FAMILY MEALS

Introducing your baby to solid foods is a trip with a destination: family meals. You start this chapter with a baby and end it with a child. It boggles the mind! Your baby graduates from cuddling and breastfeeding or bottle-feeding to sitting up with you at family meals and finger-feeding themself soft family food. To remind you of what I said in Chapter 6, by breastfeeding, I mean breastmilk fed directly from the breast. By bottle-feeding, I mean expressed breastmilk—human milk—and/or formula-fed from a bottle or from a supplemental nursing system.

During this transition stage, your baby's formula and/or breastmilk from the bottle is gradually replaced with solid food and drinking breastmilk and/or formula from the cup. After they regularly join in with family meals, your baby may have pasteurized milk from the cup at mealtime. Nipple-feeding of breastmilk and/or formula away from mealtime can be extended beyond the time they start participating in family meals. You can nipple-feed for snacks or at the early-morning and/or before-bedtime feedings. Once your child is eating family meals, the nipple feeding is an add-on to your child's eating and no longer the main event. That is, nipple-feeding is no longer your baby's primary nutritional support as it was earlier. Continue to use formula or breastmilk for bottles, even if your child takes pasteurized milk at mealtime. Taking several ounces of pasteurized milk all at one time without eating anything else at the same time can still set up a tough and hard-to-digest curd in your older baby's stomach.

Your child might take two weeks, two months, or two years for the transition from nipple-feeding to family meals, depending on whether they are coping with developmental or neuromuscular issues. The stages in oral-motor development are the same; what differs is how rapidly those stages come along. The essential bit is introducing solid food based on your child's social, emotional, physical, and oral-motor readiness.

Now is the time to start having family meals if you aren't already. Adjust your attitude! I am not talking about 18 years of broiled chicken and steamed broccoli and being "naughty" (by conventional standards) by eating pizza in front of the TV on Friday night. I am talking about having meals made up of food you truly enjoy all week long—not just food you *want* to want or have been told you *should* want. You may have pizza on movie night—or any other time—only you won't have to be naughty to do it. You will just have it.

sDOR FOR OLDER BABIES

Feed based on sDOR. As before, your child's being a Competent Eater depends on your connecting with them with feeding: by getting on the same wavelength. Your tuned-in devotion will allow you to move through this transition phase in feeding in an enjoyable and nurturing way. Because spoon-feeding lends itself to being controlling, you do have to be particularly careful to follow your baby's feeding cues and reactions to what you do. You are learning right along with them what giving autonomy with feeding is all about.

As you recall, with nipple-feeding you were responsible only for choosing breastmilk or formula and working out your mode of delivery. Your baby was responsible for *how much*—and *everything else*: how often, how fast, how continuously, how skillfully. Now you are following your baby's increasingly regular eating routine to work toward the pattern of family meals and snacks.

You are still responsible for *what* to offer your child to eat. *When* and *where* you feed your child is in transition.

Your child is *still* and *always* responsible for *how much* and *whether* to eat the foods you offer them.

Older babies eat less often and become increasingly predictable in their eating times. You support that predictability by feeding at their less-frequent intervals. As they get older, those intervals ever-so-gradually lengthen, and their hunger rhythms begin to match family mealtimes. You begin to offer sit-down snacks to tide them over for family meals and begin to let them wait briefly to eat rather than feeding them the instant they show they are hungry. Those sit-down snacks can be nipple-feedings or they can be "big child" food.

At this as at every other stage, your child's being a Competent Eater doesn't mean they enthusiastically eat everything that is put before them, including their vegetables, although your almost-toddler might. It means, instead, that they feel positive about food and eating. They eat as much as they want and need to grow well. They enjoy family meals and are comfortable with the food there—whether or not they eat it. For more, review the Chapter 1 section, "Attitudes and behaviors, not *what* and *how much*," page 3. A child who is raised well with eating can eat—and enjoy—the food that is in the world and be healthy because of it.

sDOR supports your baby's sense of agency

As before, offering solid food is far more than getting food into your child. It is about their relationship with you and about the way they feel about themself. It has to do with our universal need for *agency*: a sense of control, of knowing on a deep level that what we feel and want matters and that we can work things out with other people. From the first, you gave your baby a nonverbal sense of agency by following sDOR. Their agency is protected when you wait for them to be developmentally ready to offer solid food. Their agency is reinforced when you offer a spoonful of food and wait for them to lean forward and open up before you feed them—or when you take no for an answer when they lean back and turn away. Your accepting their message is nonverbal, but it is nonetheless a powerful message: I see and hear you, and I respect what you want.

Consider the tilt

Marsha Dunn Klein talks with parents about the *tilt* in feeding. Klein is a Tucson, Arizona, Licensed Occupational Therapist, consultant, and author of feeding therapy materials. The *tilt* is the way parents physically position themselves relative to their child during feeding. Klein points out that when parents put themselves in control, the tilt tends to be toward the child. The parent leans forward, encouraging, pushing, even forcing. The child leans back, considering, avoiding, resisting. The desirable tilt is when parent and child meet in the middle. The parent shows the food and the child gives the parent permission to feed them by staying upright or leaning forward and opening their mouth. When the parent stops leaning forward and holds their body upright, the child is freed up to come forward.

WHEN, WHAT, AND HOW

Most babies are ready to start eating solids at around age six months, but that readiness can occur anywhere from four to seven months or even months or years later. It depends on whether your baby is coping with developmental or neuromuscular issues. Wait to see signs of developmental readiness before you start, but don't wait long after that. Missing times of developmental readiness makes it harder for your baby to learn to eat and can affect their eating for years to come.[1]

With the exception of iron-fortified baby cereal, you can use family food for the whole transition from starting solid foods to your baby's sitting up at family meals and eating family food. This chapter's detail about food gives ideas about what to offer your baby to eat.

Starting solids is about letting your baby learn to eat; it is not about getting food into your baby. Keep your baby in control. Follow their lead. Wait for signs of developmental readiness to start offering solid food. Seat them so they see, lean forward and back, turn their head, open up, swallow easily, and indicate yes or no to food. Offer the spoon and wait for them to open up before you feed. Let them eat as much or as little as they want and stop feeding when they indicate they have had enough.

When to start solid food

Figure 10.1 on the next two pages gives an overview of solids feeding from first introduction to the family meal. The tilde sign (~) means that ages are approximate. Text in italics indicates oral/motor development.

Your baby's readiness cues will come along at their own pace, but they *will* come along. Offering solids will not hasten their oral-motor development. Your approximately five- to eight-month-old baby will be ready to eat semisolid food when they can sit up and open their mouth when they see the spoon coming. Your baby will give you social and emotional clues as well: They start to take an interest in what goes on outside of the two of you. That is their window of developmental opportunity. Postponing introducing solid foods beyond when they are developmentally ready can get in the way of their learning to eat.[1]

FIGURE 10.1: WHAT YOUR BABY CAN DO AND HOW TO FEED THEM

AGE	BODY CONTROL/ ORAL-MOTOR CAPABILITIES	MANNER OF FEEDING
Birth to ~6 months	Cuddles Roots for nipple *Sucks* *Swallows liquids*	Cuddling and nipple-feeding
~5 to 8 months	Sits with minimal support or alone Keeps head straight when sitting Follows food with eyes Opens mouth for spoon Takes an interest beyond you *Closes lips over spoon* *Moves semisolid food to back of tongue* *Sends food straight down their throat*	**Stage 1 Food: Semisolids** Spoon-feeding of smooth, semisolid food Cuddling and nipple-feeding
~6 to 10 months	Sits alone Chases food on high-chair tray Palms food (palmar grasp) but may not be able to let go Sucks food from between fingers or scrapes into mouth *Positions food in mouth* *Pushes food to jaws with tongue* *Munches, mashes food with up-and-down movement* *Swallows gradually* *Drinks from a cup but loses a lot out the sides*	**Stage 2 Food: Thicker, lumpier food from the spoon** Spoon-feeding of thicker and lumpier food Self-finger-feeding of thicker, lumpier food: "If it hangs together, it's finger food." Cup drinking Cuddling and nipple-feeding

AGE	BODY CONTROL/ ORAL-MOTOR CAPABILITIES	MANNER OF FEEDING
~7 to 12 months	Sits alone easily Palmar changing to pincer grasp Wants to self-feed *Bites off food* *Moves food side-to-side in mouth, pausing with food on the center of the tongue* *Chews with rotary motion* *Swallows gradually* *Begins curving lip around cup*	**Stage 3 Food: Small pieces of soft finger food; crackers and cereal; food to bite off and chew** Spoon- or self-finger-feeding of thick, lumpy food and pieces of soft food Drinks from a cup with assistance Losing interest in nipple-feeding at mealtime
~8 to 18 months	Can pick up small pieces of food (pincer grasp) Is interested in family food Wants to self-feed Wants to join in with the family meal Wants to do it themselves *Curves lip around cup* *Getting better at controlling food in mouth* *Getting better at chewing*	**Stage 4: Easy-to-chew and easy-to-swallow family food** Self-finger-feeding soft table foods Can hold and drink from an open or covered toddler cup No longer nipple-feeds at mealtime Needs a between-meal snack May be nipple-feeding of breastmilk or formula or a "big child" snack

When to offer the nipple-feeding

Feed your child when they ask to be fed and start with breast- or formula-feeding. Until they discover that solid foods are *food* and enjoy eating them, being desperate to eat will make them less patient. Later on, you can start by offering only part of the nipple-feeding. Eventually you can skip the before-solids nipple-feeding altogether and offer breastmilk or formula from the cup. You can still offer a nipple-feeding after the solids meal, but your baby will probably not be very interested. A typical pattern at this stage is to continue to offer breast- or formula-feedings at snack times as well as first thing in the morning and just before bedtime. It is all in transition.

What to offer stage by stage

Take a look at Figure 10.2. Stage 1, getting started with semi-solids from the spoon, is clearly defined as is Stage 4, eating easy-to-chew and easy-to-swallow family food at the family meal. Stages 2 and 3 are less clear and are likely to drift together as you respond to your baby's readiness. As your baby's swallowing and finger-feeding progress, you will find yourself offering thicker and lumpier food and then pieces of soft table food. Your baby will push themselves along to pick up food with their fingers and munch and later chew it with their gums. From Stage 1 through Stage 4 you will be in constant transition, and there is no predictable timetable. Depending on your baby's enthusiasm and ability to eat solid food, they will progress through these stages rapidly or slowly. By seven months, some babies are sitting up at the family meal and finger-feeding themselves pieces of soft family food; other babies get to that point at age two years or even later.

Stages 1 and 2 are for oral-motor development. Think of those stages as fun and games. Start by offering Stage 1 iron- and zinc-fortified wheat, oat, or barley infant cereal mixed with breastmilk or formula. This is a handy first offering because you can begin by making it smooth and relatively thin, then work up making it thicker and lumpier as your baby's mouth matures. Work your way together through Stage 2 thicker and then lumpy cereal and other foods that can be roughly fork-mashed, such as cooked vegetables and soft fresh, canned, or frozen fruit. A baby food mill or grinder works, but only briefly because the texture is pretty smooth. Developmentally, your baby needs lumpy food to stimulate their oral-motor development. Regular applesauce with or without sugar is ready to eat and is almost as smooth as baby food applesauce. Wait three to five days after you add each new food to see if your baby reacts to it before you introduce another. By Stage 2, you will find yourself putting Cheerios on your baby's high-chair tray and they will be happily chasing them and trying to pick them up with their palmar and then pincer grasp. A palmar grasp is holding food between the fingers and the palm; a pincer grasp is holding it between the thumb and forefinger.

Stage 3 is merely a change in texture from mashed-and-lumpy to chopped-and-small pieces. Your baby will increasingly be able to eat with their fingers, and you can offer dry cereal, crackers, and strips of toast. You can offer soft diced fresh, canned, or frozen fruit. Your baby might even enjoy eating frozen peas slightly thawed or straight from the freezer!

FIGURE 10.2: WHAT YOUR BABY CAN EAT STAGE BY STAGE

Nipple-feeding

Human and/or iron-fortified infant formula

Stage 1 Food: Semisolids from the spoon

Iron- and zinc-fortified single-ingredient baby cereal mixed thin to medium with breastmilk or iron-fortified formula

Avoid rice cereal

Breastmilk and/or iron-fortified formula

Stage 2 Food: Thicker, lumpier food from the spoon

Well-cooked, mashed, or milled vegetables and fruits

Mashed potatoes, cut-up pasta

Scrambled eggs or fork-mashed hard-boiled eggs

Soft, easily broken down dry cereal such as Cheerios or Corn Chex

Breastmilk and/or iron-fortified formula

Stage 3 Food: Small pieces (peas-sized) of soft finger food; food to bite off and chew

Chopped cooked vegetables

Chopped canned or cooked fruits

Cut-up, peeled, soft raw fruit (e.g., bananas, peaches, melon)

Tender, juicy chopped meats

Cheese

Chopped hard-cooked eggs

Mashed or chopped cooked dried beans

Strips of bread, toast, tortilla

Crackers, dry cereals

Breastmilk and/or iron-fortified formula from the cup

Stage 4: Easy-to-chew and easy-to-swallow family food

Everything from the family meal that is soft and can be cut up

Cut-up pieces of smooth foods that can cause choking: grapes, cherry tomatoes, hot dogs

Whole pasteurized milk

Stage 3 blends into Stage 4, when your baby is ready for food from family meals that can be soft and cut up. Teeth are unnecessary. In fact, your baby is unlikely to get teeth until they are 18 to 24 months old—long after they are well-established on family food. Don't add salt, but don't feel you have to avoid it, either. Your baby's sodium intake will gradually increase until they are eating the same amount of sodium as the rest of the family.

For the first time in Stages 3 and 4 your baby depends on the nutrients in solid food to supplement the nutrients in their breastmilk or formula. Developmentally, they give you a clue to this change by insisting on feeding themself: They have become what I call an *almost-toddler*. Despite the mess, it is so important to let them. They care deeply about feeding themself and will struggle or refuse to eat if you try to feed them.

Offer juice starting in Stage 4, when your child's breastmilk or formula intake decreases and they need another good source of vitamin C. Orange, grapefruit, pineapple, and tomato juice all contain vitamin C. Apple and grape juice are poor sources of vitamin C unless they are fortified, and both baby-food and regular apple and grape juice are high in heavy metals. Give juice in a cup, not the bottle. Using the bottle will contribute to getting them stuck on it. Offer juice only once a day—at breakfast or for a snack. Offer fruit *juice*, not fruit *drink*. Fruit *drink* contains a small amount of juice and is essentially sugared, flavored, and nutrient-added water.

Baby-led spoon-feeding

Take a look at Figure 10.3, "Feeding your baby solid foods," for a step-by-step description of spoon-feeding your transitional baby. It is all about keeping your baby in control when you offer them solid foods. The detail is to help you avoid doing anything that interferes with your baby's agency.

Your baby loves you as much as ever and wants you nearby. But now instead of being interested in just you, they become interested in others and in the outside world. Eating solid food is part of that interest. Your baby is ready for solid foods when they can sit up, hold their head straight, and open their mouth when they see the spoon coming. Teeth are unnecessary.

Keep your baby in control of whether and how much when you offer them solid foods. Sit them up straight so they can lean forward and open their mouth or lean back and close their mouth. Keep their head straight so they can swallow well. Give them time to show you their feeding cues. Use small spoonfuls at first. After a while, you will feed at their tempo and they may demand bigger spoonfuls. Don't make your baby fuss to get you to pay attention.

FIGURE 10.3: FEEDING YOUR BABY SOLID FOODS

Starting solids is about letting your baby learn to eat, not about getting food into your baby. At first, your baby doesn't know what a spoon is, and they don't know that solid food is—well—food! Take your time. If your baby enjoys eating solid food, feed them. If not, offer again another day.

- Respect your baby's cues to keep them in control with solids-feeding.
- At first, give part or all of a nipple-feeding before you start offering solid food.
- Seat your baby up straight in a high chair that fits them.
- Use a shallow-bowled, long-handled spoon that fits your baby's mouth.
- Sit right in front of your baby. Looking directly ahead lets your baby swallow better.
- Offer a small amount of food on the spoon—about a quarter teaspoon. Too much can make your baby gag.
- Don't crowd your baby; hold the spoon about a foot away.
- Wait for your baby to look and open their mouth before you put a bit of food on their lips.
- Only put food in your baby's mouth if they look and open their mouth wide.
- Offer spoonfuls as slowly or as fast as your baby wants to eat.
- Let your baby touch the food. Mess is all about learning to eat.
- Talk with your baby, keep them company, but don't be exciting or entertaining.
- Stop offering food as soon as your baby shows they are done. They will stop opening their mouth or turn away.

All babies are different

- Some babies learn faster than others. Your baby might love cereal right away.
- Some babies learn slower than others. Give your baby lots of chances to learn. They will.
- Some babies don't *ever* like being fed from the spoon. Keep offering but take no for an answer.
- Your baby might not eat solid foods until they can eat with their fingers.

Your baby may take to eating from the spoon right away, or they may be entirely uninterested. If they aren't interested, continue to offer a solids feeding every few days, but don't insist. If you respect their feeding cues, your baby will learn faster, not slower. Babies—like the rest of us—do better when they have a sense of agency.

Babies and young children eat as much as they want, and they don't eat much. For them, a nutritionally adequate amount is about a tablespoon. More, of course, is fine, and less is still okay. A lick or a swallow or none at all may be all your child wants to eat.

I DON'T LIKE IT, I NEVER TRIED IT

Your child will readily eat some food, experiment with others, and ignore still others. I am carefully avoiding saying they will *refuse* food. *Refuse* implies rejection. They are not rejecting food; they are just not interested. They only *refuse* in response to pressure. Don't look for ways to persuade them to eat or try to find food they *will* eat. You are giving them the opportunity to *learn*, not getting them to eat.

I copied the title of this section from a journal article by Leanne Birch, then a University of Illinois psychology professor, who established that children of all ages learn to eat unfamiliar food with time and repeated neutral exposure. *Repeated exposure* would be matter-of-factly making the food available to your child whenever it shows up at regular meals and snacks. *Neutral* would be avoiding pressure or encouragement of any kind: being absolutely willing to take no for an answer. A warning: The term *repeated neutral exposure* gets misused in control literature as "repeated neutral exposure to increase food acceptance." It is a contradiction in terms to present the food again and again with the *intention* of *getting* the child to eat it. Rather, the child is getting *accustomed* to the food and someday they will likely eat it.

Breastfed babies are less skeptical of unfamiliar food than formula-fed babies, presumably because they have been exposed to the flavors in their mother's breastmilk.[2] Babies who have been fed extensively hydrolyzed formulas are more comfortable with savory, bitter, and sour flavors.[3]

Even babies notice when they are offered something new and take time to become accustomed to it. Typically, your baby will taste the new food and not want to eat any more of it. In fact, that might be the end of the meal, as I discovered to my dismay when I offered my granddaughter Emma peaches in the midst of a successful cereal meal. Since a seven-month-old doesn't have the mental ability to say to herself, "white, cereal; orange, peaches," I couldn't think of any way to reassure her that the next bite would be cereal and more to her liking! It was tempting to slip a little into her mouth to prove my point, but I knew better: mustn't force or trick. Since then, I have learned to put a bit on a baby's lips to tell them the next spoonful will be different.

By the next meal, Emma was willing to eat again and a couple of weeks later she was eating peaches enthusiastically. Truth be told, she was also more willing to experiment when her mother fed her than when I did. Children do better with eating when they are fed by someone they know very well. The moral of the story: Don't stop offering the ignored food or your baby won't learn. They may need 5 or 10 or an infinite number of exposures in as many meals to get accustomed to the flavor, but they will get so they eat most foods. Don't limit your child's menu to what they readily accept, or they won't get the opportunity to learn to enjoy a variety of foods.

PUTTING IT ALL TOGETHER

This brings us to family meals and what to do about breast- and/or formula-feeding.

Family meals

Stage 4 children—those consuming family food—do better nutritionally than those who are dependent on baby food.[4] Nutritionists disapprove of the fact that those early family-food eaters consume pizza and French fries, but pizza and French fries provide nutrients babies need. Along with the pizza and French fries, surveys show that parents do well with providing a variety of food, even a variety of vegetables.[5]

Even though we are talking about feeding children, with respect to meal-planning, you come first. Plan and prepare meals for *yourself* and include your child in *your* meal. Your child is learning to eat the food you eat; you are not learning to eat off the high-chair tray! Have your meals be *possible, practical, familiar,* and *enjoyable* for *you.* Your child's nutritional status depends on what you routinely *offer*, not on what you *get* them to eat. In fact, trying to *get* your child to eat will spoil their eating enjoyment and impair their nutritional status. Offer regular and reliable family meals made up of the array of food *you enjoy*. Trust your child to pick and choose from what you offer and learn to eat the food you eat.

The Chapter 2 section, "Master family meals," page 56, emphasizes being realistic about planning and preparing family meals, including telling you how to be *considerate without catering*, both for your child and for adults at mealtime. Chapter 5, Discover the Joy of Eating, talks about being relaxed and positive about your own eating. You can only take another person, even an infant, as far as you have gone yourself. To trust your child to know how much to eat and to learn to eat what they need from family meals, you have to trust your own instinctive ability to manage eating.

Weaning

Weaning started when you first introduced solid food and concludes when your child is sitting up at family meals, eating family food, and drinking from the cup. You can continue to breast- or formula-feed your child beyond that point, but it's time to stop feeding on demand, where you drop everything to respond to your child's hunger cues. Now, it's time for structure. At meals offer breastmilk, formula, or whole milk in a cup. Offer any breast- or formula-feeding as a sit-down snack, or graduate to offering big-child sit-down snacks between meals. The idea of structure is to allow your child to arrive at family mealtimes hungry but not famished. Don't put pasteurized milk in the bottle, even if your child has it at mealtime. At meals, other food dilutes it and makes it digestible; on its own, pasteurized milk sets up a tough, cheese-like, hard-to-digest curd in your baby's stomach.

Weaning means giving up thinking of your child as a baby. Depending on whether things have gone well in these first few months, you will be more or less ready to do that. For a variety of reasons, it may have taken a while for nipple-feeding to go smoothly, and your baby's solids-readiness cues are slow to appear. For both of your sakes, consider delaying starting solid foods and getting in a few more weeks of cuddly nipple-feedings.

Weaning from the breast or bottle will be less heart-rending if you regard it as adding on rather than taking away. You wean more and more at each stage of solid food introduction. By Stage 4, your child will be joining in with family meals: drinking from the cup; eating a variety of foods they enjoy; and taking delight from tasting, squishing, mashing, munching, and swallowing. You are as important as ever, but in a different way. Your eating with your child is critical. They will be happier and more secure and therefore more comfortable about exploring new food.

To belabor the point, continuing to breast- or bottle-feed on demand after the transition period interferes with children's learning to eat because they aren't hungry at meals. There are reasons parents are reluctant to give up nipple-feeding. The child doesn't drink much milk and parents become alarmed. Or a bout of teething cuts down on the child's appetite for a time and alarmed parents resort to the bottle. Or parents have been in the habit of offering the breast or bottle as a way of calming the child down or putting them to sleep. Or, most poignant of all, parents simply don't want to give up this sign of infancy. Who can blame them?

Extended breastfeeding or bottle-feeding

Popular opinion is that bottle-feeding "should" be phased out as soon as possible. Prevailing thought is that extended breastfeeding "should" be supported. Let's get rid of the "shoulds" and consider the issues.

The American Academy of Pediatrics supports continued breastfeeding until two years or beyond, "as mutually desired by mother and child." The World Health Organization (WHO) recommends exclusive breastfeeding for the first six months and then continuing to breastfeed for "up to two years and beyond." WHO, of course, is addressing babies in developing countries, where breastfeeding is critical for the child's survival. Your child may or may not be interested in breastfeeding for an extended time. The same applies to you, and you have your reasons. Mothers who do extended breastfeeding find it to be rewarding, and are willing to put up with criticism, strange looks, or negative comments.

Keep in mind that this discussion about extended breastfeeding applies to the child who is in Stage 4 and capable of being well-established on family meals. The issue is *on-demand* nipple-feeding. For the Stage 4 child, nipple-feeding on demand interferes with their appetite for family meals and interest in growing up with eating. From a feeding dynamics perspective, on-demand nipple-feeding is the same as letting them have unlimited access to any other food. Continuing to feed on demand when your child is in Stage 4 makes them miss their window of developmental readiness and can negatively affect their eating for years to come.[1]

That is not to say you must give up nipple-feeding your child. You can continue to enjoy breastfeeding or feeding formula from the bottle in the morning and at bedtime and at more-or-less predictable times during the day. That treats the nipple-feeding as a planned snack and doesn't interfere with your child's eating their meals.

Nipple misuse

For the child in Stage 4, offering the breast or bottle on demand as a pacifier is nipple misuse. That teaches a child to use food for emotional reasons and, once learned, that tendency is stuck for life. Instead, older babies and almost-toddlers need to express feelings and find ways to deal with them rather than having eating be their primary response to stress. Making the shift to the Stage 4 meals-plus-snacks routine helps prevent using feeding as a pacifier. That meals-plus-snacks routine helps parents avoid falling prey to using food to cope with all the uproar and mishaps that go along with living with children. Except for emergencies. We have all resorted to cookies when we are at the end of our tether.

Letting children use nipple-feeding as a bid for attention is nipple misuse. An older baby/toddler who is being nipple-fed on demand soon learns that asking to be nursed is a surefire way of getting their mother all to themself and cutting out other children—or adults. It is legitimate for a child to find ways to get attention, but the nipple-feeding ploy is misusing food for emotional reasons. That's negative attention. While children would rather have negative attention than no attention at all, the positive kind is better.

Letting a child run around with a bottle or take a bottle to bed is nipple misuse, even if breastmilk or formula is in the bottle. Children demand too much, too often, don't eat meals, and don't get the other nutrients they need. They are also highly likely to develop baby-bottle tooth decay; sipping from a sippy cup or even an open cup can do the same.

VARIATIONS ON BABY FOOD

You may wonder if that is all there is to it. What about those little jars and pouches of commercial baby food? What about making your own? What about "baby-led weaning?"

Commercial baby food

The pureed, silky-smooth texture of Step 1 and Step 2 commercial baby foods makes them Stage 1 food that your baby will benefit from only briefly. Babies who are developmentally ready to eat solid foods progress so rapidly to family food that they only briefly need pureed baby food, either commercial or homemade. Except for iron, zinc, and vitamin D for breastfed babies, they don't need the nutrients, either. They are getting all the nutrients they need from breastmilk or formula.

I discuss this topic further in the section, "Commercial baby food," page 347.

Making your own baby food

Making baby food involves adapting family food so your baby can eat it. My recommendations for Stages 2, 3, and 4 foods are instructions for making your own baby food as you go along. However, people interested in making their own baby food are generally thinking about pureeing and freezing. There are whole books with recipes for making baby food, including keeping clean, cooking, blending, and freezing the puree in ice cube trays to provide little blocks of foods that can be thawed and fed. Those little blocks are certainly handy, and I applaud you for introducing your baby early to the lovely experiences of family food. Whether it is worth the trouble depends on how rapidly your child's oral-motor development progresses. Some babies need Stage 1 foods only a week or two.

"Baby-led" weaning

I expect it hasn't escaped you that we just discussed baby-led weaning. However, you may be wondering about "baby-led weaning" as promoted in numerous books on the topic. That would be waiting to start offering your baby solid food until they can finger-feed themself Stage 3 or Stage 4 food. "Baby-led weaning" in the book sense—let's abbreviate it as BLW—is accompanied by warnings of the perils of spoon-feeding: struggles getting a baby to accept lumpy food, coping with picky eating, mealtime battles with toddlers, having to provide children with separate meals. If you have read this far, no way will you "strap your baby into a high chair and force-feed them spoon after spoon of bland vegetables" as described in some BLW publications. BLW condemns all spoon-feeding as being force-feeding and therefore recommends skipping the oral-motor learning and nutrition of Stage 1 and Stage 2. From the first introduction of solid food, BLW assumes a child can bite off, control the position of food in their mouth, move the food to their jaws where they munch or chew it, and swallow without gagging—or choking.

Studies about BLW, even in professional journals, are not well grounded: Observations are uncontrolled and recruitment methods are not random.[6] Most mothers who set out to use BLW also spoon-fed their babies: They said their babies were not ready and/or did not cooperate.[7] Mothers who attempted to use BLW were more anxious about the food-introduction process than mothers who either started with spoon-feeding or said they were using BLW but also spoon-fed.[8] BLW-weaned 6- to 10-month-olds appear to be slower about getting the hang of eating solid foods, as they consume more breastmilk or formula and less solid food.[9]

United Kingdom researchers found infant iron intakes between 6 and 10 months at those ages to be considerably lower in BLW babies compared with "traditionally-weaned" babies, who were by then well along in eating baby cereal, fruits, and vegetables. BLW babies only began to catch up nutritionally after age 10 months.[9]

If you follow a BLW approach and want to avoid spoon-feeding, minimize choking risks by preparing food using the methods described for Stage 3 food: Make sure the pieces of food are a quarter inch or less in size so they don't plug up the end of your baby's windpipe. With respect to providing your baby with enough iron and zinc, consider mixing up baby cereal until it is thick and gluey and letting your baby eat it with their hands. Another option is to give iron and zinc supplement drops: Talk with your doctor.

HOW YOUR CHILD LEARNS TO EAT

Your baby's learning to eat is all about oral-motor development: the process of maturation that allows your baby's nerves and muscles to work together. Your baby's oral-motor readiness and willingness to learn to eat go hand in hand. Colorado public health nutritionist Virginia Beal studied babies over an entire decade and found that those under three or four months old didn't want much to do with solid foods. In fact, they and their mothers got into some real hassles over solid foods introduction. Despite earlier struggles, Beal found that the babies first cheerfully accepted solid foods at around age four months.[10] As the previous section illustrated, each child gets ready and learns to eat in their own way.

It's a back-and-forth process. To learn to eat, your baby's nerves and muscles have to have developed to the point where they can master the mechanics of eating. Offering solid foods early doesn't hasten that development. Once developed, babies still must learn to use their nerves and muscles to eat, and they do that with the food you offer. Mostly for the sheer joy of understanding more about your baby, but also to guide you in introducing solid foods, let's talk in more detail about oral-motor development.

Stage 1 oral-motor development

Babies learn to eat solid food; they don't do it instinctively. To swallow effectively, a Stage 1 child has to learn to flatten their tongue to let in the spoon, move food from the front of their tongue to the back, and swallow past the opening of the windpipe. That is totally different from the *extrusion reflex* of suckling from the nipple: They press their tongue upward against the nipple to deposit breastmilk or formula far enough back on the tongue to stimulate automatic swallowing. A just-learning or too-immature baby's extrusion reflex pushes semisolid food back onto their chin.

Your Stage 1 baby may gag if they don't swallow strongly enough, or if you put too much food too far back on their tongue. Gagging pushes the food forward in your baby's mouth and is a neurological safety mechanism that helps prevent choking. While you don't want to cause gagging with poor feeding technique or by getting pushy with feeding, it is a normal part of learning to eat. Gagging won't frighten your baby unless it frightens you. The gag reflex starts out strong and gets toned down when your baby mouths—and gags on—toys, fingers, and whatever else they get in their mouth. Ten-month-old Brenda alarmed her parents by frequently gagging herself with her fingers and even throwing up a little. After a while, she learned not to put her fingers in so far, her gag reflex became less pronounced, and her gagging and throwing up went away. Children learn instinctively and nonverbally.

Consider how the mouth works

To better understand your baby's oral-motor development, let's consider your mouth and how it works. Get a sense of the extrusion reflex by sucking on your finger. Contrast that mouth action by eating something soft like yogurt or ice cream. Notice how your tongue gets flat and lower in your mouth, your lips close over and clean out the spoon, and you use your tongue to propel the food from the front of your mouth to the back. When the food gets to a certain point on your tongue, it activates your swallow reflex and sends the food down your throat.

For you, it's automatic, but your baby has to instinctively master it all when they learn to eat semisolid food.

Still eating your semisolid food, notice your swallow when you hold your head in a variety of positions: up straight and looking straight ahead, turned to one side or another, with your chin on your chest, looking up. It makes a difference, doesn't it? It is far easier to swallow when your head and neck are straight.

Stage 2, 3, and 4 oral-motor development

Now try your mouth out on something lumpy—a mashed-up cooked vegetable, piece of soft fruit, or pasta. Put the food on your tongue and notice what happens next. You don't send it straight down as you did the yogurt but instead move the lumps of food between your jaws with your tongue, where you mash or chew it a bit before you swallow it. You may even move the food from one side to the other in your mouth.

Lumpy food stimulates your Stage 2 baby to move food between their jaws and mash it before they swallow. That is quite a complex maneuver, because they have to delay swallowing while they keep it in their mouth, move it to the side, and mash it a bit before they swallow. At first, they gag, then they learn.

Learning is such an effort that you might see your baby screwing up their whole face and concentrating on getting those little muscles to work. If you need to, you can help with the moving-to-the-jaws maneuver by putting the lumpy food on the side of their tongue.

Stage 2 lumpy food can be baby cereal mixed thick and lumpy and texture-modified family food: mashed or milled cooked fresh, frozen, or canned vegetables; mashed or milled peeled fresh, canned, or frozen fruits; finely cut-up pasta. Introduce foods one at a time to check for reactions.

Somewhere between Stages 2 and 3—lumps to soft pieces—you will find yourself offering breastmilk or formula in a cup. Notice your own cup-drinking and how you curve your lips around the edge of the cup to drink. Your baby has to learn that, too; until they do, a lot comes out the corners of their mouth.

Stage 3 food is the same food as Stage 2 except you are upping your game with texture: It is chopped or cut-up rather than mashed. Make sure the pieces of food are a quarter inch or less in size so they don't plug up the end of your baby's windpipe and cause choking. You will find yourself adding more food from family meals: hard-cooked or scrambled eggs, mashed beans, and juicy and finely cut-up meats. Your child may start feeding themself dry cereals such as Cheerios and Corn Chex, and they can learn to pick up and bite off crackers and strips of toast. In fact, they may insist on eating entirely by themself with their fingers.

Stimulated by the larger pieces of food, the Stage 3 child learns to use their jaws to chew in a rotary motion. Not only that, but they transfer food from one jaw to the other. You need to know that they pause momentarily during that transfer, when the food briefly comes to rest on their tongue. That momentary pause is risky, because anything that makes them suck in their breath, like talking or laughing, can pull the food into their windpipe.

To get a sense for that complicated mouth learning, bite off a piece of cracker. You will automatically bite off a piece that you can chew and swallow easily. Your Stage 3 baby has to learn all that with a process of trial and error. At first, they will break off the piece of cracker, then have trouble keeping it in their mouth to go to work on it. Depending on whether the piece happens to be the right size, they will be able to get it between their jaws—or not.

Grappling with all this complexity and struggling to get all those muscles working would be wildly frustrating for an adult. Your baby doesn't seem to mind or if they do, they mind the strangeness and not the difficulty getting their parts going. A child's job, after all, is getting everything to work. They will cope and even delight in the process.

Stage 4: Meals plus snacks

Stage 4 is more of the same food, now as pieces of food that your child can pick up with their fingers and eat. If all has gone well during your progression through the stages in feeding, your child is ready to join in with family meals. To be interested in mealtime food, they have to be hungry but not starved. Use sit-down snacks between meals to help them wait for mealtime or adjust mealtime a little. Consider continuing the weaning process by offering snacks made up of finger food and beverages from the cup. Alternatively, sit-down snacks can be breastfeeding or formula or breastmilk that you feed your baby from the bottle.

By Stage 4, your child has likely turned into what I call an almost-toddler, marked by their insistence on feeding themself. Your almost-toddler is likely to enjoy feeding themself so much that they eat almost anything. This is truly the honeymoon phase in child-feeding, when they enthusiastically join in with family meals and are undaunted by unfamiliar food. Enjoy it while it lasts. In a few months, your almost-toddler will turn into a toddler proper. The toddler is typically skeptical about new food (even if you know they have eaten it before), eats less (because they grow less rapidly), and says "no" to food (often at the same time as they eat it). Here is a spoiler for Chapter 11: Your toddler's erratic eating can trigger your trying to get them to eat. Don't do it! They will eat what the rest of the family eats, but it has to be *their* idea.

ALLERGIES

Introducing your child to your family's variety of food may reveal that they have food allergies. Children with undetected food allergies may be ill, their growth may falter, and their list of acceptable food may be short. They may be exceptionally reluctant to experiment with new food. Be careful: All those food avoidance behaviors can make you unconsciously try to get your child to eat. Don't do it. In fact, be particularly respectful of your child's food refusal. Children have an instinctive sense of which foods make them ill and are especially reluctant to eat them. Keep your courage, trust your child, and follow their lead with feeding.

We used to recommend early avoidance of foods that most frequently caused allergies, such as peanuts or eggs, thinking that avoidance was key to prevention. It turns out that the opposite is true: Early introduction helps *prevent* allergy. The American Academy of Pediatrics recommends early introduction.

UNDERSTANDING ALLERGIES

There are three types of food reactions: 1) IgE mediated are immediate and caused by a child's reacting to their own antibodies—their protective blood proteins. 2) Non-IgE mediated are slower in onset and cased by "cell-mediated immunity." The important difference between the two is the rapidity of onset. 3) Food intolerances, where the body has trouble digesting or metabolizing a particular food and is often a by-product of illness. The first two can be severe and long-lasting. The third is less serious and likely to be temporary.

A child with IgE-mediated allergies may have an upset stomach or vomit almost immediately after eating a food and/or have diarrhea after several hours. Other symptoms include itchy mouth and throat, rash or eczema, diarrhea, and swelling of the face or tongue.[10] To detect that type of allergy, also known as IgE-mediated allergy, introduce foods one at a time and wait two or three days to determine whether your child reacts.

Non-IgE mediated-allergies affect the esophagus, stomach, and large and small intestine and show up after a child has eaten the food a number of times.[10] Detecting your child's non-IgE-mediated food allergens may require an elimination diet that removes foods that may cause symptoms, then reintroduces foods individually to check for those symptoms.

Food intolerance causes less serious symptoms than food allergy and is likely to be temporary. An illness or emotional upset can coincide with a child reacting to a particular food. For instance, viral gastroenteritis can leave a child temporarily intolerant of the lactose or protein in milk. After avoiding lactose for a few weeks, the child can regain the ability to digest it.

Coping with allergies

Engage the services of an sDOR-committed allergy specialist Registered Dietitian to help you. One such specialist, ESI faculty member Alexia Beauregard, encourages putting the emphasis on what your child *can* eat rather than what they *can't* eat. She reassures parents that food need not hurt or generate anxiety and that mealtime, even when children have food allergies, can be a relaxing part of the day.

At the same time, work with an allergist to confirm whether or not your child is truly allergic. You don't want to make your food-to-avoid list any longer than is necessary. Many times, when children who are assumed to be allergic are challenged with a seemingly offending food, they aren't even sensitive to it.

Until your child becomes aware of what everyone else is eating, you may be able to offer them part of a meal or different food from what you eat. That is unlikely to last long! In the Chapter 11 section, "The toddler who is allergic," page 380, Beauregard recommends omitting the toddler's allergens from family menus. The Chapter 12 section, "Preschoolers with food allergies," page 443, discusses teaching your child to take responsibility for staying away from food that makes them ill.

There are always "buts" with food allergies and a big one is when the child is so sensitive to particular allergens that cross-contamination is an issue. For that child, the allergen has to be kept out of the house.

INS AND OUTS

Every parent worries about choking, so we have to discuss that. You are still changing diapers, so you will be aware of the impact of solid foods on your baby's bowel movements.

Choking

Stage 4 food—modified family food—introduces choking issues. Gagging is normal; choking is dangerous. A child chokes when they take in a breath at the same time as food moves down their throat, past the end of their windpipe. The food plugs up the windpipe and they can't breathe. As long as your child gets enough air to cough, they are probably okay. However, if they make no sound or make only a squeaky, whistling, inhaling sound, they may be choking. Have your health care provider teach you first aid for choking.

In gradually building your child's eating skills as described in this chapter, you take precautions against choking. To further prevent choking, keep mealtime calm, have your child sit straight facing forward, and stay with them while they eat. Don't let an older child feed them. If, however, your child continues to gag a lot and/or doesn't want anything in their mouth, bring it to the attention of your health care provider.

Giving a child too-challenging foods can cause choking. Hot dogs, grapes, cherry tomatoes, or cooked dry beans can slip around in the mouth and down the throat. Cut hot dogs up lengthwise; halve grapes and cherry tomatoes; mash beans. Avoid hard candy and fruit jellies. Shred or finely cut up raw vegetables, apples, and pieces of meat. Spread peanut butter thinly: a glob of peanut butter can get stuck over the end of the windpipe. For the Centers for Disease Control and Prevention (CDC) listing of potential choking hazards, do a web search for *Choking Hazards*.

Baby bowel movements

Your baby's stools will get thicker and pastier when they start eating baby cereals. Don't worry when pieces of fruits and vegetables and the stains from beets and other foods come through in diapers. Those are the waste products of normal digestion. Stools of older children and adults look the same; we just don't study them as carefully! Your Stage 3 and Stage 4 baby will be able to digest any food that they can gum well. In fact, chewing and swallowing represent the major limitation in their digestive system. Spices from particularly hot food can irritate your baby's bottom, so get out the zinc oxide when you have Tex-Mex or some other spicy cuisine!

WHAT IF YOU CAN'T HELP BUT START SOLIDS EARLY

I can understand if you have trouble accepting my advice to wait to introduce your baby to solid food. About one third of babies in the United States are introduced to solid foods before age four months. Your mother or friends or others in your neighborhood may have done it differently and their methods have seemingly worked and have stood the test of time. Our babies are so dependent on us that it is hard to take chances with something new. I would rather you stepped out of line and waited, but I know it is not easy.

You can start solids too early and still have it be okay when you pay attention to how your baby reacts to being spoon-fed. If they do their part with eating and seem to enjoy it, well, okay. On the other hand, if everything comes back out on their chin and they don't seem interested and even get upset, stop trying and wait a while. Think about those Colorado babies I talked about earlier, who got into struggles with their mothers when they were younger but willingly took solid food when they were about four months old. Here is what to consider if you start your baby on solids early:

- If your baby doesn't like eating from the spoon, don't make them.
- If you aren't enjoying feeding your baby, stop.
- Use formula or breastmilk to mix up the cereal; don't use regular milk, fruit juice, or water.
- Don't put cereal in the bottle. Your baby doesn't need it. If they are too young to eat cereal from a spoon, they are too young to eat cereal.

BE PREPARED FOR ADVENTURE

The stories below consider parents and children as they approach solid food. As you read these stories, keep an eye on love and acceptance. Most parents were able to accept their baby's eating or not eating. Some were not. Consider how that acceptance or lack of it made their baby feel. The children in the stories illustrate the oral-motor development outlined in Figure 10.1, page 308.

Sebastian wasn't interested

Clio waited patiently until Sebastian showed Stage 1 signs of being ready for solid food. Her technique was impeccable: She made Sebastian comfortable in his high chair, sat directly in front of him, and held the spoon about a foot away from his mouth. Sebastian looked quizzically at her and at the spoon. She waited. He opened his mouth ever so slightly. She put a dab of cereal on his lip. He closed his mouth and turned away, squeezing the cereal out on his chin. She waited, spoon suspended. He hung his hand over the arm of the high chair and looked at the floor. This routine was repeated over the next several weeks. Even though he didn't eat a bite, Sebastian still learned because Clio brought him to the table when she ate and put thick baby cereal and then other Stage 2 foods on his high-chair tray. Sometimes Sebastian accidentally got his fingers in the food and into his mouth, but he had no aha moments. Clio gave him a spoon and a cup, and he enjoyed handling and mouthing them. When he began to struggle to pick up food, Clio progressed to Stage 3 food: small pieces of finger food and food to bite off and chew. He gagged a bit at first, but quickly developed Stage 3 oral capabilities so he could munch and swallow. From there, he rapidly learned to eat family food. Pam Estes, Registered Dietitian who works with children who have functional needs, says, "Children don't do, don't do, don't do. Then they do." Sebastian was learning in that invisible way that children do.

I start with Sebastian not to discourage you but to make a critical point: In order to successfully introduce solid foods to your baby, you *must* take no for an answer. Eventually, even uninterested babies get around to eating. The drive is built into them the same as with smiling, rolling over, and sitting up. It's more rewarding for us when they eat, but you still do your jobs with feeding by exposing them to food and to the possibilities of eating by including them in family meals.

Essentially, Sebastian's reactions and Clio's accepting responses led to the "baby-led weaning" method of going straight to Stage 3 and then Stage 4 food. The "baby-led weaning" folks insist that spoon-feeding is controlling and disrespects information coming from children. Review the stories in this section. Are the spoon-feeding parents ignoring and overruling information coming from their children? Some are, some aren't.

Jatta ate the first time

You can see Stage 1 in action with Jatta's first introduction to solid foods in the Transitional Child section of the *Feeding with Love and Good Sense II* video. (Do a search for the parents' version on the Ellyn Satter Institute website. I know those videos are old but feeding dynamics do not change.) Jatta's mother, Megan, first gives him part of a breastfeeding, then puts him in the high chair, where he sits up straight and looks interested while Megan stirs up baby cereal for him. When she offers him the spoon, he shows Stage 1 oral-motor capabilities: He opens his mouth, mostly closes his lips over the spoon, keeps much of the cereal in his mouth, and swallows. He even reaches for the spoon. Jatta gains eating skills as that first feeding goes on: He closes his upper lip more completely over the spoon and keeps more of the cereal in his mouth. Jatta and Megan are having a good time, and Megan's tempo is great: She gives Jatta time to see the spoon coming before she tries to feed him. When Jatta fusses, Megan picks him up, puts him on her lap, and again offers the spoon. He is interested—until he is not. He begins to ignore the spoon, and Megan stops the feeding. Jatta is worn out. This is all new to him, and it takes a *lot* of concentration and energy.

Michelle was *not* ready for solids

On the first *Feeding with Love and Good Sense Videotape* (search for the exact title on the Ellyn Satter Institute website), an oldie but still goodie, we see part of a spoon-feeding with Sarah and four-month-old Michelle. Our first clue that Michelle is not yet in Stage 1 is that she is reclining on her mother's lap. She also does not open her mouth for the spoon. Sarah, a clearly loving mother, nonetheless ignores Michelle's unwillingness to eat. Michelle squirms, turns her head away, and fusses, and Sarah takes advantage of her open-mouthed protests to shovel in food. She scrapes the food off Michelle's chin again and again and puts it back in. Michelle is not keeping the food in her mouth, and she is not swallowing. Finally, Sarah stops, but only after Michelle sets up quite a howl. Why, I asked Sarah after the taping, did she continue to try to feed when Michelle clearly didn't want to eat? "Because she has to have it," she answered, with real concern. "It's time she starts to eat solid food." It wasn't. Michelle was getting her nutritional needs met from her formula. Ironically, Sarah's determination to get cereal into Michelle was likely getting in the way of providing for Michelle's needs. Michelle's experience that eating is unpleasant will stay with her and make her less interested in eating later on.

Ella, an experienced spoon-eater

Ella, on the *Feeding with Love and Good Sense II DVD*, is seven months old and experienced with eating Stage 1 and Stage 2 solids from the spoon. She eats her cereal readily, is cautious but willing with avocado, and regains her enthusiasm with pureed carrots. Ella's attention wanders to the video camera, but her mother reminds her, "Hi, I'm right here, look at me" and waits to feed Ella until she pays attention. Toward the end, Kathy asks, "Are we done? Everything's coming back out." Kathy has observed that when Ella gets enough to eat, she still enjoys having food in her mouth, but she doesn't swallow. Her mother calls a halt, cleans her up, and offers a breastfeeding. Ella isn't interested. Kathy could skip the mealtime breastfeeding and offer breastmilk or formula in a cup along with the meal. Ella is ready for thicker, lumpier Stage 2 food and she would likely enjoy chasing Cheerios around her high-chair tray. Cheerios are a good early finger food: They are small enough not to cause choking and break down easily in the mouth.

Alex is ready for family food

Ten-month-old Alex, also on the *Feeding with Love and Good Sense II DVD,* is sitting in his high chair while his mother, Marcella, and his older brothers eat dinner. He shows all the signs of being ready to eat Stage 3 and likely even Stage 4 food: He struggles to pick up the finger food on his high-chair tray and struggles again to get it out of his hand and into his mouth. He moves the food to his jaws and munches before he swallows. While Alex feeds himself, Marcella slips a spoonful of baby-food bananas into his mouth. Alex tolerates it, but he is not interested. Marcella and Alex aren't playing their parts of sDOR. Her job is to engage Alex in the feeding process and go by his signals. His job is to pay attention and say yes or no to food. Alex is far more interested in his brother's spaghetti than in those bananas. About the time they are ready for Stage 3 or 4 food, many children suddenly refuse to eat from the spoon and insist on feeding themselves with their fingers. Alex's way of refusing is to ignore the spoon-feeding. Why not cut up the spaghetti and let Alex feed himself with his fingers? A finger food is anything that hangs together long enough to get it from the high-chair tray to the mouth.

Madison and Daniel can join in with family meals

Year-old twins Madison and Daniel, also on the *Feeding with Love and Good Sense II DVD,* are having their first family dinner with their parents, Alan and Pam. Until now, their parents fed them separately, spoon-feeding them Stage 2 food and letting them have cereal and crackers on their high-chair trays. Like Alex, Madison and Daniel show oral-motor readiness for feeding themselves Stage 4 food. They can pick up finger food, get it into their mouths, move the food to their jaws, munch, and swallow. Dinner is pizza; their parents cut it into bite-sized pieces, and the children enthusiastically feed themselves. Maddie gags but can breathe so she isn't choking. Alan's phone rings but he ignores it—answering it would take away from this lovely meal. Daniel eats enthusiastically and struggles to do it. Daniel is chubby and eats a lot, but that's okay. He knows how much he needs to eat. Trying to get him to eat less will make him eat more. Maddie puts food in her mouth, samples it for taste and texture, then lets it fall into her lap. This is typical toddler eating behavior. But Maddie isn't finished with the food in her lap and goes after it. This time, she chews it up and swallows it. Alan and Pam help the children drink from the cup, and somewhere during the meal, both children lose their plates. Finally, they are finished. Their parents are surprised at how enthusiastically and how much they ate.

Children with functional needs

All the children we just discussed are healthy, neurotypical children. The story is somewhat different when a child is ill or has a condition that complicates getting their nerves and muscles working smoothly together. Then, introducing solid food takes even more sensitivity and restraint. A child might have been born prematurely or have Down syndrome, muscular dystrophy, or other cognitive or muscular limitations. For such children, signs of readiness are slower to appear. This could be at six months adjusted age for a prematurely born child, or considerably later for a child with cognitive or neuromuscular limitations. Include your child in family meals and be prepared to go slowly with respect to introducing new food experiences.

A child who has had medical procedures applied to their mouth will find the introduction of solid foods to be threatening. It can take months for them to get accustomed to eating semisolid cereal from the spoon, then more months to accept gradually thicker cereal and then lumps. Advancing from pureed to mashed bananas or peaches can constitute another threat that also has to be approached slowly. There is something to be learned at every step. There are subtle differences in mouth motions to swallow thinner and thicker semisolids, and lumps stimulate movement of the tongue to the side. There are differences in the smoothness, slipperiness, and flavor of cereal versus mashed bananas versus mashed carrots. It isn't easy but be patient. When you move slowly and patiently through this learning-to-eat process, eventually your child will learn to eat. Remember the tilt: Your sitting upright lets your child lean forward to show you they are interested in eating. And remember what my ESI colleague and functional needs dietitian Pam Estes says: "Children don't do, don't do, don't do. Then they do."

Variations on the theme

Those are the basics; the surprises will be your own. You will have your own adventures as you watch your child make use of the learning opportunities you offer them. At first, children express what they want as yes or no—eating or not eating. Surprisingly soon, they express what they want as the drive to do it themselves. At times, their drive to feed themselves outstrips their capability and demands their parents' considerable ingenuity.

From the first, Nicolas insisted on feeding himself—and he couldn't. He could get his hands into the bowl, smear the food on his face, and get a few grams into his mouth. He could grab the spoon and wedge it in his mouth. Nicolas loved it all, but his parents were frustrated because he wasn't eating much. They need not have worried. He didn't really need the solids, and he was learning to eat—in his own way.

Clara's father pulled her high chair up to the table and gave her spoonfuls of food while he ate his own dinner. He filled the spoon and handed it to her. She struggled until she got the spoon into her mouth and sucked it off, then let him take the spoon back so he could fill it again and hand it to her.

India was developmentally ready to eat semisolid food but totally uninterested in the spoon. Her mother prepared Stage 2 food for her by thickening the baby cereal and putting it on the high-chair tray. Baby cereal can be thickened to the gluey stage, and instant mashed potato flakes make a good thickener for other food. India put her mouth on the edge of the tray and shoveled the cereal into her mouth with her hand and arm.

Kent's parents provided him with thick, gluey, hang-together food and Kent used his palmar grasp to feed himself: He folded his fingers into his palm and captured the food. At first, he could close his fingers but not open them, so he squeezed the food out between his fingers and sucked it off.

UNDERSTAND SOCIAL/EMOTIONAL DEVELOPMENT

With breast- and bottle-feeding, paying attention and responding to your baby's cues supported your baby's processes of homeostasis and attachment. Now, paying attention and responding to their cues supports their separation-individuation. Your baby continues to work on the earlier developmental stages—being engrossed with eating helps them stay calm and focused; being respected with feeding lets them give and receive love. Based on their secure sense of your love, your baby now begins to explore and try themself out on the world around them and discover they are separate from you.

You may have heard about the "terrible twos," when the toddler's drive to explore and be oppositional come to the fore. As we will discuss in more detail in the next chapter, that behavior comes from the toddler's developmental task of separation-individuation: The toddler needs to discover that they are a person separate from you, the people they love best. They need to say no, to learn and explore, and to be independent. But most of us don't realize that separation-individuation can start about midway through the first year.

Five to nine months: Separation-individuation

Your older baby is interested in *things*, and they want to see what is going on around them. That is the start of separation-individuation. Until then your baby has no sense of where they start and where you leave off. Your baby loves you as much as ever and wants you near, but their process of discovery means their attention is no longer focused one-on-one. Your baby will suddenly sit up and look around in the middle of a nipple-feeding. They drain a bottle or breast in a hurry because they have things to do! Your introducing solid food goes right along with their interest in *things*.

Seven to fifteen months: Separation-individuation

Your older baby becomes an almost-toddler—probably suddenly, when they refuse the spoon, grab at it, and refuse to eat food they have happily let you spoon-feed them before. It is easy to miss this transition because it is so abrupt. One day—or one feeding—you and your baby are contentedly doing the spoon routine. The next, the refusal business starts. Unless you know what is going on, it would be natural to respond by trotting off after second and third spoons and playing feeding games. Not a good idea. Your almost-toddler will be happiest—and you will be too—if you let them feed themself. Let them keep the spoon. Put thick and gluey food or soft pieces of food on the high-chair tray and let your almost-toddler eat the best they can. Do not try to feed them, or they will fuss and not eat. They are not being naughty. They still love you and need you and will eat most happily when you are near. They still enjoy the food. In fact, they enjoy feeding themself so much they eat almost everything.

Almost-toddlers want to do it *themselves*!

My granddaughter Emma demonstrated what the almost-toddler is all about. Emma had moved along very nicely, communicating back and forth with her parents and learning to eat solid foods. By age eight months, she had worked her way up to finger-feeding herself soft, cooked fruits and vegetables, cereals, breads, and toast. She was in Stage 4. Her favorite was gnawing on strips of toast. Being a bit rusty on infant feeding, I handed Emma a too long strip of toast. She gripped it at the very end and proceeded to stick it so far into her mouth that she gagged herself. Naturally, Emma's mother reached over to adjust her grip. Instantly, Emma jerked the toast as far away as she could get it and glared at her mother. Words could not have said it more clearly: "I want to do it myself." Amazing. Eight months!

Dr. Irene Chatoor, a child psychiatrist specializing in infant feeding problems at Children's Hospital Medical Center in Washington, DC, emphasizes that a baby's need for autonomy is not a trivial matter. Chatoor has observed that the highest incidence of nonorganic failure to thrive happens around age nine months, during the early blooming of the separation-individuation phase of development. Nonorganic failure to thrive is serious growth failure, far beyond the point of a downward blip on the growth chart. Babies with nonorganic failure to thrive are so undernourished that they are thin and short, lack energy to play and explore, and show behavioral distortions.

Parents often misinterpret their children's bids for autonomy as food refusal and put pressure on feeding. Children react by resisting eating. Parents feel they *must* get food into their child and feeding struggles severe enough to affect growth are hard to watch. Desperate parents push, children resist, parents push harder, and children resist all the more. The child cries and protests, getting so upset that they don't even know they are hungry. In most cases there is nothing the matter with the child—or the parent. They are just caught up in the struggle.

CHOOSING FOOD

With the exception of baby cereal, let your baby eat the foods you enjoy. The only limitation is texture: Depending on their developmental readiness, your baby needs their food to be mashed, diced, or chunked. Throughout these chapters, I have done my very best to combat good-food/bad-food thinking. This section gives you the detail of why it is *all right* to give your baby foods you enjoy.

You choose food for your older baby for both developmental and nutritional reasons. The developmental part, learning to eat, has to do with oral-motor development. The nutritional part is building up their list of accepted foods in preparation for when they go off breastmilk or formula. For most of the transition period, they can safely depend on breastmilk or formula to give them the nutrients they need. It is only when they eat so much solid food that their breastmilk or formula intake decreases that the solid food becomes equal in nutritional importance.

Introduce one new food at a time, waiting three to five days to check for reactions such as stomachaches, diarrhea, skin rashes, or wheezing. Then go on to the next food. If your child is not interested in eating something, take no for an answer, and offer it again in a few days. Everything is new to them, and it takes a while to get used to all the tastes and textures.

Adjust your expectations of how much your child will eat. Even when they enjoy a food and eat it enthusiastically, it is likely they will eat a tablespoon or less. More is okay.

Iron and zinc-fortified baby cereal

The six-month-old, breastfed baby is near the end of their iron and zinc stores, so they need a good source of iron and zinc in their diet. Unless you have been using a non-iron fortified formula, which is not recommended, the formula-fed baby is getting iron and zinc. As a consequence, the formula-fed baby's learning to eat infant cereal is strictly for developmental reasons and you can skip it, although baby cereal is handy for adapting semisolid food to make it thicker and lumpier. For breastfed babies, start with one cereal feeding daily and work up until your baby is taking two to three meals daily. Keep in mind that if your baby refuses cereal initially, it is because they are skeptical, not rejecting. Spoon-feeding is so new and such a drastic change that it takes some babies a while to get the hang of it. If your baby is particularly skeptical, be particularly slow and cautious about offering the food.

During Stage 1, offer your baby the breast- or bottle-feeding first, before you offer solids. Since at six months it's still too early to use pasteurized milk, mix infant cereal with iron-fortified formula or breastmilk. If you don't have enough expressed breastmilk, using iron-fortified infant formula for mixing up cereal makes sense. It contains well-absorbed iron and zinc and will supplement your baby's nutrition. Why not purchase a container of powdered iron-fortified infant formula and mix it up as you need it? If you keep it in the refrigerator, it will stay fresh longer. Read up on your formula choices in the Chapter 9 section, "Infant formula," page 274. If you are concerned about cow milk allergy, choose one of the extensively hydrolyzed formulas. Don't use juice to mix up baby cereal: It makes the cereal taste like juice and your baby won't learn to enjoy the good flavor of cereal.

Why I don't recommend other first solid foods

Meat as a first solid food is high in iron but the texture is difficult to adapt for beginning eaters. Some first foods that are fine developmentally, such as yogurt, cottage cheese, and pureed fruits and vegetables, don't contain as much iron and zinc. Yogurt and cottage cheese simply offer more of the same milk nutrients your baby has been getting all along. Vegetables and fruits give a little iron and zinc, but not enough, and are low in energy. Some vegetables are high in heavy metals and/or nitrates. When you introduce vegetables, protect against heavy metals and nitrates by keeping the totals your baby eats down to around two to three tablespoons a day.

The low-calorie content of fruits and vegetables is generally not a problem because babies eat more of other food and get the calories they need. But if your baby is a particularly slow gainer, you may want to go easy on the fruits and vegetables on the general principle that there is no sense in making it more challenging than necessary for them to get enough calories. Fruits and vegetables are interchangeable nutritionally and developmentally, so if your baby lacks interest in one, you can offer another. People make elaborate arguments for starting with one or the other, but don't worry about it. No particular order is better than any other, and there's no rush for your baby to eat fruits and vegetables.

"Adult" cereals that advertise being good sources of iron for babies, like Cream of Wheat, Maltomeal, and oatmeal, have only two to three milligrams of iron per threeounce serving. Furthermore, the iron is in the form of iron phosphate, which is poorly absorbed. In reality, the iron is there more for the label than for the nutrition! However, if you hate the idea of infant cereals and if your baby is on iron-fortified infant formula, you have some flexibility: You could start them on adult cooked cereals. Avoid Cream of Rice—like other rice products, it is high in arsenic.

Don't sweeten your baby's cereal and, in particular, avoid honey until your baby is a year old. They may accept cereal more readily if it is sweet, but it is better for them to learn to enjoy the unadulterated taste of grain. Honey may be contaminated with botulism spores and your baby's digestive system is too immature to defend against them.

Baked goods containing honey have the same shortcoming: Even baking doesn't destroy botulinum spores.

Water

Generally, a breastfed or formula-fed baby isn't too interested in drinking water. Since both are relatively diluted, babies' fluid needs are satisfied with the nipple-feeding. Certainly, it is good to offer water, but don't be surprised if you get turned down. Your baby will likely be more interested in drinking water from a cup after they are eating solid foods. When you carry them around and have a glass of water yourself, offer them some as well. Offer them a drink of water to clean out their mouth after they get finished eating. Getting your child in the habit of drinking water now will contribute to their good health for a lifetime.

Fruits and vegetables during Stages 2 though 4

Your job is to *let* your child enjoy fruits and vegetables. Your job is not to *get* your child to eat them. Fruits and vegetables are important, but they are no more important than any other food group, and they are definitely *not* worth having feeding struggles about. It is only in Stage 4, when your child's breastmilk or formula decreases, that your child actually needs fruits and vegetables. Even then, it is unnecessary to worry about or even keep track of how many fruits and vegetables they eat. Your child will eat enough fruits and vegetables when you offer them every day at a meal or two and enjoy them yourself.

As I discussed in the Chapter 1 section, "sDOR frees you from the numbers," page 23, the key to your child's eating enough fruits, vegetables, and other "healthy" food is *routine plus trust:* routinely having them as a part of family meals, trusting your child to learn to eat them. In other words, following sDOR. Children whose parents follow sDOR do well nutritionally. Routine plus trust also provides for your nutritional welfare. Read about the research with Eating Competence discussed in the Chapter 1 section, "Consider your Eating Competence," page 15. That research makes it clear that people do well nutritionally when they provide themselves with meals and snacks where they eat as much as they want of food they enjoy.

The fruits and vegetables you eat can be adapted for your baby at Stage 2, Stage 3, and Stage 4, starting with fork-mashed or milled, progressing to finely cut-up pieces, then arriving at bigger pieces that your child can pick up and gum. You can offer your Stage 2 child potatoes, carrots, sweet potatoes, and tomatoes, all of which can be easily fork-mashed or, later on, diced or chunked. When your child reaches Stage 3 or Stage 4, they can have diced or chunked cooked asparagus, cabbage, cauliflower, brussels sprouts, peppers, and zucchini. Stage 2 fruits might be bananas and applesauce. Stages 3 and 4 offer more options, such as diced or chunked grapes, strawberries, raspberries, melon, mandarin oranges, fresh or canned peaches, plums, and apricots. Of course, seeds come through in the diaper, but that's all right.

One of the most popular segments of my *Feeding with Love and Good Sense Video* (the old one) is of eight-month-old Elsa sitting at the table with her parents, eating pieces of watermelon and green beans. Elsa is absolutely intent as she chases the food around the high-chair tray with her awkward little fingers, capturing a green bean between her palm and fingers and scraping it off the heel of her hand into her mouth. Sometimes she drops food and has to chase down another piece, and sometimes she gags, but it doesn't bother her—she keeps right on eating. Elsa's parents keep her company, but they don't interfere, even though they could do it quicker and cleaner. With feeding and parenting, the developing child requires parents' support and self-restraint.

Juice

Offer juice starting in Stage 4, when your child's breastmilk or formula intake decreases and they need another good source of vitamin C. Orange, grapefruit, pineapple, and tomato juice have vitamin C. Offer fruit *juices*, not fruit *drinks*, which contain a small amount of juice and are essentially flavored and nutrient-added water. Give juice in a cup, not the bottle. At the end of the first year, your baby is depending less or not at all on nipple-feeding and letting them have a juice bottle prolongs their dependence. Regular juices—fresh, canned, or frozen concentrate—are all fine and are just as nutritious as baby juice. Juice is a good breakfast or snack beverage, but get in the habit of giving milk, breastmilk, or formula, in a cup, for lunch and dinner. Don't give apple juice, even if it is fortified with vitamin C. It contains indigestible sorbitol, which attracts fluids into the intestine and makes stools more liquid. It is also high in arsenic.

Children generally like fruit juice and are willing to drink more than they need. But children fill up from too much and aren't hungry for meals. Overdoing juice can also cause stomachache or diarrhea. You can avoid overdosing by offering juice at only one eating time daily—say breakfast or a snack—and give it from a cup, not a bottle. If your child is simply thirsty, offer water.

Parents who give too much juice are aided and abetted by their children, who appealingly point to the refrigerator and say "juice" as their first word. That is powerfully hard to resist but resist it you must. Strange though it may seem, given the chance, often children would rather drink than eat. While children push themselves along to learn and grow, they also take the easy way out if it is offered. Unlimited juice is definitely the easy way out. I wish I had a nickel for every poorly eating toddler I have evaluated to find that they were taking 12 or 16 or 20 ounces of juice a day, often from a bottle, often apple juice. Frequently the child had diarrhea and tooth decay as well. Too much juice too frequently made available, even from a cup, can damage teeth and impair the nutritional adequacy of the diet.

Nitrates in fruits and vegetables

For the time being, limit potentially highnitrate vegetables such as beets, carrots, and spinach to one or two tablespoons per feeding. Because of their low stomach acidity, the young infant may convert nitrate to nitrite, which can displace oxygen in hemoglobin. The rapid breathing, lethargy, and shortage of oxygen that results is called methemoglobinemia, or blue baby, and can actually be fatal if the dose of nitrate is very large. A while back there was a report of twin boys who were fed bottles of homemade carrot juice made from a batch of carrots that happened to be very high in nitrate. One of the babies refused the bottle, but the other took a lot and became very ill from methemoglobinemia. By age six months, babies' stomach acidity increases and nitrate overload is less of a problem, but I still wouldn't take chances with carrot juice.

Carotenemia

Both you and your baby can turn yellow if you eat a *lot* of dark green and deep yellow vegetables and fruits, such as broccoli, sweet potatoes, carrots, squash, apricots, watermelon, and peaches. This condition is called carotenemia, caused by the excess accumulation of the yellow coloring in food, carotene. Carotene is good because it converts to vitamin A, but giving so much that it causes carotenemia is unnecessary. It doesn't hurt you or your baby and it goes away if you eat highcarotene vegetables and fruits about every other day.

Breads and cereals

The Stage 4 baby can control the position of food in their mouth and munch or chew it before they swallow. They have a serviceable grasp—either palmar or pincer—and they delight in clutching pieces of food and gnawing away. At first your baby may be able to grasp but not let go. Your baby's chewing, swallowing, and finger-feeding themself breads and cereals opens up new possibilities.

Cheerios, Corn Chex, cornflakes, and other dry cereals make great finger foods as do low-salt versions of cheese crackers, saltines, and wheat thins. I know I said let your baby eat anything you eat, but at first it is worth being conservative. Your baby will gradually eat more sodium until, by the time they are a toddler, they will eat the same amount as the rest of the family. Choosing low-sodium versions of transitional foods eases young children into increased sodium intake.

To go on: Shredded wheat crackers such as Triscuits are a bit tough. Graham crackers (not the honey ones) and animal crackers work, as do strips of tortillas and toast. Eating bread makes pizza possible; eating noodles and other pasta lets your child eat the family lasagna or spaghetti and meat sauce. Cut your child's serving into half-inch pieces to start. To let your baby eat rice, halve its arsenic content by cooking it as you do pasta in a large amount of water, draining the cooked rice, and throwing away the water. Basmati rice is lower in arsenic and cooks faster than regular rice.

Cheerios, wheat thins, and graham crackers introduce whole grains, a worthwhile addition for your child. It is a good idea to include whole grains, but no more than about half the time. Whole grains are bulky and can fill up your young child before they get enough to eat. To be sure you are getting whole grain products read the label: The first listed ingredient should be whole wheat or whole some-other-grain.

If you can manage it, continue to offer your baby iron- and zinc-fortified baby cereal for the first three or four months they are eating family food. I realize that advice seems strange in the scheme of things, and your baby might just lose interest. Not to worry. Depend on regular meals and snacks of wholesome food to support their iron and zinc nutrition.

Milk, yogurt, and cheese

You can begin offering formula or breastmilk from the cup any time during the transitional period from all breast- or formula-feeding to eating family foods. Your child may have whole pasteurized milk when they are a year old, eating family meals and snacks, and drinking from a cup. Continue to use breastmilk or formula for any bottle-feedings: Do not put pasteurized milk in a bottle. Or juice. Do not bother with toddler formula. The best toddler formulas are simply relabeled infant formula; the worst ones are nutritionally inferior to pasteurized milk.

Offer your child *whole* pasteurized milk in a cup at mealtime at least twice a day. Nutrition policy makers and professional organizations recommend low-fat milk, presumably to keep children's weight down. It doesn't and, in fact, it may do the opposite. A survey of 11,000 children aged two to four years found that those who drank whole milk were *less* likely to be "overweight" than those who drank 1 percent or skim milk.[11]

In addition to the above research, I recommend *whole* milk because young children are more inclined to drink it than lower-fat milk, and they need the fat to get enough calories. The fat in whole milk is an important source of nutrients for building nerve and brain tissue. Definitely do *not* use low-fat milk if you use mostly lean meats *or* use low-fat food preparation techniques *or* limit the butter or salad dressing your child uses at the table.[12]

Only half of toddlers are offered whole milk, which is reflected in the fact that the fat content of the average toddler diet is too low.[13] Young children who eat too little fat are hungry frequently and find it difficult to wait for family meals and snacks. This is a particular problem with vegetarian family food, which tends to be low in fat. Two percent milk isn't too bad, provided you include a good source of fat with meals and let your child eat as much butter and other fatty food as they want. One percent and skim milk are *way* too low in fat.

Beyond offering milk as the mealtime beverage twice a day, don't worry about how much milk your child drinks. Children's milk intake usually drops off just after they are weaned, then increases when they are two or three years old.[14] Children depend on milk to get enough calcium and vitamin D, as do grown-ups. A few children are allergic to milk or, following a bout of gastroenteritis, temporarily can't digest milk sugar (lactose). True lactose intolerance generally doesn't show up until a child is five or six years old. Fortified soy milk gives as much protein, calcium, and vitamin D as dairy milk but is lower in fat—about equivalent to 2 percent milk. Almond, oat, and other non-dairy milks are fortified, but have a considerably lower nutrient content than dairy milk. Almond milk is shockingly low in protein, even though it is made with nuts. Dairy milk has eight grams of protein per cup; almond milk has one gram.

Pasteurized milk sold in regular grocery stores is safe and wholesome for your child. It is subject to strict regulation. If you have doubts about your child's nutrition or they haven't yet made the transition to family food, it is wise to offer your child breastmilk or formula for a while longer. However, to avoid getting stuck on the nipple, put mealtime formula in a cup. Read the section, "Extended breastfeeding or bottle-feeding," page 317.

Why is it all right to give pasteurized milk at age one year but not before? By that time, the other food your child eats makes up for the nutrients lacking in milk, such as iron and vitamin C. Also, other food dilutes the pasteurized milk, dilutes and softens the milk curd in their stomach, and makes it digestible. As I explained in the formula-feeding chapter, even when cow and goat milk are pasteurized, they set up a tough, hard-to-digest curd in your baby's stomach. Younger babies get intestinal bleeding from drinking pasteurized milk; older babies do not. Don't feed *unpasteurized* milk of any type at any age.

To support your child's milk drinking, make milk the family mealtime beverage, pour your child a small glass of milk for them to drink or ignore, and drink milk yourself. If you can't drink milk, drink water. Whatever you drink will be appealing to your child, so if you drink soda, Kool-Aid, or juice, your child will want that too. There is no need to promote milk: Promotion risks turning it into something your child would rather avoid. It's okay to occasionally put flavorings in milk but be mindful of your intent. If you are so invested in getting your child to drink milk that you are willing to go to a lot of trouble to make it happen, your child will know that. They will make drinking milk *your* thing, not theirs, and they will use it to manipulate you.

Even the child who drinks milk will go through periods when they don't drink much. Don't make a fuss about it; just wait. And drink your milk. They will go back to drinking milk when they are ready. After all, if you drink it, they will figure out on their own that that is the thing to do.

I realize that some cultural traditions don't support milk as a mealtime beverage. If that is the case for you, take special care to offer other good sources of calcium and vitamin D, such as yogurt, cheese, or soy yogurt. Read yogurt labels to be sure they contain vitamin D. Calcium-fortified orange juice gives calcium but not vitamin D and/or protein.

The child who drinks too much milk

Occasionally a Stage 4 child will seemingly fill up on milk to the exclusion of other foods. I wouldn't worry about it, and I certainly wouldn't restrict their milk intake. Remember the Chapter 1 section, "The Clara Davis studies," page 26. The transitional infants she observed often ate in "waves," where they consumed eight to ten eggs, three or four bananas, or five to seven potatoes in a single meal. Milk consumption ranged from 11 to 48 ounces. Be sure to do good Stage 4 feeding: Let your child join in with family meals, finger-feed themself, and drink milk from a cup. Consider offering big-child foods at snack time.

Meat, poultry, fish, eggs, dry beans, nuts, and seeds

Protein foods can come last because your child doesn't need them for quite a while. They have been getting iron and zinc from infant cereal, plenty of protein from breastmilk or formula, and have been developing their oral-motor skills by learning to enjoy fruits, vegetables, and breads and other grains.

The problem with meat and poultry, of course, is that it cannot be gummed. It doesn't help much when your child gets molars at about 18 to 24 months because even preschoolers have trouble chewing meat or poultry unless it is particularly juicy and tender. Some protein foods such as fish, eggs, lentils, split peas, mashed cooked dried beans, and tofu are easy to gum. Be careful to take the bones out of fish. Do a web search for *Advice about eating fish* for guidelines about which fish to avoid or have only once in a while. Cheese is in the milk group, but it's still a protein food, and you can give your baby pieces of cheese.

Use good sanitary techniques when you handle raw meat in general or raw poultry in particular: Do a web search for *poultry safety guidelines*. To make meat and poultry more palatable for your young child, cook it in liquid at low temperature with a cover on the pan until it is tender. Chop or cut it up very finely across the grain, and moisten it a bit with gravy, broth, or cooking liquid from vegetables. Consider a well-cooked but still-juicy ground beef patty, meatloaf, or casserole. Because casseroles are easy to chew, they make wonderful food for young children—once they have been introduced to all the ingredients. Cut up the noodles to about a half inch in length so your baby can eat them well.

I will bend my stance on commercial baby food and say baby meat sticks occasionally come in handy. They are a lowsalt, lownitrate, convenient (if expensive) meat source for lunches. Because of the salt and nitrate, wait a while to use lunch meat. When you offer hot dogs, cut them into quarters lengthwise.

Don't forget eggs

Eggs can be a mainstay of feeding a family. Eggs are nutritious, easy to enjoy, easy to chew and swallow, easy to keep on hand, and easy to cook in a variety of appealing ways. Your Stage 2 child is ready to be offered a fork-mashed or soft-scrambled egg. Don't worry about the cholesterol in egg yolks. Cholesterol in the diet has been proven not to raise your child's—or anybody else's—blood cholesterol. We used to recommend early avoidance of foods that most frequently caused allergies, such as peanuts or eggs, thinking that avoidance was key to prevention. It turns out that the opposite is true: Early introduction helps prevent allergy. A review of 32 studies indicated that infants introduced to peanuts and eggs before 11 months were less likely to develop allergic reactions to them than children who were exposed when they were toddlers and preschoolers.[15] The American Academy of Pediatrics recommends early introduction.[16]

Cooked dry beans, seeds, and nuts

Lentils, hummus, and refried beans are great for beginning eaters. Some white beans are very soft when they are cooked, but if beans keep a firm shape, mash them a bit before you offer them. Chickpeas are just the right size and shape to cause choking, so make sure to mash them. Nuts such as peanuts, cashews, and almonds belong in the protein group. They are hard to chew so they definitely need to be chopped up. Spread peanut butter and other nut butter thin on bread or crackers so they don't cause choking. Chop up pumpkin seeds, they could be big enough to cause choking. Sesame seeds and pine nuts are smaller and less likely to cause a problem. Think of sesame seeds in tahini and pine nuts in pesto.

Fats

In addition to whole milk, provide for your almost-toddler's calorie and fat needs by using fat in cooking and offering spreads and sauces at mealtime. In addition to whole milk, let them have vegetables you have seasoned for the family with butter or other fats. Moisten meat and poultry with sauces or gravy. Experiment to see what your child does with pats of butter and regular salad dressings. Some children eat butter by the handful, and that's all right. They stop doing that once they get the fat they need from other food.

Sugar

Sugar is not evil. Adding sugar to tomatoes takes the rough edge off the flavor. Adding sugar to peas makes them taste fresher. Your child doesn't have to have cookies or other desserts. However, when the rest of the family has dessert, your almost-toddler will want it too. That is just fine. See Figure 11.7, "Regularly offer 'forbidden' foods," page 366.

NUTRIENTS AND YOUR OLDER BABY

This section might be more for me than for you! It can't hurt and it might help, provided it doesn't turn you into a nutrition fanatic. Instead, as with the previous sections about choosing food and putting together family meals, I hope it supports your feeling good about food and taking an interest in it.

Iron

Iron in red blood cells carries oxygen to all parts of the body. When children don't get enough iron, they may look pale, act cranky, and not have much energy. Iron-deficiency anemia is one of the most common nutritional problems in children. You can, however, prevent anemia without much trouble by:

- Breastfeeding or using iron-fortified formula.
- Starting to offer your breastfed baby iron-fortified infant cereal by around age six months. By then, the natural supply of iron your baby had at birth is near to being used up.
- Supporting your child in learning to eat so they don't get stuck on milk. Dairy products have little iron.
- Including meat, poultry, fish, and nuts. Clams, oysters, and liver are particularly high in iron. Fruits and vegetables have some iron. Peaches are especially rich in iron.
- Having sit-down snacks and avoiding regularly giving food handouts. Foods eaten on the run tend to have mostly calories and few other nutrients.

Zinc

Dietary zinc supports your child's growth and immune function. Breastfed infants tend to have inadequate zinc intake after age six months. Most iron-fortified infant cereals are fortified with zinc as well: Check the label. A lot of foods are high in zinc, so by the time your child is in Stage 4, chances are their zinc intake will be just fine. Good food sources of zinc include meat, shellfish, whole grains, cooked dried beans, seeds, nuts, dairy, and some vegetables. Dark chocolate is high in zinc.

Vitamin E

Vitamin E is important for immune function and to protect body cells from damage. Children's intake of vitamin E, like their intake of zinc, may be low when they are first weaned.[17] Vitamin E is found in plant-based oils, nuts, seeds, fruits, and vegetables. When you offer your child meals and snacks choosing from all the food groups, they are likely to get enough Vitamin E.

Vitamin C

Your breastfed or formula-fed baby gets enough vitamin C. Vitamin C strengthens bones, cartilage, and other connective tissues, and helps the body absorb iron. Offer your Stage 4 child a good vitamin C source every day. It is in most fruits and vegetables and concentrated in oranges, grapefruit, strawberries, cantaloupe, tomatoes, mangos, papaya, pineapple, peppers, broccoli, and cauliflower. Apple and grape juices have vitamin C only when they are fortified, and they are also high in arsenic and lead. Apple juice contains sorbitol, which can cause diarrhea.

High levels of vitamin C do not protect against colds. At most, extra vitamin C acts as a mild decongestant to relieve cold symptoms. Since dosing with high levels of vitamin C can cause negative side effects, it is better to avoid giving it to your child in amounts above the Daily Value.

Vitamins A, folic acid, phytochemicals

Fruits and vegetables are most notable as sources of vitamins C and A and other nutrients such as B vitamins, folic acid, and phytochemicals. Fruits and vegetables are important nutritionally, but not more important than foods from any other food group. Moreover, they are not important enough to justify trying to entice, force, reward, guilt-trip, or trick your child into eating them. Offer fruits and vegetables regularly, enjoy them yourself, and sooner or later your child will eat them, too. Offer a good vitamin A source three times a week. That would be dark-green and deep-yellow vegetables and fruit: apricots, peaches, mango, pumpkin, squash, carrots, sweet potatoes, broccoli, spinach, and other greens. Offer a good vitamin C source every day.

Fruits and vegetables such as peas, beets, bananas, potatoes, and apples contain less vitamin A and C, but contribute other nutrients. For example, bananas have folic acid, and fruits and vegetables in general are good sources of potassium. Most will give some trace elements such as zinc and copper. All have fiber.

B vitamins

Children usually get enough B vitamins (thiamin, riboflavin, niacin) because they like vitamin B-rich foods like enriched and whole-grain breads, cereals, and pasta. Your physician may recommend a vitamin B12 supplement if your child follows a pure vegan diet.

Vitamin D

Vitamin D works with calcium and phosphorus absorption and metabolism to build and maintain strong bones and teeth. Modest vitamin D deficiency weakens the bones and extreme deficiency causes rickets, thinning of the bones characterized by bow legs and bumps on the ends of the ribs. Formula has plenty of vitamin D; human milk is not a good source. The American Academy of Pediatrics recommends supplementing breastfed babies with no more than 400 IU vitamin D per day.[18] Too much vitamin D can weaken bones the same as too little: Be careful not to give your baby more than the recommended dose. Stage 4 babies can get enough vitamin D from fortified pasteurized milk. Egg yolks, salmon, and trout naturally have vitamin D. So does cod-liver oil, but I would be surprised if you use that! Your older baby will need a vitamin D supplement only if they don't drink vitamin D fortified pasteurized milk. Skin makes vitamin D when exposed to the sun—unless it is always well-slathered with sunscreen. If you are curious, do a web search for *How much sunshine for enough vitamin D.*

Calcium

The bones of children who don't get enough calcium aren't as strong as they could be and therefore break more easily. Calcium is, of course, necessary for the formation of strong teeth and bones, and vitamin D is essential for utilizing calcium. Pasteurized milk is the major and most dependable source of calcium and vitamin D. Supplementing calcium can be done, but that requires two or more doses of syrup or tablets distributed throughout the day. Calcium lactate and calcium carbonate supplements are absorbed reasonably well. Avoid bonemeal and dolomite because they may be contaminated with lead and other trace elements.

Fluoride

Fluoride, of course, is important for strong teeth. It promotes and protects tooth enamel and inhibits caries-producing bacteria. Children who get recommended amounts of fluoride from birth have two-thirds fewer cavities than children who do not get recommended amounts. Applying fluoride varnish to teeth is now part of routine dental care for young children.[19]

It is easy to get too much fluoride, so give your child a fluoride supplement only on the recommendation of your health care provider. It is hard to know how much fluoride your child gets, and too much can cause fluorosis: white mottling of the tooth enamel and colored mottling and even demineralization in extreme cases. Your child will get fluoride from municipal drinking water, formula made up with fluoridated water, foods and drinks that use fluoridated water in processing, and fluoridated toothpaste and mouth rinses. Be stingy with fluoride toothpaste because your child will swallow it. Bottled water that contains fluoride is labeled. Properly treated municipal water is fluoridated to a level of somewhere between 0.3 and 1.0 parts per million. Check with your local health department to see if your water is fluoridated.

COMMERCIAL BABY FOOD

The staged approach to adapting family food for your baby I describe in this chapter allows you to sidestep the whole issue of commercial baby food. Your baby won't need it.

Having said that, let me reassure you that feeding commercial baby food won't hurt your baby. Just don't get stuck on it. Some parents enjoy giving their cooperative babies little meals of meat and vegetables, topping things off with a baby dessert. Baby food desserts taste good and if you use them, you may find yourself eating them right along with your baby. Unlike grown-up desserts, they don't have that much to offer nutritionally.

If you are seeking convenience, keep in mind the earlier suggestions for adapting family food.

Nutrition and safety

Baby food companies' advertising pitches would have you believe that commercial baby food is essential. They claim that commercial baby food provides your baby with needed nutrients, supports your baby in learning to eat, is safer, and gives your baby early exposure to fruits and vegetables so they eat them later on. None of that is true.

Commercial infant foods are generally diluted with water and thickeners so the food doesn't taste the same as home-prepared food. With respect to nutrition, the key word is *needed*. Babies ages 6 to 12 months who are "consumers" of commercial baby food do get more nutrients than those who are not.[20] They don't *need* them. With the exception of iron from iron-fortified baby cereal, the nutrients end up in their diapers. By Stage 4, when your child actually needs the nutrients, children consuming family food do better nutritionally than "consumers" of baby food.[4]

The safety of the basic ingredients in even-organic baby food is the same as both organic and nonorganic adult foods. Both "adult" and baby carrots, sweet potatoes, apple juice, grape juice, and rice contain high levels of heavy metals. Sweet potatoes and carrots absorb lead as they grow, and rice pulls arsenic in preference to other heavy metals from the soil. Apple and grape juice contain high levels of inorganic arsenic and lead.

Learning to eat

Baby-food manufacturers claim to offer babies early exposure to and greater acceptance of fruits and vegetables. However, commercial baby foods don't taste much like the foods at family meals. High-temperature processing and diluting with water affects the flavor, making it hard to tell what the food actually *is*.

The baby-food business categorizes their foods in *steps*. Truth be told, that's where I got the idea of categorizing weanling foods into *stages*. Step 1 commercial foods are the same in texture as Stage 1 foods: smooth and similar to smooth, thin-to-medium baby cereal. After that, baby food Steps and my Stages diverge. Stage 2 food gives your baby experience with thicker, lumpier food and stimulates them to use their tongue to push food between their jaws. Commercial Step 2 are still silky smooth and offer no oral-motor learning beyond Step 1 foods.

Babies eating Stage 3 foods learn to pick food up with their fingers, bite off and chew. Babies eating Step 3 foods learn to suck semisolid food from a food pouch. Babies eating Stage 4 food learn to feed themselves soft and easy-to-chew food from family meals. "Mealtime for toddler" foods are similar to Stage 4 food: They are shelf-stable, low-sodium versions of grown-up TV dinners. They are handy at times but not a substitute for including your child in family meals.

What does commercial baby food contain?

Today's baby peas, peaches, and other single-ingredient baby foods are better than before in that they generally contain half or more of the named ingredient and half or less water. Manufacturers don't have to tell you how much water. Dinners are likely to have fillers and preservatives.

Because they are made from white rice flour, baby snack foods such as baby wafers and puffs are high in arsenic; they also have no fiber or protein. [21]

Both baby food and grown-up carrots, spinach, and beets are potentially high in nitrate, so let your baby eat only two to three tablespoons altogether a day. Commercial baby food companies say they screen for nitrate, but they don't necessarily *remove* it.

GOOD FEEDING IS A CONVERSATION

Good feeding is a nicely flowing nonverbal conversation, a conversation that happens again and again when you follow sDOR in feeding your baby. Not only are good feeding conversations intensely satisfying, but they also make a fundamental contribution to your baby's nutritional, social, emotional, and intellectual development. You have a good conversation when your baby is excited and wants to eat fast and you feed them fast and maybe even reflect their pleasure and excitement. You have a good conversation when you accept your baby's lack of interest in eating and let it go rather than trying to get them to eat. The two of you are on the same wavelength, and you both have a good time. But if you insist that your baby eat or suddenly stop feeding them for no apparent reason, you have broken a basic rule of conversation. You might know you have run out of food, but your baby will not, and they will feel upset. It happens to us all sometimes, but if it keeps happening, you are not going to be a favorite conversation partner, and feeding is not going to be a favorite activity for either of you.

Some babies' messages are difficult to figure out. Some parents have difficulty letting go of control and trusting their baby to take the lead. If either holds true for you and your baby, get help. It is that important.

WHAT COMES NEXT

Give yourself a lovely pat on the back. You have come through the constant changes of the transitional feeding period to arrive at a family-meals-plus-sit-down-snacks routine. From now on, your little one will be polishing their skills—getting better at drinking from the cup, chewing, eventually learning to use a spoon and fork. If all goes well, you will even get a breather before your enthusiastically eating almost-toddler turns into a *real* toddler and shows the more limited appetite and contrariness of that stage. Then, your respecting your child's wishes early on will pay off: Your toddler is more likely to listen to you when you have listened to them when they were younger.

REFERENCES

1. Coulthard H. Delayed introduction of lumpy foods to children during the complementary feeding period affects child's food acceptance and feeding at 7 years of age. *Matern Child Nutr*. 2009;5:75–85.
2. Sullivan SA. Infants, dietary experience and acceptance of solid foods. *Pediatrics*. 1994;93:271–277.
3. Mennella JA. Early milk feeding influences taste acceptance and liking during infancy. *Am J Clin Nutr*. Sep 2009;90:780s–788s.
4. Briefel R. Toddlers' transition to table foods: impact on nutrient intakes and food patterns. *J Am Diet Assoc*. 2004;104:S38–S44.

5. Welker EB. Room for improvement remains in food consumption patterns of young children aged 2-4 years. *J Nutr*. 2018. doi:10.1093/jn/nxx053
6. D'Auria E. Baby-led weaning: what a systematic review of the literature adds on. *Ital J Pediatr*. 2018;44:49.
7. Białek-Dratwa A. Use of the Baby-Led Weaning (BLW) method in complementary feeding of the infant: a cross-sectional study of mothers using and not using the BLW method. *Nutrients*. 2022. doi:10.3390/nu14122372
8. Tabangi M. Maternal anxiety during solid food introduction: insights from a comparative feeding practices study. *BMC Pregnancy and Childbirth*. 2025. doi:10.1186/s12884-025-07859-8
9. Rowan H. Estimated energy and nutrient intake for infants following baby-led and traditional weaning approaches. *Journal of Human Nutrition and Dietetics*. 2022;35:325–336.
10. Beal VA. On the acceptance of solid foods and other food patterns of infants and children. *Pediatrics*. 1957;20:448–456.
11. Scharf RJ. Longitudinal evaluation of milk type consumed and weight status in preschoolers. *Arch Dis Child*. 2013:335–340.
12. Sigman-Grant M. Dietary approaches for reducing fat intake of preschool-aged children. *Pediatrics*. 1993;91:955–960.
13. Bailey RL. Total usual nutrient intakes of US children (under 48 months): findings from the Feeding Infants and Toddlers Study (FITS) 2016. *J Nutr*. 2018;148:1557S–1566S.
14. Beal VA. Dietary intake of individuals followed through infancy and childhood. *American Journal of Public Health*. 1961;51:1107–1117.
15. Soriano VX. Complementary and allergenic food introduction in infants: an umbrella review. *Pediatrics*. 2023. doi:10.1542/peds.2022-058380
16. Greer FR. Effects of early nutritional interventions on the development of atopic disease in infants and children: the role of maternal dietary restriction, breastfeeding, timing of introduction of complementary foods, and hydrolyzed formulas. *Pediatrics*. 2019. doi:(4): e20190281
17. U.S. Department of Health and Human Services. *Dietary Guidelines for Americans. 8th Edition*. 2020.
18. Simon AE. Adherence to Vitamin D Intake guidelines in the United States. *Pediatrics*. 2020. doi:10.1542/peds.2019-3574
19. Clark MB. Fluoride use in caries prevention in the primary care setting. *Pediatrics*. 2020. doi:10.1542/peds.2020-034637
20. Reidy KC. Food consumption patterns and micronutrient density of complementary foods consumed by infants fed commercially prepared baby foods. *Nutr Today*. 2018;53:68–78.
21. Loria K. Are there still heavy metals in baby food? *https://www.consumerreports.org/babies-kids/baby-food/are-heavy-metal-levels-in-baby-foods-getting-better-a1163977621/*

PART III

How to Feed: The Toddler and Preschooler

CHAPTER 11

Feeding Your Toddler

Toddlers are called toddlers because they—well—toddle. Physically, your almost-toddler becomes a toddler when they can crawl, walk, or scoot on their backside to explore the world. Emotionally, socially, and cognitively, they become a toddler when they demonstrate that they are separate by roaming out and checking back in, saying no, and testing what is and isn't okay.

Now that your child is a toddler, their eating honeymoon—and yours—is well and truly over. If they haven't already, your child will soon replace their almost-toddler enthusiasm about eating practically everything with the toddler's typically unpredictable eating pattern. Courage. When you follow sDOR your child will learn to eat your food, they will be well-nourished, and they will eat the amount they need.

We are working toward your toddler's coming to meals willingly, enjoying being there, being pleasant enough to be allowed to stay most of the time, and not having anything expected of them that they can't deliver. Do not expect your toddler to neatly eat everything that is before them including their vegetables. In terms of the toddler's food consumption, being Eating Competent means a spoonful of this, a fingerful or possibly a lot of that, and squishing or ignoring everything else.

As summarized in Figure 11.1, your toddler's Eating Competence looks like anything but. While toddler food skepticism looks like a step in the wrong direction, it grows out of their cognitive development. The toddler is wary, and justifiably so. They have developed mentally enough to become suspicious of unfamiliar food, but not enough to use thinking and reasoning to get comfortable with what they consider to be new food. As a preschooler, your child's food skepticism will decrease because they can talk about it and help cook it or grow it. It will, that is, provided you haven't panicked earlier and tried to get them to eat.

FIGURE 11.1: THE TODDLER'S EATING COMPETENCE

Here is what to expect from your toddler's eating attitudes and behavior:

- Toddlers are skeptical of unfamiliar food—or food they regard as unfamiliar.
- In spite of their skepticism, toddlers learn to eat new food with time and repeated neutral exposure.
- Toddlers are erratic. They eat a lot one day and hardly anything the next. What they eat one day, they ignore the next.
- Toddlers don't eat some of everything at a meal like grown-ups do—they eat only one or two foods.
- Toddlers will stop doing what you don't want, such as causing a ruckus at mealtime, but they won't do what you do want—such as eat.

IN THIS CHAPTER

To raise a Competent Eater, your job is to hang in there with family meals and not get discouraged by your toddler's skeptical, opinionated, erratic eating. You have roughly two years of feeding adventures, pitfalls, and fun. Or not fun, depending on your attitude. If you enter this period with a healthy dose of curiosity about your toddler and the assumption that on some level they know what they are doing, then I promise you fun. But if you have even the tiniest desire to get your child to eat certain amounts of certain foods, I promise you won't have fun.

This chapter lays the foundation for everything that comes afterwards with feeding. The version of the Satter Division of Responsibility in Feeding (sDOR) that you establish with your toddler is appropriate—with minor modification—throughout your child's growing-up years. The same as the last chapter, about two thirds covers the feeding relationship: understanding and addressing toddlers' quirky behavior; translating routine plus trust in feeding into managing family meals and snacks; solving feeding problems. The last third is about food and nutrition: choosing food and deciding about supplemental nutrients. For a sneak preview of what to expect in feeding your toddler, skip ahead to some stories that pull it all together: "Toddler feeding skirmishes," page 385.

THE TODDLER DIVISION OF RESPONSIBILITY IN FEEDING (sDOR)

Who does what is critically important for your toddler. Consider the story of a powerful Norse god who boasted he could get anyone to do his bidding. A woman responded that she knew of someone whose will was stronger than his. She was referring to her two-year-old daughter. Foolish god, he didn't believe it, and it was left to the girl to prove the truth of the mother's words. That mother knew what you and I know. You can't force a toddler to do your bidding.

It is a tricky balance, and sDOR helps you maintain that balance. Following sDOR gives your child warm, kind leadership with feeding and provides room for independence with eating. As with any other stage in feeding, your child needs to have their emotional needs met in order to eat well.

- You are responsible for the *what, when,* and *where* of *feeding.*
- Your child is responsible for the *whether* and *how much* of *eating.*

sDOR gives your child *repeated neutral exposure. Repeated exposure* is having food show up from time to time at family meals. *Neutral* means *no pressure.* That means being absolutely willing to take no for an answer and reassuringly clear with your child that they don't have to eat anything they don't want to eat.

Figure 11.2 elaborates on following sDOR with the toddler. Don't worry that sticking to your feeding jobs will make you rigid and bossy. These are reasonable limits, and your toddler will feel most secure and free to explore when you provide this guidance.

FIGURE 11.2: YOUR FEEDING JOBS AND YOUR TODDLER'S EATING JOBS

<table>
<tr><td colspan="2">Your toddler eats best when you follow sDOR by doing the what, when, and where of feeding, then trust them to do the whether and how much of eating.</td></tr>
<tr><td>Your feeding jobs
• Choose and prepare the food.
• Provide regular meals and snacks.
• Make eating times pleasant.
• Step by step, show children by example how to behave at family mealtime.
• Be considerate of children's food inexperience without catering to likes and dislikes.
• Not let children have food or beverages (except for water) between meal and snack times.
• Let children grow up to have bodies that are right for them.</td><td>Your child's eating jobs
• Your child will eat.
• They will eat the amount they need.
• They will learn to eat the food you eat.
• They will grow predictably.
• They will behave the way you want them to at mealtime.</td></tr>
</table>

TODDLER DEVELOPMENT

sDOR supports the toddler's primary developmental task of separation-individuation. Toddlers are about the business of demonstrating to themselves and others that they are a separate person. They have a tremendous need to be independent, to be successful, to explore, and to have limits. They experience themselves as separate when they insist on doing it themselves and when they say *no*. Insistent as they are on having their own way, they feel ambivalent about it all. They need to know that they are their own person, but they also need to know that they can't dominate you.

Your toddler can direct their energy to self-assertion because they are securely grounded in your love. They can take chances with defying you because they are pretty sure you won't give up on them. With infants it's easy to see what love looks like because you gratify their every wish. But what does love look like with a toddler, where gratifying their every wish will fail them utterly? It looks like keeping them safe and teaching them to be successful; socializing them so they can get along with other people; showing them what is and isn't okay; keeping the size of their world down to what they can manage.

Your toddler is learning to retain their sense of self at the same time as they experience the rewards of being part of the family. That all happens when you follow sDOR. While giving up the conviction that they are the star of the family may seem a wrenching loss, it is a necessary one. Without it, the child can go through life having to work overtime to be the center of attention and only then feeling included.

Sorting out feelings and sensations

If all that isn't complicated enough, consider the toddler task of *somatopsychological differentiation*. That mouthful term means learning to distinguish among emotions and differentiate emotions from sensations. In order to make those distinctions, your toddler depends on you to apply the appropriate response to their dilemmas. Clear as mud? Perhaps this example will help. Say your toddler is angry and frustrated because you have said no. How do you react to their anger? Do you tolerate their upset while not letting them get destructive, maybe even say, "You are angry?" Do you try to jolly them out of it? Do you give them a cookie?

You tolerate their upset, keep them from being destructive, and hang in there with them until they cool off. That teaches your toddler to identify their upset as anger and discover what to do about it. It is not easy, and you may mess this up a few times—even quite a few times—before you get it right. Take heart. Children are resilient little creatures who give us lots of chances to learn. Being able to feel anger is important for letting us know when something is going on that is not in our best interest. The important learning is how to *respond* to anger. Joking with your child confuses anger with happiness and humor, which is not good. Feeding them confuses hunger with anger and teaches them to eat for emotional reasons. In fact, it is during the toddler period that learning to eat for emotional reasons becomes deeply embedded. Again, relax. A single cookie handout or even a few won't teach your child to eat for emotional reasons. That's a good thing, because what parent hasn't resorted to cookies when they are at the end of their tether?

Your toddler depends on routine and autonomy

With all that going on, no wonder your toddler is touchy. Your toddler needs sDOR to accomplish their developmental tasks. You help by following sDOR and, in fact, applying routine and autonomy to all things parenting. Despite their protests, your toddler feels most secure when boundaries are in place. It demonstrates to them that you are stronger than they are and that they can depend on you to take care of them. They are like the security guard, checking all the doors but not really wanting to find any open. Of course, this is all nonverbal and has to do with their innate sense—a sense that we all have—of what is good for us and what isn't.

SORT OUT CONTROL ISSUES

Raising a toddler sets the stage for years to come in the way you manage control issues with your child. Being clear about what is yours to control allows you to do authoritative parenting. You can be warm and confident with providing structure and clear expectations. Then you can be open, trusting, and supportive of your child's independence and individuality.

Because control issues in feeding are so critical and so nebulous, I have devoted three figures to the topic. Figure 11.2 gives details of following sDOR with toddler and older children; Figure 11.3 details crossing the lines of sDOR; and Figure 11.4 discusses toddler moves and countermoves as you sort out control.

FIGURE 11.3: CROSSING THE LINES OF sDOR

These feeding errors are common. They are typical of what parents do when they feel it is their responsibility to get their child to eat and grow in certain ways.

You aren't doing your jobs with feeding if you . . .

- Are inconsistent about providing sit-down meals and snacks.
- Let your child have food or drink handouts between times.
- Let your child misbehave at mealtime.
- Limit the menu to "healthy," low-calorie, low-fat food.
- Limit the menu to what your child will eat.

You are intruding on your child's jobs with eating if you persuade or trick them to . . .

- Eat their vegetables or anything else.
- Clean their plate.
- Insist they take a bite of everything.
- Eat other food, even their vegetables, before they can have dessert.
- Eat less than they are hungry for.
- Eat more than they are hungry for.

The Figure 11.3 *intruding* tactics are controlling by virtue of being pressuring and manipulating. Children behave poorly when they are on the receiving end of such tactics, and their nutritional welfare suffers. Your child doesn't need pressure from you because they already feel pressure within themselves. They want to grow up. They push themself along to learn to crawl, walk, talk, and ride a tricycle. Why wouldn't they push themself along to grow up with eating? Because we don't expect them to or let them, that's why. Somehow, we have gotten the notion that children won't eat unless they are pushed or prodded into it. A child's eating becomes our investment, and then it loses its appeal for the child.

Avoid the one-bite rule. Insisting on even one bite and/or even one taste or smell constitutes pressure and interferes with your child's jobs with eating.

Don't cater. If you make it especially for your child, you will expect them to eat it, and they know it. Instead, let them experience the consequence of being hungry before snack time. Again, we are not starving them into submission; we are teaching them to take eating at mealtime more seriously.

Be prepared for toddler experiments

Figure 1.3, "Trust is a two-way street," page 12, illustrates how trust with feeding depends on everyone staying in their own lane. That means sticking with what they can control and not intruding on what is someone else's to control. Toddlers resist being controlled and continually strive to take over what you control. It sounds diabolical, but that is simply what growing up is all about. Resist the enticement by holding firm with your jobs. Over and over and over again.

Figure 11.4 illustrates some of the finer points about staying in your lane with feeding. Your toddler's erratic food acceptance entices you to cross the line of sDOR and try to get them to eat. Their quirky mealtime behavior entices you to relax the structure of meals and snacks and just feed them on the run. Your toddler is *experimenting*, not being naughty: "Is this all right?" "What about this?" ". . . and this?" "I couldn't do—be—touch—this yesterday, how about today?" It can be exhausting. But hang in there, keep your sense of humor, and enjoy it while it lasts. At some point your toddler's experiments will end, they will be satisfied that they are their own little person, and they will turn into a cooperative preschooler. Most of the time.

sDOR and finishing the meal

Hungry toddlers behave well at meals and snacks. They eat with focus and attention until they get full. That can take anywhere from 5 to 15 minutes. After that, they are all done and ready to get down. Let them. Keeping them there after that point will likely create misbehavior on their part and frustration on yours.

Teach them to say "may I go" in whatever language they can manage. Consider having them clear their plate from the table as a signal they are finished. Teach them to respect your needs by playing quietly while you finish eating. Have some books and toys nearby and direct their attention to them. Continue to include them by looking and responding to what they say. They will test by wanting to come back to the meal, but say, "It's time for you to play while we finish eating." Be prepared for them to get upset, cry, and even have a tantrum. Ignore it.

Saying no isn't easy, and you may find yourself experimenting with alternatives. Reminding: "You said you were finished." Reasoning: "Wouldn't you rather play with your trucks?" Bargaining: "You can come back just this once." Warning: "Stop bothering or I will give you a time-out." If all goes well, it won't take you long to catch on: Your toddler learns from what you *do*, not from what you *say*.

FIGURE 11.4: TODDLER EATING MOVES AND YOUR COUNTERMOVES

Your toddler will test to find out what is and isn't all right. Here are some of the finer points of staying in your lane with feeding.

YOUR CHILD'S MOVE	YOUR MOVE
They say, "I am not hungry."	You say, "You do not have to eat; just sit with us for a while."
They are too worked up and busy to eat.	Spend a few minutes with them just before the meal reading a book or washing hands. Set a five-minute timer.
They cannot take time to eat.	Arrange for them to be hungry at mealtime by not allowing eating between times.
They are too hungry to wait for meals.	Have sit-down snacks between meals.
They do not want to stay at the meal until you finish eating.	Let them leave when they get full. They will stay at the meal longer as they get older and enjoy conversation.
They are messy on purpose, naughty, or otherwise disruptive at the meal.	Give one warning, then have them leave. They are full or they would eat—and behave! Don't let them come back.
They come right back begging for food or to be allowed to join in.	Tell them there will be more food at snack time. Ignore their tantrums.
They leave, but they want your attention, to sit on your lap, or to eat off your plate.	Pat them on the head and send them away. Keep toys nearby and interest them in playing. Look, smile, nod, or comment but don't interrupt.
They do not eat "enough" at mealtime.	Only they know how much is enough. Arrange for them to be hungry by not giving food or beverage handouts between times, except for water.
They beg at mealtime for peanut butter, cereal, or other food.	You say, "You do not have to eat anything if you do not want to, but this is what we have."

PLAN MEALS FOR THE WHOLE FAMILY

Figure 11.5 elaborates on your jobs with feeding your toddler. Instead of feeding toddlers immediately when hunger strikes as you have done before, let their hunger rhythms adjust to match family meal- and snack-times. It's quite revolutionary, in terms of your toddler's young life. Now instead of having the family cater to them, the toddler begins learning to fit into the family without losing their sense of independence.

Following mealtime basics gives your child choices within limits. You offer structure and safety by making your child's world small enough so they can manage it. Instead of turning them loose to choose food in the grocery store or even in the kitchen, you turn them loose at the family table to choose whether or not to eat from what you provide. Your toddler will test and resist your *what, when,* and *where* limits, but that is how they learn.

Do your feeding jobs and don't worry when your toddler goes through the long warm-up of 20 (or 40 or 80) meals to get around to eating a particular food. As long as they are positive and relaxed at meal-time, your toddler will get there. It is all part of the learning process. Not-worried parents raise children who are less inclined to be picky eaters—as long as parents continue to follow sDOR.

FIGURE 11.5: TODDLER MEALTIME BASICS

- Have three meals a day with planned snacks in between. Don't give food or beverage handouts between times, except for water.
- Manage the timing of sit-down snacks to help your child be calm, well-rested, and hungry but not famished at mealtime.
- Include your child in family meals. Eat with them. Don't feed them separately.
- Present foods in a form your child can manage relative to shape, texture, and temperature.
- Let your toddler look, feel, mash, and smell to explore—but not to get a rise out of you.
- Don't try to get them to eat or even smell, lick, or taste anything they don't want to.
- Don't make them clean their plate. Even adults have trouble knowing what and how much they will eat.
- Make family mealtimes pleasant. Don't argue, fight, or scold.
- Talk and pay attention to your toddler, but don't make them the center of attention.
- Turn the TV off and put away the phone and tablet: They distract from eating and interfere with family social time.

However, not worrying can go too far and become negative if you don't do your jobs with feeding.

Make family meals *manageable*

Allow me to quote my colleague Jennifer Harris, "No meal is perfect. Eat together anyway." Allow me to quote myself, "Even the most reprehensible family meal is better than no meal at all." While some days you will have the time and energy to prepare your dream home-cooked family meal, most days you won't. Researchers in Atlanta found that for most parents of young children, "resource depletion" is the name of the game. Parents have too much to do and too little time to do it in. Resource-depleted parents were more likely to try to get their child to eat more or less than they ate voluntarily.[1]

Do not make boring food, even if it is nutritionally superior. Think back to the story about Annie in the Chapter 2 section, "Lighten up on 'healthy' food," page 55. Annie would only eat at the neighbor's house because their food tasted good. This was in contrast to her parents' broiled poultry and fish, vegetables without added fat, fresh fruit, bread with a dab of diet margarine, and nonfat milk. Annie's parents started to include more fat and sugar in their meals, and Annie started eating at home. She even stopped telling her parents about the food next door.

Be considerate without catering

As Figure 11.6 outlines, don't try to please every eater with every food at every meal, but do plan meals that let your little and big eaters be successful. Provide one or two side dishes that family members *generally* eat. You have done your feeding job by making the food as accessible as you can without sacrificing structure. It doesn't undo your job when others decide not to eat.

Include generally enjoyed foods—what my readers call "safe" foods—in quantities large enough for everyone. Then let eaters—including yourself and your partner—eat what tastes good at that very meal. Have your child's favorite foods sometimes—but not all the time. Other family members have rights, too.

Trying to produce a meal your child will eat is a common trap and one you can avoid. Back in the day, I did lots of magazine and newspaper interviews. Often writers approached me on the topic of getting children to eat, and almost without exception, they began by asking for a list of foods children like.

FIGURE 11.6: BE CONSIDERATE WITHOUT CATERING WITH MEAL PLANNING

Cook one meal for everyone. Don't offer substitutes. Instead, plan the meal to reassure yourself that you are giving your child and other family members every chance of finding something they will enjoy eating.

- Let everyone pick and choose from food offered at the meal.
- Serve dishes in parts so your child can eat or not eat each part. Children often eat the rice but ignore the stir-fry, eat the spaghetti but ignore the meat sauce. Eventually, they get around to eating the whole dish.
- Settle for providing each eater with one or two foods (milk can be one) at each meal they generally enjoy. If the main dish isn't too popular, include well-received side dishes that everyone shares, such as bread, pasta, fruit, etc.
- Pair unfamiliar with familiar food: foods your family members have enjoyed before with those they have not yet learned to enjoy.
- Settle for one main dish. Don't offer even easy-to-prepare alternatives such as pizza, hot dogs, chicken nuggets, cereal, or peanut butter. When you do serve pizza, chicken nuggets, etc., make them the main dish for everyone to share.
- Include high-fat spreads and sauces with the meal such as butter, salad dressing, dip, or gravy and let your child eat as much as they want. Children and others who need a lot of calories eat more fat, those who need fewer calories eat less.

"We can't know that," I would say firmly and, after hundreds of interviews, no doubt somewhat impatiently." Only the child knows that and it changes constantly. Adults are not to cast about looking for something that children will eat. They are to offer a variety of food and let children pick and choose from what is available."

Don't hide vegetables in other foods

It is all right to include vegetables in soups, casseroles, and other foods, but don't *hide* them. Cut the vegetables into large enough pieces so your child can see them and put them aside if they don't want to eat them. Keep in mind that trust flows both ways. Just as you need to trust your child to do their part with eating, your child needs to trust you to do your part with feeding. Being trustworthy includes you being honest with your child about what is in the food that you offer them to eat.

Sooner or later, they will discover you have been pulverizing carrots and putting them in the brownies or sneaking beets into smoothies. They will become suspicious of all food and particularly negative about vegetables. In a child's mind, it goes something like, "That can't be too good if they are doing all that to get me to eat it."

Consider milk as the primary mealtime beverage

Milk is important. It is children's main source of calcium and vitamin D. Young children don't eat that much meat, and they get much of their protein from milk. Children who get enough calcium[2] and vitamin D[3] have stronger and more fracture-resistant bones; children who avoid milk have more broken bones.[4] Depending on your cultural background, you and your family may not routinely drink milk. If that is the case for you, include the other good sources of calcium and vitamin D. More about that in the "Celebrate food" section.

Even the child who drinks milk will go through times when they don't drink much, especially right after they are weaned from the nipple. Don't make a fuss about it, and don't push milk. Instead, put a small glass of milk at your child's place, and let them drink it or not. Chocolate or strawberry milk are fine once in a while, but regularly flavoring milk to get it into your child is pressure, and pressure backfires. Drink milk yourself. If you are lactose intolerant, make it a small glass of whole milk or use lactose-free milk. If you cannot drink milk, drink water. Your child is unlikely to become lactose intolerant until they become a preschooler or older.

When parents complain that a child drinks "too much" milk, I check out feeding. Are parents following sDOR? If they are, I encourage them not to worry about it, remind them about toddlers' erratic eating, and tell them a child's milk consumption can range from none at all to over a quart a day. Just to be sure, we tease apart whether they are trying to get their child to eat certain foods. If they are, it is likely the child is getting turned off to the foods parents are trying to get them to eat and resorting to drinking milk because nothing else appeals.

Serve dessert along with the meal

You may be familiar with mealtime hassles about dessert. "Finish your vegetables and then you can have dessert" say generation after generation of parents. Thereby they ensure that generation after generation of children learn to love dessert and despise vegetables. Not only that but making dessert a reward for eating pressures a toddler twice to eat more than they want, once to eat the meal to get the dessert and once to eat dessert when they are already filled up on the meal.

Make dessert an ordinary part of the meal by putting a single, child-size serving at your child's place setting. At mealtime, let them eat the dessert when they want to. Your child might eat it first, still be hungry, and go on to eat the rest of the meal. Or they might eat a bite of dessert, then a bite of something else. Or they might do it the standard way of eating the meal and saving the dessert for the end. Tell them ahead of time there is only one serving of dessert but also know that your toddler will try to get you to give them more dessert. The answer is no, even if your toddler leaves the meal after eating only their dessert.

"One serving of dessert" violates sDOR—for a good reason. Children push themselves along to learn and grow. They also take the easy way out when it is offered. Since sweets are so much easier to learn to eat than other mealtime food, children are likely to fill up on dessert when it is available in unlimited amounts and not learn to eat mealtime food. Treat chips the same as other mealtime food by providing enough so everyone can eat as much as they want. At first, family members may eat a lot of them, but after the newness wears off, they will just eat them.

Include sweets

To make up for being restrictive (and violating sDOR) with the one-serving-of-dessert strategy, occasionally offer unlimited sweets for sit-down snacks. I talked about "forbidden" food in the Chapter 2 section, "Help your child be comfortable with family meals," page 46. Here it is again in Figure 11.7 to let you know I really mean it.

Figure 11.7 gives strategies for finding a balance between too much and too little "forbidden food." Include sweets such as cookies, candy, or cake as part of your regular meal- and snack-time routine. Do the same with chips and other savory snack-type food. Consider soda. Your child will want it if you drink it. If you can't give it up, maintain a double standard: Tell your toddler it is a grown-up drink, which it is. If they still want it when they get older, let them have soda occasionally for snack or along with a particular meal such as pizza or tacos. Even when your child is older, include it as part of a meal or snack rather than letting them drink it on the run. Maintaining structure holds down on overall consumption and protects teeth.

Conventional nutrition advice is to totally avoid or do bare-minimum consumption of sweets and chips.[5] Certainly *too many* sweets and chips dilute the nutritional quality of the diet. But parents don't let children eat sweets and chips as much as they want, whenever they want. If you are like most parents, you are looking for moderate, realistic, and practical ways to include sweets and chips.

FIGURE 11.7: REGULARLY OFFER "FORBIDDEN" FOODS

Take the "special" and "forbidden" out of high-fat, high-sugar foods by including them regularly.

- Put one serving of dessert at each person's place when you set the table. Let children and others eat it before, during, or after the meal. Children are less likely to eat more than they want when they are allowed to have dessert first rather than having to earn dessert by eating the rest of their meal.
- Don't allow seconds for dessert. Unlimited sweets at mealtime compete unfairly with other mealtime foods.
- Include chips or fries at mealtime. Arrange to have enough so everyone can eat their fill. Unlike sweets, fatty foods don't compete unfairly with other food.
- To make up for limiting sweets at mealtime, periodically offer unlimited sweets at snack time. For instance, put a plate of cookies or snack cakes and a carton of milk on the table. Let your child (and yourself) eat as many cookies as they want. At first you may both eat a lot. But the newness will wear off, and you won't eat so many. Having as many cookies as they want at snack time is different from the mealtime-dessert strategy because eating cookies for snack doesn't interfere with eating other nutritious food.
- Don't be afraid of even food you consider particularly delicious. You and your child will get enough, and it will stop tasting as good—until the next time you have it. Paying attention lets you enjoy it and know when you are satisfied.
- Be strategic about soda.

Experience shows that restricting sweets and chips doesn't work. Parents who restrict find candy wrappers and chips packages under the couch. As my colleague Peggy Crum observed when she read this chapter, when you put chips and sweets on a pedestal, children just jump higher to get them. Even when they try really hard not to eat them, sweets-and-chips-deprived children (and adults) just can't help eating a lot of them when they get the chance. Then they feel bad about eating them. They also tend to be fatter.[6]

Having sweets and chips regularly at meals and sit-down snacks is the happy medium. At first, children eat a lot, but after a while those foods lose their special appeal, and children don't eat so many of them.

HELP YOUR TODDLER BE SUCCESSFUL WITH MEALS

Along with strategies for making food accessible to your toddler, consider these strategies for helping them participate in family meals.

Help your toddler take time to eat

Help your toddler be calm, rested, and ready to eat. Toddlers play hard and have a lot on their minds; they need help getting their mind on food and eating. Give your child a five-minute alert before the meal. Help them settle down by washing hands with them and even letting them play in the water a bit. If you can find the time, sit down and read a short book. After you sit down at the meal and before you start to eat, interrupt the hurry-up of getting there and focus everybody's attention on eating by sharing a quiet moment of relaxation, saying bon appétit or grace, or singing a little song.

Let your toddler serve themself

Parents are often startled with the recommendation to serve family-style and allow their two-year-old to serve themself. This seems to be a big step, but it is a worthwhile one. Toddlers relish independence and are more interested in eating when they feel they are in control. Put the food in smallish serving bowls with soup spoons or teaspoons and let your child serve themself. Have a number of backup spoons to start with, as your toddler will forget to put the spoon back in the serving bowl or lick it off before they do. Let them pass the dish after they serve themself—or after they don't take any.

Hang on to your curiosity and your sense of humor. As with everything else, your child will have a lot to learn. Don't expect your child to eat all or even some of what they take. They are learning to eat the food, even if they take it and it sits on their plate. Small serving dishes and small plates encourage them to take a bit less so there isn't so much waste, but there *will* be waste.

If you serve your child, ask if they want the food, and then ask how much they want. If you serve plates in the kitchen, reassure your child that they don't have to eat what is on their plate if they don't want to, and that there is more of everything if they want more.

Give your child a comfortable chair

If you eat at a table, a comfortable chair will help them stay put during the meal. Taking the tray off the high chair and pulling it up to the table might work or do a web search for *youth chair for dining table*. Your toddler will do best if their elbows are at table height. That lets them see the food, use their fingers and utensils, and reach their glass. Support their feet—dangling feet are uncomfortable. A chair is best—booster chairs tend to wiggle around and are both less safe and less effective at helping settle a child down to eat.

Use child-size plates and utensils

A small plate with a low, sticking-up rim works well because it gives a bang-board for pushing the food onto the fork or spoon. Child-size silverware is great, or a broad salad fork and teaspoon work well. Consider a cup with handles or a glass with a broad base that sits firmly; choose one that is small enough so they can get their little hands around it. Use a covered junior cup if you want to, but keep in mind that specialists in children's oral-motor development say it is better to let a child learn to drink from an open cup. If you are concerned about your floor, protect it, as there will be spills and food droppings.

Occasionally children ask to be allowed to sit at their own small eating table and chairs. That is fine once in a while and also comfortable for them, as long as they don't abuse the privilege by getting up and running around during the meal. However, doing the little table routine too often takes away the specialness of it and deprives your child of eating with you.

Be easygoing about manners

Developing positive attitudes about eating is more important than mastering the niceties of mealtime manners. Provide your child with silverware, but don't insist they use it. Letting them use their fingers to feel and mash food helps them gain experience with the food and get comfortable with it. You'll be able to tell if your child is truly exploring food or just playing or messing around. Toddlers eat with attention and focus until they get enough, then they start messing around. Let your child leave the meal when they show they are finished and teach them to play quietly nearby while you finish your meal.

Sooner or later your child will begin to imitate your mealtime behavior. Do you consider that a promise—or a threat? Reminding your child to sit properly, eat neatly, and use the napkin interrupts their eating. Interrupted children either become rebellious or so preoccupied with the mechanics that they lose interest in food. As children mature, the spills, dropped food and utensils, and general mess decrease. In the meantime, keep a roll of paper towels handy.

Avoid the no-thank-you bite

In case you are among the uninitiated, the rule of the no-thank-you bite is that every child has to take a mouthful of every food at the meal. Or two. Or three. Or sometimes even a no-thank-you *helping*! I don't like that rule and I don't recommend it. It is a control tactic that interferes with rather than enhances children's food acceptance. Why? Because it overlooks the fundamental point that children *want* to grow up with eating. Children do get around on their own to taking bites. *Insisting* they take bites takes away their initiative and makes their eating your thing, not theirs.

Don't you just hate it when somebody tells you to do the very thing you are just about to do? Toddlers feel the same way. Even the most slow-to-warm-up or uptight child has within them the driving need to experiment and master. That need pushes them along to experiment and master with food the same as with everything else.

Understand gagging and choking

To protect your child against choking, take the precautions listed in Figure 11.8.

FIGURE 11.8: PROTECT YOUR CHILD FROM CHOKING

Avoiding choking is about choosing and adapting food so your child can safely eat it. It is also about managing eating times so they are low key and well supervised.

- Build your child's eating skills. Let them work up slowly to more difficult foods.
- For the child under age three, avoid nuts, raw carrots, hard candy, gum drops, jelly beans, and other hard or firm foods of about that size and shape.
- Adapt foods that may cause choking hazards. Cut hot dogs lengthwise, quarter grapes and cherry tomatoes, peel and grate raw apples and carrots, finely chop nuts.
- Pay attention while your child eats so you can be sure they aren't choking.
- Have your child sit while they eat; don't let them wander around.
- Keep things calm at eating time.
- Have your health care provider teach you first aid for choking.

Young children gag. The gag reflex is a neurological safety mechanism that helps prevent choking. When food slips to the back of a child's tongue before they are ready to swallow it, the gag reflex shoves the food back out again. If you don't react to your child's gagging, they won't either. They will go right on eating. But if your child continues to gag a lot and doesn't want anything in their mouth, bring it to the attention of your health care provider.

While gagging is to be expected, choking is dangerous. How do you tell the difference? As long as your child exchanges enough air to cough, they are probably okay. However, if they make no sound or only a squeaky, whistling, inhaling sound, they may be choking. During swallowing, food moves down your child's throat past the end of their windpipe. They choke when they inhale and suck food into the windpipe. Laughing or catching their breath while they eat can make a child choke. So can being upset in general during mealtime. Slippery round foods like hot dogs and grapes are difficult for an inexperienced eater to control with their tongue and push between the jaws. When such foods slip down your child's throat, they are just the right size and shape to plug up the windpipe. Children also have an increased risk of choking on foods that are difficult to chew, such as tough meats and hard nuts and candies. Children have also choked on sticky foods, like large wads of peanut butter.

HAVE SIT-DOWN SNACKS

Sit-down snacks are essential for making family meals work. Consider the scenario where your toddler leaves lunch having eaten little or nothing. Ten minutes later they are begging for food. You say, "That's it until dinner time." Yikes! That could be five or six hours of food-begging and tantrums! What if instead you say, "That's it until snack time." Whew. Two or three hours—or even less if your toddler is just getting into the meals-plus-snacks routine and you move snack time up a bit. You still have to put up with begging and tantrums, but the end is in sight.

A snack just *is*. It is not a reward or prompt for *anything*. Do not use snacks to leverage your child's mealtime eating, as in "If you want your snack, you had better eat your dinner." Offer the bedtime snack even if it seems to come up pretty soon after dinner and your toddler hasn't eaten much. Toddlers often don't eat much at dinner because the food tends to be more grown-up and therefore more challenging, they are tired, and they have been eating all day. Your child is doing the best they can; they are not holding out for snack. Have the snack be filling but not thrilling—for instance, crackers and milk rather than ice cream. Children will skip dinner to wait for the ice cream, but not for the crackers and milk. But maybe your child will do it the other way around!

Manage snack timing and food

Even if your toddler takes time to eat at mealtime, their energy needs are high, their stomach is small, and they need to eat often. Let your child eat as much as they want at snack time, the same as at mealtime. Have snacks be your idea and bring them out as reliably and matter-of-factly as you do meals. Have your child sit down for snacks and sit down with them. Offer the snack even when your child seems to forget about it. They need to trust you to feed them.

You do not, of course, want your toddler's snack to fill them up so they don't eat at mealtime, but the way to manage that is with timing rather than restricting how much you let your child eat at snack. Have the snack long enough after the meal to give your child time to get hungry but not too hungry. Have snack long enough before the next meal so they have time to get hungry again but not starved.

Put another way, to manage snacks, get there first. If you plan on a reasonably consistent snack time and get the food ready, you will be able to manage food selection, timing, and location. If you offer snack before your child is too hungry, they will eat a moderate amount. On the other hand, if you wait until they are hungry and committed to what they want to eat and where they want to eat it, you will be asking for trouble.

Snacks are little meals

A snack is not a treat. A snack is not an apple or some carrot sticks. To be filling and last a while, a snack needs two or three of the food groups—protein, grains or other starches, fruit or vegetables, whole milk. For staying power, make one of the choices a source of protein and fat, such as cheese, peanut butter, or whole milk. Any food that you consider appropriate for a meal is appropriate for a snack. Often at snack time, children are more willing to try new foods. That might be a time to trot out some vegetables and dip. Consider these filling and sustaining snacks:

- Crackers and whole milk
- Peanut butter or cheese with fruit or fruit juice
- Raw vegetables, regular (not low-fat) dip, milk
- Breakfast cereal and whole milk
- Buttered toast strips, whole milk
- Fruit smoothie made with whole milk or whole-milk yogurt
- Raisins and cheese
- Sunflower seeds and fruit juice
- Cookies and milk
- Hummus and raw vegetables, pretzels, or pita chips
- Snacks and your child's mealtime routine

Don't be concerned if your family eats at an unusual time—such as having the evening meal quite late or quite early. The child this age is fitting into the family's routine instead of having the routine fit around them. You can help your child be hungry but not famished for a late dinner by offering more than one afternoon snack. Consider having a filling and sustaining snack two or three hours after lunch, and then a lighter snack, such as raw vegetables, fruit or fruit juice, or crackers, later in the afternoon. Such hors d'oeuvres can help tide your child over while you get dinner ready. Or, if it fits better into your family's schedule, you can do it the other way by substituting an early dinner for your child's afternoon snack. Then offer a substantial bedtime snack.

CHOOSE CHILD CARE THAT FOLLOWS sDOR

At child care as at home, children eat best when adults follow sDOR, use family-style meal service, eat with children, and enjoy time together. In such settings, I have seen children who don't eat much or take much interest in food eat more, selectively eating children start to experiment with food, and food-preoccupied and seemingly voracious children become relaxed about food.

When you are choosing a child care program, try to visit to get a sense of the program, and observe a snack or mealtime. Are they doing family-style feeding? Is there an adult sitting with the children and eating the same food? Does the group look happy and relaxed? If you see something that seems a little off, ask the person in charge about it. Why do they do it that way?

Child care providers are important partners

Your child care provider not only can support what you do at home with feeding, they can extend it. They give your child the experience of eating other food with other people. As long as there is no pressure on your child to eat, they will do just fine. Unfortunately, child care providers have challenges with doing optimum feeding. Busy child care providers and teachers may find it difficult to find time to eat with children. If they are in the Child and Adult Care Food Program (CACFP), they get financial support for meals, but along with that support comes guidelines and regulations.

How can you support sDOR in your child care setting? Upon enrollment, child care centers typically ask questions about your child's food and eating in addition to finding out about medications, chronic illnesses, allergies, and so on. That gives you an opportunity to talk with them about how you manage feeding and what they can expect from your child's eating. You will likely have a receptive audience. Child care providers want to be successful with your child, and they want you to be comfortable with having your child in their care.

Begin by sharing that at home you practice sDOR and tell them what that is. As a consequence, your child is comfortable with unfamiliar food, but they may or may not eat it. You do not consider your child to be picky but rather to be taking their time with learning to eat new food. Sometimes they don't eat much and other times they eat a lot, but overall, they eat as much as they need.

Second, share that at home you depend on repeated neutral exposure to allow your child to learn to eat new food, both at meals and when you cook or garden with them. That is, you don't pressure, persuade, or encourage them to eat and you don't talk about good or bad foods and what they should or shouldn't eat.

Tell them about research with sDOR.2-6y, the inventory for measuring parent adherence to sDOR, which shows that children do better nutritionally when parents follow sDOR. The same research shows that parents who follow sDOR do not pressure or encourage their child to eat certain amounts or types of food. Parents simply provide their child with repeated neutral exposure to the foods they, themselves, enjoy.[7] For more about sDOR.2-6y, see the Chapter 1 section, "Research with sDOR.2-6y," page 28.

The portion size requirement

I mentioned CACFP regulation and guidelines. CACFP is a United Stated Department of Agriculture-sponsored program that provides funding for nutritious food as well as guidelines, inspection, and training. My colleagues and I *love* the training part because we get to present to child care and Head Start workers. They are good observers of children, have great senses of humor, and really *get* sDOR. However, the *guideline* part includes a portion size requirement that regularly trips us all up.

CACFP specifies how much of each food each child should be provided. Depending on the way the CACFP inspector and even the child care licensing agency interprets the regulation, that can mean *in the child*, *on the plate*, or *all together* in the serving bowl. From the trust perspective, there is only one right interpretation. Number three—the serving bowl—reflects the love and autonomy that child care providers are so good at giving. Number one takes away love and autonomy. I am reminded of my colleague's son who came home *starved* from his lovely new child care center. After a few days and a good bit of sleuthing, his mother discovered that the rule was, "If you take it, you eat it." The rule overwhelmed his hunger and interest in food, and he was forced into his solution of not taking it.

Clearly, parents, child care providers, inspectors, and licensing agencies share the common goal of supporting children's eating nutritious food. They all benefit from being reassured that achieving that goal will be best accomplished by following sDOR. The same as at home, children who are pressured or persuaded to eat their vegetables might eat them today or in the short run, but they don't learn to enjoy them for a lifetime.

ADDRESS FEEDING ISSUES

Below are some strategies that I hope will allow you to address your feeding issues. Remember, children change rapidly. If you change what you do and make your changes permanent, your child will change right along with you.

In considering your child's feeding issues, consider their history with eating—and your own. When my Ellyn Satter Institute colleagues and I evaluate a toddler or preschooler with eating problems, we generally find struggles with feeding that have started in infancy and become more and more complex as the child has gotten older. The child may have been temperamentally perplexing, seemed vulnerable, or been difficult to feed. The parent might have been particularly anxious about the child's welfare, alarmed that the child seemed small or ill, or had a certain notion about what the child should eat and/or how they should grow. Often, parents' own struggles with eating have made it challenging for them to trust their child to determine whether and how much to eat.

If your feeding struggles with your child have been going on for a while, you are often upset about them, and if despite your best efforts and multiple helpers, you can't resolve the problem, get help from a professional who fully understands sDOR. An expert assessment and informed help working your way out of your dilemma can make all the difference in years to come. Neither parents nor children who struggle with feeding get their needs met. Parents don't feel like good parents, and children don't feel like good children.

Cautious children and those with oral sensitivity

Feeding the cautious, orally-sensitive child is the same as feeding the easygoing, adventurous child. However, hanging in there with sDOR is a lot more difficult because you get so little positive feedback. For the longest time you have to trust your cautious child to eventually get around to eating a variety of food. Continue to follow sDOR, be friendly and supportive, and give your child the opportunity to learn to manage their own caution and sensitivity.

It isn't much fun to cook for cautious children, so remember you are planning and preparing meals for the whole family and inviting your child to join you. Make food accessible for your child, not by planning menus around what they do and don't eat, but by being considerate without catering with meal planning. Get the emphasis off what and how much your child eats and, instead, emphasize your child's positive eating attitudes and behaviors. The good eater enjoys family meals, picks and chooses from the food provided, and eats as much or as little as they want. While they poke along at a snail's pace learning to eat new food, remind yourself that because your child is Eating Competent you have done everything you can to support them in doing well with food consumption.

Dietitian Jane Fowler, who for years taught parent education classes in Walnut Creek, California, talks a good bit with parents about understanding their child's temperament as it relates to their eating. She observes, for instance, that cautious, slow-to-warm-up children seem so uninterested in new food that parents often fall into the trap of not challenging them—not giving them opportunities to learn. "It isn't much fun feeding him," said a mother who loved to cook and wanted her son to enjoy what she prepared. After she stopped trying to get her son to eat her wonderful food, she was able to see how he pushed himself along to learn. He looked at the food, watched her and other family members eat it, asked for the serving dish to be left near his plate, put some *on* his plate but ignored it, put some in his mouth and took it out again. You get the drill. Children have their own ways of sneaking up on new food.

Picky eating

Do your feeding jobs and don't worry when your toddler goes through the long warm-up of 20 (or 40 or 80) meals to get around to eating a vegetable or any other food. This is all part of the learning process. Unworried parents raise children who are less inclined to be picky eaters—as long as parents continue to follow sDOR. However, not worrying is negative if it means not taking responsibility for the tasks of planning, cooking, and orchestrating pleasant meals. Not worrying amounts to neglect when a parent gives up on offering regular meals and snacks and just lets the toddler have a bottle or beg for food throughout the day.

We have discussed preventing picky eating by following sDOR and being appropriately unconcerned about what and how much your child eats. Now let's reinforce your resolve by taking a look at what happens when parents don't do that. Researchers Pelchat and Pliner surveyed families from an upper-middle-class Canadian suburb and found that it was all about the feeding. Mothers offered only foods that children readily accepted, prepared substitutes when children asked for them, and prodded, rewarded, and punished their children to get them to eat. The mothers complained that their child dawdled or was messy at mealtime, refused to eat new foods, and preferred junk foods. They did not understand that their child's eating grew out of the way they managed feeding.[8]

Here is a little test. What makes a child dawdle and be messy at mealtime, refuse new food, and prefer junk food?

This is a difficult one and I am sure you have a number of correct answers. The one I am thinking of is that the *parents'* belief about what and how much the child *should* eat leads to those negative child eating behaviors. Those Toronto parents may have been keeping the child at the meal after the child said they wanted to leave in hopes they would eat more. Whereupon the child dawdled and was messy. Parents may have tried to get their child to eat certain foods. Whereupon the child didn't simply ignore those foods, they applied pressure right back by refusing to eat. Parents may have become desperate to get their child to eat something—*anything*. Whereupon the child took the only avenue open to them and filled up on high-fat, high-sugar food.

Food jags

Food jags take two people, the child to demand the food and the parent to produce it. Following sDOR means you don't cooperate with food jags.

A food jag is when a child wants to eat the same foods, prepared in the same way, every day or at every meal. A typical food jag is a toddler wanting hot dogs at every meal. Typical food-jag behavior is refusing to eat or having a tantrum when they don't get their hot dog. You may decide to go along with your child's food jag until they get tired of hot dogs but be prepared for them to go on another food jag with something different. I predict tater tots or chicken nuggets.

Let's consider the food jag from the child's point of view. Demanding a particular food could simply be the toddler's experiment to find out whether they can control the menu. Your response? "We will have hot dogs soon. For now, this is what we have." In the meantime, provide a considerate-without-catering menu that includes food your toddler generally eats. However, your toddler could be caught up in holding out for hot dogs. They may leave the meal without eating. So be it. Snack time will come soon.

Your toddler could have a genuine hankering for hot dogs. You can have hot dogs for lunch and occasionally include them in the family dinner menu. Sometimes your toddler gets lucky and sometimes someone else in the family does. If you ban hot dogs from your menus, your toddler has a point. It's time to lighten up and include food they enjoy.

The child who is "too big" or "too small"

The Chapter 3 section, "Your child may be bigger or smaller than average," page 75, addresses predictable variations in eating and growth. Chances are there is no problem. Some children are just big, and they might have big appetites. Some children are just small, and they might have small appetites. That is normal for them. Following sDOR will allow your child to grow up to get the body that is right for them.

From the perspective of the trust paradigm, growth is proceeding well when it is consistent. By that I mean their weight or BMI follows generally along a particular percentile curve or makes a smooth and gradual shift across percentiles. Growth is concerning when it abruptly and considerably accelerates—diverges upward across percentiles—or falters—diverges downward across percentiles. Growth is *not* concerning when it is above the 85th or below the 15th percentiles, unless it has accelerated or faltered to get there.

Do a bit of soul-searching. It wouldn't be surprising if you were on some level concerned that your child is "too big" or "too small." That concern can creep into feeding. Ask yourself, "how would I do this [let my child eat this or that food, this or that amount] if I weren't concerned about their size?" Your concern could also come from outside interference by others who think your child should grow in a certain way. Courage.

Diagnosing causes weight acceleration

The Chapter 4 section, "More about BMI cutoffs," page 120, reviews research showing that children grow better, meaning more consistently, when parents *do not* accept an "overweight" or "underweight" diagnosis. On the other hand, children gain too much weight when parents accept the verdict that their child is "overweight/obese," along with the underlying message that they should do something about it.

It takes a lot to derail a child's growth. Poor food selection will not do it but struggles around feeding *will*. Abrupt weight shifts across percentiles indicate that something is amiss medically, nutritionally, emotionally, and/or in terms of the feeding relationship. Getting to the bottom of that *something* could require professional help.

For support in holding steady in feeding and raising your unusual child, read my book *Your Child's Weight: Helping without Harming*.

The toddler with constipation

Before I launch into the topic of constipation, let me remind you that your child's toileting habits also require a division of responsibility. That is, you provide the toilet, and your child makes use of it. If you make your child's toileting your business, your child can withhold their bowel movements. They can become more invested in the struggle with you than in doing their toileting job.

Normal bowel habits are extremely variable. One child will have a bowel movement more than once a day, another not for several days. Neither hurts your child nor causes problems as long as you are casual and accepting.

For some children, constipation can be a medical as well as a behavioral and nutritional concern. Some children have underactive intestinal tract muscles, and children with an irritable bowel can have periods of alternating diarrhea and constipation. If your child's bowel habits are of ongoing concern to you, consult your health professional.

The toddler with diarrhea

Diarrhea caused by gastroenteritis is a medical condition to address with your health care provider. Usually, children's loose stools aren't diarrhea at all but simply a change in bowel habits. However, some toddlers and preschoolers develop chronic nonspecific diarrhea. These are bowel movements so urgent that a child has trouble getting to the bathroom, and stools so runny you have to change their socks as well as their pants. That is a nuisance, not a physical ailment. The child isn't ill, and the diarrhea doesn't indicate that they are absorbing nutrients poorly.

An extremely high-fiber diet can give a child loose stools, but the main culprit seems to be too much juice. Most children and many adults poorly digest and incompletely absorb fructose, or fruit sugar. Leftover fructose in the large intestine attracts water and liquifies the stools. Fructose also feeds intestinal bacteria that, in turn, cause gas and intestinal irritation. Juices or fruits that also contain sorbitol such as prune, pear, peach, and apple are particular culprits. Sorbitol can't be digested or absorbed, but attracts water, makes the stools loose, and can also contribute to intestinal gas. A low-fat diet contributes to loose stools by leaving children hungry and prone to depend on sugar to get enough to eat.

Unless your health care provider indicates otherwise, continue to include your child in family meals and snacks and let them eat what and as much as they want. Offer them juice at only one meal or snack a day. Ignore old-fashioned advice to follow the BRAT diet, an acronym that stands for bananas, rice, applesauce, toast, and tea. It doesn't work.

The toddler with functional needs

The Chapter 7 sections, "Vulnerable babies; controlling advice," page 210, and "Babies who require tube-feeding," page 212, discuss in more detail feeding issues with children who have functional needs. Given positive eating attitudes and behaviors, once their medical and nutritional issues are managed or resolved, such children are able to push themselves along to eat a greater variety of food and, if all goes well, eat enough to provide for their nutritional needs. If not, the amount they *can* eat can be supported by tube-feeding. They can even have blended family food by tube instead of their formula.

Making the transition from tube- to oral-feeding

Your child may be a toddler by the time they are ready to finish learning to eat. If all has gone well, you will have been able to establish a positive feeding relationship from the first even if they have been fully tube-fed by holding them and giving them a chance at the nipple and, later on, including them in family meals and letting them have experience with food. See the Chapter 7 section, "Consider trust-based tube feeding," page 213, and sections following.

Your tube-fed toddler will get around to eating when they are given repeated neutral exposure to stage appropriate food in the context of pleasant family meals. The Chapter 10 section, "Children with functional needs," page 330, addresses oral-motor issues that might or might not pertain to your toddler during their transition to family food. It may make logical sense for your toddler to be gradually introduced first to pureed food then to thicker, lumpier food before they are allowed to finger-feed themself soft pieces of food. But those semisolid foods may be unappealing for them, and they will know perfectly well that it is baby food. Children who miss achieving previous developmental tasks do best when they are provided with opportunities that fit their current stage in development. They fill in the gaps on their own.

Keep in mind that the previously tube-fed child may be coping with a particular kind of oral sensitivity. Adults who have had their jaws wired say at first food feels uncomfortable and even painful in their mouth and they have to ease back into eating. Your child will take care of that on their own, but knowing what they are experiencing will help you give them all the time they need.

Children will be slower in learning to eat if they have been traumatized with traditional feeding therapy or forced to eat in other ways. They require regular reassurance in word and deed that they don't have to eat if they don't want to. Eventually, they get their anxiety under control and eat. For reassurance, remember that we can apply the definition of *Competent Eater* to your child even if food does not regularly pass their lips. They enjoy family meals and they are comfortable with being exposed to the food there.

The toddler who is allergic

Your toddler's food allergies are likely to be a continuation of allergies that appeared when they were making the transition to family meals. See the discussion in the Chapter 10 section, "Allergies," page 323. It is particularly important to trust your toddler's lack of interest in certain foods, even if they have a very short list of foods they eat. Children instinctively learn to avoid foods that make them ill, so it can be difficult to tell the difference between a toddler's natural skepticism about new food and the allergic toddler's food avoidance. It doesn't really matter. Either way, trust them to eat and not eat. At the same time, be aware of pitfalls. Because you have seen your child become ill and unhappy as a result of their food allergies, it is easy to become overprotective and fall into the traps of limiting the menu too much, catering too obviously, or manipulating your child in order to get them to eat what *is* available to them.

If all goes well, you will also be able to work with an sDOR-committed dietitian specializing in food allergies. Dietitian Alexia Beauregard, Ellyn Satter Institute faculty member, is one such specialist. In the process of helping many parents of allergic children, Beauregard has found almost without exception that the feeding relationship is distorted. It need not be so. She firmly believes that food doesn't have to hurt or generate anxiety and that mealtimes, even when children have food allergies, can be a relaxing part of the day. Beauregard emphasizes what you know all too well. Your child's food allergies are not just your child's issue, but an issue of your feeding relationship and, indeed, of the whole family.

The most common allergens—foods that cause allergic reactions—are milk and wheat; others are peanuts, eggs, tree nuts, fish, shellfish, soybeans, and sesame. Your child is likely to have their own distinctive list. Work with an allergist to be sure your child's list of foods-to-avoid is as short as possible. Beauregard recommends putting the emphasis on what the toddler *can* eat rather than what they *can't*. Omit your toddler's allergens from family menus so the whole family can eat right along with the allergic child. Do web searches to find, for instance, wheat-free and/or dairy-free foods. Plan meals substituting hypoallergenic food and be considerate without catering. Follow sDOR and trust your child to eat as much as they need and bring themself along with respect to learning to eat new food, just as you would any other toddler.

Omitting your child's allergens from family meals won't last forever. When your child is a preschooler, you can begin to teach them to distinguish between "okay" and "not-okay" foods at family meals, and they can begin to take responsibility for staying away from food that makes them ill. Until then, it works best if the whole family is offered a diet that avoids the offending allergens.

Beauregard gives siblings special consideration, both to avoid having the allergic child get more than their share of attention and to allow siblings to be exposed to a wider variety of food. She says school lunch is an important source of variety for siblings of allergic toddlers, and of course, visits to relatives and friends help a lot. She suggests taking older siblings out to a meal or snack where they can eat regular food but more importantly have the parents' undivided attention. Parents can also get out the regular food—Goldfish or regular ice cream, for instance—during the toddler's nap time, then be careful to wash hands and clean up afterwards so the toddler doesn't get any lingering allergens.

Beauregard has found that the parental attitude of matter-of-factly taking leadership with feeding and giving the child autonomy with eating is all-important. So true. In my experience, children with chronic health conditions do best in the long run when, with their parents' support, they take stage-appropriate responsibility for themselves and for the condition. I certainly acknowledge that dealing with such health conditions is difficult and represents a loss for the child as well as for the parents. At the same time, with any health, physical, cognitive, or behavioral attribute, your child will do best if you can continue to do authoritative parenting. Accept the condition, help them as much as you can, and teach them to be increasingly responsible for managing their condition as they grow up.

The toddler with diabetes

I won't try to address the details of diabetes management for your child. That is for you and your child's health care team. I will, however, introduce you to the possibilities of continuing to follow sDOR in parenting your child with diabetes.

Having your child develop diabetes can feel like a loss. Put on top of that loss your responsibilities for managing your child's condition, and it can be quite a blow. Be reassured that your child's diabetes need not spoil your feeding relationship. You can still follow sDOR. Your part with the *what, when,* and *where* of *feeding* is the same, and your child with diabetes can still be trusted to do their part with the *how much* and *whether* of *eating*. You can even follow the "Enjoy Sweets" guidelines (page 402).

Following sDOR is authoritative parenting, and children with diabetes do best long term when parents do authoritative parenting.[9] Parents do better, too. Parents who follow sDOR have better quality of life. They feel better, sleep better, and have lower stress levels.[7] The principles of feeding and the principles of parenting are identical. Parents provide leadership—structure and clear expectations—at the same time as they give their child warmth, respect, independence, and realistic mastery opportunities. That is, parents show the child in a stage-appropriate way what they have to learn—both overall and with managing their diabetes.

Your child has diabetes because their pancreas doesn't make enough insulin at any one time to metabolize the carbohydrate their body makes from food. To balance out the available insulin, the best thing you can do is offer them regular meals and snacks. Eating regularly helps avoid peaks and valleys in food consumption. Offering meals that contain protein, fat, and carbohydrate, with particular emphasis on fat, also helps to smooth out peaks and valleys by releasing food into the system gradually so available insulin can match it. Including any sweets at meals or snacks that offer that combination slows the rate at which the sugar gets into the system. These are the exact principles that I laid out for adult diabetes in Chapter 5. What is different is that your child's food intake is likely to be highly variable, and they may only rarely eat a combination of protein, fat, and carbohydrate at any one time. Their blood sugar is likely to be more variable, as well, since it is affected by illness, growth spurts, activity, medication, and other factors.

You can't get your child to eat certain amounts or types of food at those regular meals and snacks, so don't try. It isn't any more possible when a child has diabetes than for any other child! Instead, standard practice with child diabetes is to first let the child eat, then adjust their insulin to match their food intake. That's where today's world of diabetes care shines, in that providing that insulin can be flexible and personalized.

Rapid-acting insulin, multiple injections, and insulin pumps that measure blood sugar and administer insulin can mimic the body's response to food intake. You can follow sDOR, let your child eat at meal- or snack time, then give the insulin afterward to cover the food they have eaten. You do rough carbohydrate counting to estimate how much insulin to inject or let the insulin pump do it. As a result, whether your child eats a little or a lot isn't critical because you adjust the insulin dose to let them make use of a little or a lot of food. Doing eating-first-insulin-afterwards lets you keep things in balance for your child through growth spurts, variations in physical activity, illnesses, and birthday parties.

There is one caveat. When a child is given a daily dose of long-acting insulin, not eating at all is not an option. You may have to treat a small glass of milk or other food as medicine, and insist your child consume it before they can leave the meal or snack. Distinguishing between food as *food* and a set amount of food as *medicine* keeps the expectation from spoiling the feeding relationship.

Work with your provider to establish your child's target blood range, realizing that that range may vary as your child goes through illness, growth spurts, or puberty. You know your child best, and you will pick up on their signs of low blood sugar: They act tired and are crabby and even irrational. You know they need food; they may be too upset to eat. Too-low blood sugar can be caused by too much insulin, too little food, a peak in activity, or all three. Keeping the target blood sugar close to "physiological" level—the level you would see in a child without diabetes—makes a child more vulnerable to having an insulin reaction; keeping the target range somewhat higher cushions them. A higher target range cushions you, as well, in that you don't have to be as vigilant.

Continuous glucose monitoring systems, linked to parents' cell phones, can be used with children as young as two years. There are still decisions to be made. Practitioners who promote keeping blood sugars lower feel strongly that it protects children with diabetes from the long-term degenerative consequences of the disease. Practitioners who set target blood sugars somewhat higher consider avoiding insulin reactions a priority and point out that the reactions themselves contribute to degenerative consequences. From the perspective of the feeding relationship, having a higher target blood sugar range is less likely to distort feeding.

If you feel your current approach to managing your child's eating and diabetes is distorting your feeding relationship and making your child less capable with eating, talk with your health care team. They may be willing to work with you on your child's behalf. Consider looking for a dietitian who is expert with sDOR to help you parent well while managing your child's diabetes.

The toddler with cystic fibrosis

From the trust-paradigm perspective, feeding the child who has cystic fibrosis is the same as for any other child. Follow sDOR and raise your child to be Eating Competent. That is *way* more easily said than done, because cystic fibrosis is a life-threatening condition. Children with cystic fibrosis have lung dysfunction and malabsorption, which is difficulty absorbing nutrients from the intestinal tract. Because of that, they have high energy demands. U.S. guidelines estimate calorie requirements at 10 percent above to nearly twice that of a child without the disease.[10] That malabsorption is assumed to render children incapable of regulating their food intake—of knowing how much they need to eat—but that isn't true. It is just that the demands of the disease may be so great that the child simply can't keep up.

Being afraid for your child means pressure almost inevitably creeps in to feeding. We have talked before about the hot potato of feeding pressure that gets tossed down the line until it ends up in the child's lap. In this case, the disease itself is the hot potato that puts pressure on the medical team managing the disease, on parents, and on the child. While advances in medication and equipment have revolutionized cystic fibrosis management, the reality of the disease remains. It is a serious condition, management is complicated, and it is all too understandable for everyone concerned to let pressure creep in to feeding, often despite their best efforts to avoid it.

You and your child will likely receive comprehensive care from a team located at a cystic fibrosis care center. With respect to feeding, professionals in those care centers tend to be either *trust*-paradigm-oriented or *control*-paradigm-oriented.

For professionals following the *trust* paradigm in feeding the child with cystic fibrosis, nutritional management means teaching and guiding parents in following sDOR and tracking growth. Consistent growth indicates that the child's hunger and appetite are keeping up with their energy need. Growth faltering indicates they need help consuming enough calories. Rather than trying to get the child to eat more food or higher-calorie food and put the feeding relationship at risk, trust-oriented practitioners recommend supplementary tube-feeding. Generally, that feeding is via a gastrostomy tube (G-tube) inserted through a surgical opening in their stomach.

Parents of children on tube-feedings continue the routine of family meals and planned snacks. They discover they don't have to be afraid of tube-feeding but rather feel enormous relief at not having to worry about how much their child eats. Children are generally tube-fed at night, then trusted with *whether* or not to eat and *how much* to eat at meals and snacks during the day. Children who are fed following the trust paradigm are likely to be Eating Competent as they grow up. As a consequence, they are less likely to have the distorted eating attitudes and behaviors and even eating disorders that appear common with cystic fibrosis.[11]

On the other hand, professionals following the *control* paradigm may instruct parents to *get* their child to eat a high-fat, high-calorie diet rather than trusting the child to eat based on their hunger and fullness cues. Growth faltering is likely to be addressed by working with parents to get their child to eat more food and/or higher-calorie food. Control-based practitioners may be less likely than trust-oriented practitioners to routinely use tube-feeding to supplement the child's voluntary food intake. Control-oriented professionals may instruct parents to follow a division of responsibility in feeding but still encourage parents to get their child to eat more in response to growth faltering.

You have a tough decision to make in seeking care for your child, particularly if you don't have a fit between your preferred approach to feeding your child and that of your local cystic fibrosis care center. I can only encourage you that finding that fit—and feeding in the best possible way for you and your child—is well worth the effort.

TODDLER FEEDING SKIRMISHES

Now that we have all the pieces, let's have some fun by talking about typical skirmishes with toddler eating. As you read these stories, consider that parents show their love by keeping their child safe, socializing them, showing them what is and isn't okay, and keeping their world down to a size where they can manage it.

Soon you will have your own stories of your toddler's erratic and entertaining eating. Struggles about control are a normal part of this stage. On the other hand, if you feel uncomfortable with setting reasonable limits, if the struggles are prolonged or continuous, and if you can't seem to get things to go right with your child, get professional help. It is *that* important and has everything to do with your relationship with your child and the way your child grows up feeling about themself. An ounce of prevention now is worth many pounds of cure later on.

Curtis wasn't hungry

My younger son Curtis, then about two years old, climbed eagerly into his high chair, apparently prepared to do his usual thorough job of eating his dinner. This time, however, he had another idea, and he couldn't wait to try it. He sat back in his chair, crossed his arms, and announced, "I won't eat." I was puzzled, because he was my third child, and I had long since given up on getting any of them to eat. Then I realized that, being a toddler, he was likely running a little experiment to find who was in charge of his eating.

At any rate, I had my cue. I was supposed to say, "Oh, dear, you have to eat." But I could see that little glint in his eye that I had come to recognize as his making an opening move. I did some quick thinking. It scared me that he might not eat, because when he was hungry, he got crabby, impulsive, and super hard to be with. He also refused to eat. I considered what I could do to get him to eat: beg, plead, threaten, bribe, play "here comes the airplane." None appealed. So, I said, "That's all right, you don't have to eat. Just keep us company for a bit, then you can go." He looked absolutely crestfallen. It seemed like such a good game, and I just wasn't playing. He sat a minute, and then he said, "I want some of that." He ate it, and asked for something else, and so on until he had eaten his meal.

Curtis gave me an engraved invitation to cross into his lane. Had I had taken it, that meal would not have turned out well for anyone. Here are some other moves you may recognize.

I'm not hungry (I can't take time to eat)

This is a slight variation on the previous theme, the difference being when it happens. You call your child to dinner, they are busy playing, don't want to be bothered, and probably don't even know they are hungry. A five-minute warning may help, but even then, a child may insist they aren't hungry. If you say, "Oh dear, you must be hungry, you haven't eaten for hours," you lose. You have crossed the line into their territory of *how much* and *whether*. However, you can recover. You can say, "You don't have to eat, but come and keep us company for a few minutes while we eat." Chances are when your child gets to the meal, gets their mind off playing, and settles down a bit, they will eat. But maybe not.

Then you have to deliver and let them leave when they want to. If you keep them there in hopes they will eat, they won't trust you the next time. They will also misbehave. When you let them down, say, "That's all until snack time." Keep in mind that saying that is for you, not for them. They will be back, probably immediately, likely more than once, wanting to rejoin the meal and, later on, begging for a food handout. Hold firm, even if they have a tantrum. They are learning that mealtimes are for eating and other times are for doing something else, and they learn from what you *do*, not what you *say*. Keep in mind that you are not trying to starve them into submission, as in "If they get hungry enough, they will eat." They really won't, and the philosophy is cruel. Instead, you are maintaining structure which, in turn, allows your child to get their needs met. At first, you can fudge a bit by offering snack a little earlier, but you get the idea.

Now I'm hungry

Let's say this wily toddler we just talked about leaves the meal and goes back—briefly—to playing. Now they return, begging to rejoin the meal. Tough talk aside, you are tempted. Here is your poor sweet little child, large eyes trained on you, wanting another chance. What hard-hearted parent wouldn't give such an appealing waif that chance? Keep in mind that they are not an awful child. This is just an experiment to see if you really mean it about no food until snack time. So you say, "You said you were done. Now run along and play."

Your child will not say, "Oh, excuse me, I was confused about that." They are likely to get upset, whine, or cry. That is your cue to ignore them until they stop fussing. Then help them find something else to do as in, "That looks like a nice book/car/puzzle."

Chances are you will have to run your own experiments before you can do this. The issue of food makes it particularly difficult for parents to set these sorts of limits. Chances are that you will let your toddler come back to the meal. Chances are that once they get back, they still won't eat and will do something to annoy and upset you and spoil your meal. If you learn quickly, it won't take too many repetitions. If you learn slowly, take heart, you will get there. If you don't learn at all, get help. These nonproductive struggles take on a life of their own and spoil eating, feeding, and parenting. They can even make you give up on family meals.

Argh! I don't like that

Don't get bogged down in *like—don't like*. Think instead of *eat—doesn't eat*. Labeling a food as "liked" makes you expect your toddler to eat it every time it shows up at the meal. They won't. Labeling a food as "disliked," especially if you let your toddler hear you telling others, "They don't like that" condemns that food to permanent rejection. Say nothing at all and teach your child to do the same. All they need to do is ignore the food. If they must, they can say, "I don't want that." "Okay," is a good response. You may also say, "You don't have to eat it—there is plenty of other food."

It's all right to give your child some encouragement, but know your audience, and be prepared to take no for an answer. My older son, Lucas, would look at a new food and say, "I don't want that." I would say, "Try it, it might taste good." He knew I was willing to take no for an answer, and he generally tried it and often ate more of it. He also knew he didn't have to try it if he didn't want to. Curtis taught me that even that gentle encouragement and being willing to take no for an answer can come across as pressure. *One time*, I said to him, "Try it, it might taste good," and he gave me a glare that left no room for misinterpretation.

When you include a new food at mealtime, endorse the food by eating and enjoying it. If you enjoy it. If not, don't eat it. Period. Do *not* make a big deal of eating it because your child will see through you and conclude there is something wrong with the food. If your child tries a food, give tacit approval by pleasantly watching them and saying nothing at all. Children seem to understand tacit approval and give it to each other all the time. Or you can say, "I see you tried it." Do not say, "Oh you brave and wonderful child—I am so proud of you—you are Daddy's little angel." I exaggerate, of course. You *wouldn't* say that. Recognition is fine, but praise detracts. It turns their eating into *your* thing.

Nonproductive moves include saying, "It's good, you'll like it," "It will make you big and strong," and "You have to take a bite." All of these moves involve your putting pressure on your child to eat and crossing the lines of sDOR. You are already doing all you can to "get" your child to eat. The food shows up on the menu every so often and you demonstrate it tastes good by enjoying it yourself (but not raving about it). Children don't care if food is good for them; they care if it *tastes* good.

I want cereal, please

Now we have the toddler who has surveyed the meal and made an alternative request. Not only that, but they use the magic word. So you ask yourself, "What's the matter with a little cereal? I don't have to cook anything, it's right there handy. We could just keep cereal on the table in case they don't eat." As you no doubt expect, I will tell you what is wrong with it. It says to your child louder than words can say, "I don't expect you to learn to eat your meals." As I have said probably too many times before, your child wants to grow up with eating, but they will also take the easy way out if it is available. When it is not on the menu, peanut butter on the table is also the easy way out. The justification, of course, is that peanut butter gives the child protein if they don't eat the main dish. The message to the child is still "I don't expect you to learn to eat."

Granted, learning to manage unfamiliar food creates a certain amount of anxiety for children—for all of us, really. However, that anxiety is part of growing up. Trust your child to manage their anxiety. They will ignore the unfamiliar food until they are ready to begin sneaking up on it, then gradually learn to eat it. Beyond being considerate without catering with menu planning, if you make an alternative readily available, they won't learn. It interrupts the repeated neutral exposure children need to learn to enjoy new food.

See what a good eater I am?

A mother consulted me about what she considered her 18-month-old daughter's too-hearty appetite. I evaluated the little girl's growth, and it *was* going up from her percentile curve. She and her husband had gone to China to adopt their daughter when she was four months old. To their considerable relief, the infant had been well cared for and appeared to have had plenty to eat and plenty of affection. From the first, she ate a great deal. She enjoyed her formula, enjoyed solid food, and later on, enjoyed family food. The problem? The mother said that family and friends were so relieved at what good shape the little girl was in and at how well she ate that she got a lot of attention for her eating. Her aunts, uncles, and grandparents clustered around her, exclaiming at the gusto with which she attacked her food. I had my answer. The little girl was a pleaser, and she had learned to eat for her audience. They had been inadvertently getting her to eat more than she was hungry for.

This was quite different from a common adoptive- and foster-parent experience with children who seemingly grew up not getting enough to eat. At first, those children eat enormous quantities of food and can't seem to get filled up. Parents understandably react by trying to slow or restrict children's eating, but that further frightens children and makes them put all the more pressure on eating. Instead, parents have to do the opposite of what seems right, that is, reassure their child that they may eat all they want and that there will be enough. When parents can do that and really mean it, it isn't long before the child stops eating so desperately. Offering a child enough to eat is the strongest possible message of love.

Layla vomited her lunch

A child care provider approached me about three-year-old Layla, who regularly threw up at lunch time. Layla was well but cautious about eating, and the provider had been gently encouraging her to eat what the other children were eating. My theory was that the throwing up had a couple of causes. First, Layla couldn't tolerate being encouraged to eat. Second, she was getting attention for her throwing up. When she started to gag, the provider grabbed her out of her chair and rushed her to the bathroom.

I told the provider about sDOR and we agreed the first step was reassuring Layla she didn't have to eat if she didn't want to. The provider was to stop her encouragement. She was doing a great deal already by sitting with the children, enjoying their company, and eating the same food they were eating. Layla immediately became more comfortable at mealtime, but after a couple of weeks, she was still throwing up and the provider was still rushing her to the bathroom. Time to take away the attention. They were near to the bathroom, so when Layla started to gag, the provider encouraged her to go there on her own to throw up. After that, she was to ignore Layla's leaving, vomiting, and coming back. After a while, Layla stopped vomiting.

Because Layla reacted so strongly to her provider's gentle encouragement to eat, we wondered whether at home she was being pressured to eat. The provider had a conversation about sDOR with the parents, but they weren't convinced that unless they kept after her, Layla wouldn't eat. Nonetheless, at child care Layla continued to be able to eat well and not throw up.

Keep in mind that the voluntary vomiting of an otherwise healthy child is far different from forceful vomiting accompanied by pain and discomfort. That is a medical issue that needs to be addressed by a health care professional.

Chipmunk cheeks

Children develop strange behaviors if they get attention for enacting those behaviors. Eating a lot for an audience is no more far-fetched than a child's voluntarily vomiting or packing so much food into their cheeks that they look like a chipmunk. The vomiting or packing starts out as a chance behavior, but if parents react, the child can learn to do it again. How satisfying is it for a toddler experimenting with control to stand proud and unbending while a parent wheedles to get food out of their mouth? Routinely cleaning out the cheek pouches, then ignoring the behavior, keeps it from getting exaggerated. The take-home message? Be casual and matter-of-fact about your child's eating and about their strange behaviors around eating. By the way, check yourself to be sure you aren't putting pressure on your child to eat. Throwing up and cheek-packing are ways children defend themselves against pushy feeding.

I want to do it myself

Thirteen-month-old Tobin was developmentally divergent, but he had the same burning need for autonomy as any other toddler. Tobin had been born with cognitive limitations and skeletal malformations. He had done just fine on nipple-feeding, but when his mother tried to introduce solid foods, it went so poorly that she stopped trying and Tobin was put on tube-feeding.

Indiana public health nutritionist Pam Estes worked with Tobin's family as part of a zero to three program for children with developmental divergence and functional health care needs. When Pam met Tobin as a two-year-old, his mother was putting him in a reclining infant seat and feeding him mashed table food. Tobin wasn't really interested, but he would mouth and swallow. He gagged a lot, and his mother complained that feeding him was "an all-day job." His weight had been dropping off his percentile curve, and he had been put on what Pam called a "super formula"—a formula containing 30 calories per ounce—on the grounds that the formula was higher in calories than solid foods. Pam doesn't like those formulas and neither do I. We also don't like Pediasure, Instant Breakfast, or other high-calorie formulas. They are a poor substitute for letting a child learn to eat and the families learning to feed. Tobin didn't seem to like the formula either, because he was taking less and less of it.

Pam's approach was two-pronged. She encouraged gradually cutting back on the super formula and tube-feeding, especially at mealtime. She encouraged including Tobin in family meals by taking the tray off his high chair and letting him sit at the table. Imagine his parents' surprise when Tobin's face brightened up, he focused his attention on the food, and he began to struggle to pick it up. At first, he just chased food around, but his mother helped by putting it where he could easily reach it. Tobin quickly developed the muscle control he needed to feed himself, chew, and swallow. Gagging stopped being a problem once he was sitting upright and feeding himself. You can imagine Tobin's breathless parents and how they had to positively sit on their hands and zip their lips to keep from cheerleading. Awed and a little tearful, they could only admire their determined son as he struggled to do it himself. Tobin knew what he needed to do, and once he was allowed, he did a good job with feeding himself.

Pam found her work with children who had functional needs to inform her practice with all children and their families. She points out that all parents benefit from understanding that the child has capabilities, and that parents and professionals can help best by looking for and enhancing those capabilities. "Having that attitude makes all the difference between handling feeding difficulties with dread, concern, and frustration or with confidence, practicality, and even joy," she said. "So many children surprise us when we back off and allow them to manage their own eating."

PUTTING A FAMILY MEAL TOGETHER

Following sDOR gives your child choices within limits. Your toddler will test and resist your *what*, *when*, and *where* limits, but that is how they learn. In the Chapter 10 section, "Choosing food," page 333, I introduced you to the possibilities of what to eat by giving you lists of family foods you could adapt for your transitional child. Now, choosing food is about feeding yourself and your partner, with consideration of your child as a family member. To reassure you that you can eat what you enjoy, this section outlines the possibilities of choosing family food and tells you more about nutrition and food composition.

The Chapter 2 section, "Master family meals," page 56, coaches you in developing the meal habit, starting with eating what you eat now and working your way up—if you can and want—to planning and preparing meals based on the food groups: a protein, one or two grains and/or starchy vegetables, fruit or vegetables or both, milk, and fat. My colleague Jennifer Harris advises "a main dish and two sides." Use the guideline that works for you. A nutritionally complete meal might contain only two food items, such as a tuna noodle casserole with peas and a glass of milk. Or everything could be separate, as with meatloaf, mashed potatoes, broccoli, bread, and milk. Vegetables might be part of a combination dish, as in spaghetti and meat sauce or stir-fry with rice. Fruit can be served as part of dessert, as in oatmeal raisin cookies, or given as juice along with a snack. Here are a few other dinner suggestions from *Secrets of Feeding a Healthy Family*:

- Swiss steak, mashed potatoes and gravy, gingered broccoli
- Chicken and rice, glazed carrots, apple custard
- Spaghetti carbonara (made with eggs and bacon), mixed vegetables, fruit salad
- Braised pork chops with sweet potatoes, chunky applesauce
- Hamburgers on buns, tomato slices, potato chips, fresh fruit
- Mostaccioli with spinach, feta cheese, and scalloped corn
- Chicken soup with noodles and vegetables, fresh fruit, ice cream
- Marinated chicken stir-fry, rice, fresh or canned fruit
- Black beans and rice, corn pudding, orange rounds with parsley
- Hot dogs, potato chips, vegetables with ranch dressing, cookies

I haven't written it, but each menu also includes milk and bread of some kind—even when it makes for an odd menu. The point of this varied list of appealing food? That you don't have to make your menus boring to feed your toddler. They can eat what the rest of the family eats. The mostaccioli menu is a little odd—scalloped corn doesn't really *go*—but most toddlers find scalloped corn accessible and can fill up on it if the main dish is too challenging.

Prepare food once and serve twice—or three or four times. Each of these menus has features that, with preplanning, allow you to make dinner in a hurry and provide good-tasting leftovers for lunches and other meals and/or for the freezer. For more help getting meals ready, consider pre-prepared foods or ingredients and convenience foods such as canned or frozen dinners or hearty soups. Evaluate the nutritional quality of a one-dish canned or frozen dinner by reading the nutritional label to see if it contains a vegetable and starch and has enough protein to consider it a main dish. An adequate level of protein would be about 10 grams of protein from a one-cup serving of main dish or hearty soup. Your toddler will likely eat about a fourth of a serving.

Hamburger, fried chicken, pizza, taco, and other fast-food and take-out places offer nutritious meal options. These fast-food meals may not provide many fruits and vegetables, but you can make up the fruits and vegetables at snack time or at another meal.

Make food easy to eat

Earlier, I talked about being considerate without catering with menu planning by providing one or two foods that your child generally eats so they can be successful with the meal. Those principles still hold. Within that context, Figure 11.9 addresses modest food preparation adjustments that make food easier for small children to eat.

FIGURE 11.9: MAKE FOOD EASY TO EAT

These strategies take into account your child's limited oral-motor ability and inexperience with eating. They do not cater. Catering is making special food for your child or limiting the menu to foods they readily accept.

- Make some foods soft and creamy. If you have dry meat, offer creamed peas.
- Make the mashed potatoes a little softer than you would for adults.
- Allow children to eat foods at room temperature.
- Prepare salad greens without dressing and serve them as finger food.
- Make soups thin enough to drink from a cup or thick enough to spoon easily.
- To tone down the flavor of a strong-flavored vegetable such as broccoli, cook in about an equal volume of cooking water, leave the lid off the pot while you cook, and then throw away the water. You will be throwing away nutrients, but children are more likely to be able to eat them.
- Prepare food well. Children accept foods better when they are properly cooked with natural colors and textures preserved.
- Add a little extra color. Children are interested in a little parsley in the casserole, or some carrot grated into the coleslaw.
- Cut foods into bite-size pieces, preferably before you serve. Toddlers can't handle knives and are likely to get upset about not being allowed to try—and upset again when they try and fail.
- Keep ground beef patties in the freezer to substitute when you have roasts or steaks that your child truly can't eat.
- Cook patties until all the pink color on the inside goes away but stop cooking before they dry out.

Let me tell you the story behind these suggestions. During World War II, dietitian Miriam Lowenberg saw to it that Rosie the Riveter's children got their lunches. Child care centers were set up in the huge Kaiser plant and shipyard in Portland, Oregon, for fathers in the military and mothers working in the World War II factories. Children came from all over the country, with many cultural backgrounds and all sorts of family food ways. Lowenberg found that certain food preparation techniques helped the children in her care succeed with eating. Toddlers and even many preschoolers can't chew tough and fibrous food, such as meat, and too-dry food seems to get stuck in their mouths summarizes her suggestions.

While it is worth going to some trouble to make food well-prepared, attractive, and accessible, don't feel you have to make food cute. You may delight in making little orange section boats and gingerbread man sandwiches. That's great for a party or special occasion, but not on a regular basis. If you routinely go to a lot of trouble to make food adorable for your child, you are putting in more effort than they are. They will sense that and eat less well, not better.

CELEBRATE FOOD

As I have said before, both you and your child will be better served when you take a positive interest in food than when you are afraid of it. Feed yourself faithfully; give yourself permission to eat and invite your child to join you for family meals and snacks. Remember, people who are positive, joyful, and reliable with eating—who are Competent Eaters—do better medically, nutritionally, emotionally, and socially.[12] Children whose parents follow sDOR do better nutritionally.[7]

The discussion in this section about food groups is intended to free you to eat food you enjoy. Your child might eat what you enjoy—or not. Either way, give yourself a pat on the back and relax and enjoy mealtime. Provided you follow sDOR and keep mealtimes pleasant, you can trust your child to do the rest. You can find a website to tell you how much your child should eat from each of the food groups, but *don't*! You can even get an app for tracking how many of the foods your child *should* eat, but *don't*! No child ever ate according to a formula. Keeping track will only upset you and make you controlling. The word "should" is the tipoff. Any time "should" enters, it brings pressure right along with it.

Enjoy bread, cereal, rice, and pasta

Enriched and whole grain breads and cereals offer B vitamins, including folic acid and iron. Read your bread label to be sure the white flour is enriched and whole wheat flour listed as such, not merely as "wheat flour." Whole grain gives fiber and other nutrients in trace amounts like zinc. Use whole grain about half the time or less. While whole grains support healthy bowel function, too much can cause bowel problems.

Somewhere in the back of your mind, you may have the lurking conviction that starchy foods are "bad" for you and even, horrors, *fattening*. Simply not true. Foods high in complex carbohydrates are bulky, filling, and for the most part, relatively low in fat and therefore relatively low in calories. High complex carbohydrate foods—starchy foods, if you will—help you and your child eat as much or as little as you need because they are good foods to fill up on.

For each meal, include bread or a "bready" food such as tortillas and one other complex carbohydrate, such as rice, pasta, or potatoes. Children can usually manage to eat starchy foods when everything else seems just too strange and overwhelming. Making starchy foods available at every meal means children generally eat more than the five servings a day they need from this group, and that's fine. They may even eat mostly white bread at every meal for *weeks*. That's fine, too. A serving is about a quarter of the adult serving—two tablespoons of rice or a quarter-slice of bread. Don't worry if your child eats the rice but skips the stir-fry or eats the spaghetti but skips the meat sauce. Eventually, they will get around to having the whole dish, but only if you let them do it at their own rate.

Ready-to-eat breakfast cereals are on this list. It is up to you whether you depend on the relatively unadorned cereals such as Cheerios, Wheaties, Kix, and Oatmeal Squares or the sugar-coated and flavored cereals such as Frosted Flakes or Fruit Loops. Sugared and flavored cereals offer the same B vitamins and iron as the other cereals. In fact, these frosted cereals can be like a vitamin/mineral supplement—they advertise and really do give 100 percent of the daily requirement of many essential vitamins and minerals. But children don't have to depend on breakfast cereal or any other food to give them 100 percent of *anything*. Cereals need to make only a partial nutritional contribution to the overall day's intake, the same as any other food. They don't have to carry the full load.

Crackers are fine for children, and can add nutrients, variety, and pleasure to meals and snacks. The bread group also includes buns on hamburgers, pizza crust, tortillas, and bagels. Tortilla chips could be here, but they are so hard and tough that toddlers may choke on them. For more ideas, do a web search for *bread food group list*.

Enjoy fruits and vegetables

Fruits and vegetables offer many of the same nutrients: vitamins A and C, B vitamins, fiber, carotene, folic acid, phytochemicals, and protective nutrients. Include five a day. Within those five, try to offer a good source of vitamin C every day such as orange or grapefruit juice, broccoli, tomatoes, or peppers. Try for a dark-green or deep-yellow fruit or vegetable about three times a week, such as apricots or broccoli. Do a web search for other fruits and vegetables but ignore the shoulds and oughts. If you provide fruits and vegetables at meals and snacks and refrain from promotion, you and your child will eat enough of them to be healthy. Depending on whether you can afford the time and cost, it is okay to seek out organic and/or non-GMO fruits and vegetables, but not essential. The nutrients are there, either way.

After that, your job will be done. Don't get caught up in counting how many fruits and vegetables your child eats or even tastes. Keeping track will only worry and frustrate you. Sometimes your child will eat fruits, sometimes vegetables, some days neither, some days both. In all cases, you still get your points for providing a meal and your child gets their points for remaining calm in the presence of foods that they may not yet enjoy. Your including fruits and vegetables at meals and snacks lets your child become accustomed to them and eventually eat the variety that adds up to nutritional excellence. But don't hold your breath. It could take *years*.

Including five a day is not as difficult as it may seem. Fruit and vegetable juices count, and we all get vegetables from French fries, potato chips, and tomatoes in spaghetti sauce, pizza sauce, and salsa. Consider pre-washed salads and ready-to-cook or ready-to-eat fresh vegetables and fruits. Fruits and vegetables don't have to be fresh to be nutritious. Use canned and frozen vegetables and fruit to cut down on preparation time and to vary the taste. Sweetened applesauce and fruits canned in syrup are fine. If you don't like the syrup, drain it off. One hundred percent juice counts as fruit, such as orange, grapefruit, and pineapple juice, and apricot and peach nectar.

Include vegetables and fruits for breakfast by making an omelet with spinach or putting fruit on cereal. Snacks are another way to add to the day's offerings. Consider a banana, sliced apple, raw vegetables with dip, a pear with peanut butter, frozen peas eaten frozen like little ice cubes. Notice the word *offerings*. Your job is done when you provide it.

Make fruits and vegetables more interesting by dressing them up with butter and sauces. Use dips for raw vegetables—the full fat, not the diet, kind. Choose main dishes that contain vegetables, such as pizza and tacos. Make casseroles and soups that contain vegetables, such as tuna-noodle casserole with peas. Bake fruit pies, cobblers, crisps, and make fruit sauces to serve over ice cream. Consider dried fruit, such as raisins or dried apricots, being careful to observe whether their toughness is within your child's chewing-swallowing ability. Certainly, do not let your child wander around eating these or any other foods—the risk of choking is increased and constant munching on sticky, sugary dried fruit increases the risk of tooth decay. Besides, stepped-on raisins stick to the floor like glue.

Then, even though the fruit or vegetable is as delicious as it can possibly be, back off. Generations of parents have somehow been taught that children don't eat vegetables, and generations of parents have created that very reality by forcing, enticing, and rewarding their children to eat vegetables. Let your child learn to eat vegetables at their own speed and in their own way. The same goes for you—learn to enjoy a food experiment the way your child does. Give yourself an out by looking but not tasting, tasting but not swallowing, swallowing but not forcing yourself to take another bite. Giving yourself an out means you will be more interested in the food the next time it shows up at the meal. Perhaps later rather than sooner, like a new song, it will grow on you.

Because it is so important, allow me to belabor this point. You can use all your ingenuity to come up with a variety of fruits and vegetables prepared in delicious and groundbreaking ways, but you must not try to force your child—or yourself—to eat them. Take it slowly and trust your child—and yourself—to learn to enjoy them. Good intentions aside, you will continue eating fruits and vegetables only if they truly give you pleasure. Forcing them down either yourself or your child may work for a while, but eventually you will give it up as a bad job.

Enjoy meat, poultry, fish, dry beans, eggs, and nuts

There is a vegetarian section coming up, so don't take this discussion of meat, poultry, or fish to mean you should eat them. Note this category also includes dry beans and nuts.

Include proteins at two or more meals and/or snacks a day. Your toddler will eat small amounts, but an ounce a day of meat, poultry, fish, or the equivalent in other high-protein foods is enough. An egg is equal to an ounce of meat, as is ½ cup cooked dried beans or 2 tablespoons of peanut butter. As with fruits and vegetables, don't keep score. If you regularly have them on the menu, they will get enough. Some days they will eat more, others less.

Include red meat if you can. People nowadays have the idea that red meat is bad and actually take pride in avoiding it. Red meat is good for you, and it is particularly good for your child because it carries more than its nutritional weight. National statistics show that from beef alone, on which we spend only about 5 percent of our calories, we get 14 percent of our protein and disproportionately large amounts of B vitamins and iron.[13] Moreover, the iron in meat is very well absorbed, far better than that in vegetables and grains, and eating meat with a meal improves iron absorption from vegetables and grains. Red meat and, to a lesser extent, poultry and fish contain *meat factor*, which improves iron absorption overall.

Consider pre-prepared ingredients to save time and mess such as lean ground beef, stew meat (plan to cook it with liquid at low heat for a couple of hours), breakfast steaks (thin, quickly sauteed steaks), cutlets, chicken legs or thighs, boned chicken breasts, stir-fry chicken, canned chicken, frozen fish fillets, canned tuna or salmon, boneless pork chops or stir-fry, small ham roasts and slices. Hit the frozen food or deli case or fast-food restaurant for prepared chicken breasts or drumsticks, chicken tenders, or fish sticks. Other fast choices from the protein list include canned baked beans, cans or jars of pre-cooked navy beans, garbanzos, black beans, refried beans, hummus, and tofu.

Don't forget eggs and all the wonderful ways you can cook them. Luncheon meats, sausages, hot dogs, and bacon are all okay. There is lingering worry about such processed meats because they contain nitrate and sodium nitrite. Sodium nitrate used in processed foods retains color and prevents spoilage. A couple of decades ago there was a nitrates-and-cancer scare, but the theory has since been questioned. The same as anything else in the environment, it depends on dosage. Eaten in moderate amounts, nitrates won't hurt your toddler.

Parents complain that toddlers don't eat much meat, and toddlers do seem to find meat challenging. It is often drier and chewier than other foods. Your toddler won't have molars until 18 months of age at the earliest, and even then, they won't chew very well. Cook meat and poultry so it is juicy and tender, then cut it into thin slices across the grain. Also consider a juicy ground beef patty, meatloaf, casserole, or hearty soup. Because casseroles are relatively soft and easy to chew, toddlers can generally do better with them than with plain meat. But don't knock yourself out to find what your toddler will eat. It won't work and your toddler will experience it as pressure.

Enjoy milk and other high-calcium foods

Milk is good for children. The rumors (and even press conferences by seeming authorities) that get hyped every so often saying that milk is bad for people in general and for children in particular, are simply wrong. Such ideas about milk are based on flimsy evidence by people on crusades. Charges against milk do not hold up to careful examination. Buy organic milk if it makes you feel more comfortable and if you can afford it. Otherwise, pasteurized milk sold in regular grocery stores is safe and wholesome for your child. It is subject to strict regulation. Do not use milk that is not pasteurized.

Milk and milk products contribute important amounts of protein to most children's diets and provide everyone's primary source of calcium and vitamin D. Calcium is necessary for formation of strong teeth and bones, and vitamin D is essential for your body making use of calcium. The fat in whole milk is an important source of energy for young children. The toddler needs 16 to 24 ounces of milk per day and more won't hurt. As with the other food groups, don't keep score. Have milk available at meals and your child will drink it when they need it.

Adults and older children from some ethnic groups are lactose intolerant, meaning they can't digest the sugar in milk. That generally is not a problem for toddlers because they keep making lactase—the lactose-digesting enzyme—until they are a bit older. The Chapter 12 section, "Lactose intolerance," page 451, discusses this in more detail. I also realize some cultural traditions don't support milk as a mealtime beverage. If that is the case for you, take special care to get other good sources of calcium and vitamin D in your child's diet such as cheese and yogurt.

Enjoy fats and oils

Fats and oils provide essential fatty acids for brain and nervous system development and health. Your child's stomach is small and energy needs are high, so they depend on fat to make food taste good and to get enough long-lasting calories for activity and growth. Current pressure to avoid fat seems to have—inappropriately—reached the youngest set. Infants, toddlers, and even preschoolers benefit from having as much as 40 percent of their calories come from fat. Surveys show that young children get only about 30 percent of their calories as fat.[14] Toddler calorie intake decreases when they go off breastmilk or formula, and they instinctively make up for it by eating fatty foods. It's up to you to give them the opportunity. However, be wary of the current weight-reduction fad of emphasizing high-fat food and lots of meat at the expense of carbohydrates. There is nothing to be gained by going to either extreme. Enough fat gives essential nutrients and enhances the pleasure of food. Too much just wastes calories and unbalances the diet.

Fat makes food appealing and easier for beginning eaters to chew and swallow. For your cooking to have enough fat, consider methods that are moderate rather than low in fat. Sauté or fry meat, poultry, and fish along with air-frying, roasting, and stewing. Use sauces, cream, or canned soups in casseroles. To make it possible for your toddler to get enough fat, offer high-fat food at meals and let your child eat as much or as little as they want. Think high-fat spreads, sauces, gravies, dips, and salad dressings. If your child is particularly hungry and needs a lot of calories, they will eat more high-fat food. If they aren't so hungry and need fewer calories, they will eat less. The same holds true for adults. Notice that while you and your child eat and enjoy fatty foods, a steady diet of them is not pleasant. The same appetite mechanisms that promote eating a variety of foods provide guidance with low- and high-fat food as well. If you pay attention, you will observe that you can get enough of even luscious, high-fat food.

I endorse butter, but when I say butter, I mean butter or margarine. Butter's wonderful taste adds greatly to good food flavor and, because it tastes so good, you may use less than if you try to settle for margarine. You may find your toddler eating plain butter or scraping butter off their bread and asking for more. Give it to them. They likely need that butter to get enough fat in their diet. When they don't need so much fat, they will stop eating so much butter.

Nutrition policy makers say to avoid saturated fat to keep from getting degenerative diseases such as heart disease, stroke, and cancer; although the evidence isn't strong. Just in case eating the "right" fat and avoiding the "wrong" fat helps, use a variety of vegetable and animal fats to hedge your bets. Emphasize monounsaturated fats in your cooking, frying, and salad dressings—olive, peanut, and canola oils. All animal fats contain monounsaturated fat as well as stearic acid. Chemically, stearic is saturated fat, but research shows that, like monounsaturated fat, it neither raises nor lowers blood cholesterol. Artificial trans fats are generally regarded as being undesirable, and manufacturers are not allowed to use artificial trans fats in food.

It is okay to include polyunsaturated fats such as corn, sunflower, and soybean oils; just don't emphasize them as much as the monounsaturated ones. If you use margarine, consider choosing one that has as the first listed ingredient one of the monounsaturated fats. Hardened or hydrogenated oils in vegetable shortenings don't have the nutritional advantages of liquid oils. They work great for baking, but for frying and cooking, the oils are better for you. I am puzzled by the coconut oil fad, because it contains 90 percent saturated fat.

If you enjoy unusual fats for cooking and baking, I have you covered. Chicken and goose fat are high in monounsaturated fat. Lard, fatback, and bacon are about 40 percent each saturated and monounsaturated fat. Tallow comes from red meat and contains 40 percent monounsaturated fat and 25 percent stearic acid.

Enjoy sweets

As I said earlier, allow a single serving of dessert at mealtime and let your child eat it before, during, or after the meal. Periodically offer cookies, cakes, or other sweets for snacks along with milk and let your child eat as many sweets as they want at that time.

With the exception of tooth decay, no disease is caused by sugar. Eating too much sugar doesn't make children hyperactive,[15, 16] although letting a child have a sugar-only snack can soon leave them hungry and cranky and likely to behave poorly. In a study of 25 three- to five-year-olds described by their parents as sensitive to sugar, children were given a three-week trial with a high-sucrose diet, followed with a three-week trial with a diet matched for sweetness with aspartame, and then three weeks with saccharine. Teachers, parents, and behavioral experts observed and tested children in each of the dietary trials and found that there were no differences among the three diets in children's mood, behavior, or cognitive performance.[16] An analysis by the same authors of 16 excruciatingly well-controlled studies found the same. There was no relationship between children's sugar intake and their mood, behavior, or thinking.[15]

The common wisdom is that neurodiverse children, such as children with ADHD, shouldn't have sweets because "sugar can disrupt the balance of neurotransmitters in the brain." That doubtful "wisdom" comes straight out of the "don't trust the body" thinking of the control paradigm and can make the child sneak to eat a lot of sweets and even gain too much weight. It is true that the brain chemistry of neurodiverse children makes them crave sweets. On top of that, it is hard for them to pay attention to how they feel, and the sweets craving can sneak up on them and become strong before they are aware of it. Depriving them of sweets isn't the answer. It makes sweets all the more appealing and can lead to a perfect storm of cravings and impulsive eating.

Instead of depriving your neurodiverse child of sweets, manage them the way you do with other children. Let your neurodiverse child have a single serving of dessert at mealtime and offer unlimited sweets at snack time. Address their particular craving for sweets by having them frequently at snack time. Eventually your child will enjoy sweets regularly, matter-of-factly, and not in excess.

Beverages for thirst

Do your child a nutritional favor and teach them to drink water. Offer them water when they swing through the kitchen, when they get up from a nap (and go down), or after you come home from a walk. You are not trying to force-feed water but only reminding your child to notice whether they are thirsty. Consider offering water as well as milk at mealtime. Many of today's families give their child water bottles to carry with them and bring to meals. That's just fine and a good way to remember to drink water.

Consider your child's lifelong bone health. Overconsumption of soda, fruit *drinks* (which contain mostly water and sugar), and even fruit juices along with underconsumption of milk can be related to not getting enough calcium and vitamin D. While the problem is greatest among children ages five years and up, now is the time to begin heading it off. I don't lean on you much, but on the beverage issue I will lean on you. At meals, offer milk. At snacks, offer juice or milk. The rest of the time, give your child water. Save soda and fruit drinks for certain occasions, then have them as part of a meal or sit-down snack. Don't let your child carry soda and/or fruit drinks around between times. Young children do not need sports drinks, and particularly avoid energy drinks that contain caffeine.

Vegetarianism

There is nothing about the vegetarian diet that is inherently superior to diets that include meat and other animal protein foods. In fact, unless you have chosen to eat a vegetarian diet for philosophical, aesthetic, or moral/ethical reasons, you might consider drawing on the best features and enjoyable qualities of both dietary patterns. At the same time, you can moderate your meat consumption. Include legume-based main dishes and include a small amount of meat to add flavor as well as nutritional value. Consider Mexican tortillas with shredded chicken and refried beans, Brazilian black beans and rice with bits of bacon or sausage, and navy bean soup with bits of ham and crackers.

Vegetarian children can do fine nutritionally, but the diet does need to be well planned and include milk, cheese, eggs, and fat. Legumes, seeds, and nuts, in proper combination with grains, provide nutritionally complete protein. However, to get a certain amount of protein from, for example, a bean and rice dish, a child would have to eat four to six times more food than from an animal source. The solution, of course, is to include cheese, eggs, or milk at each meal. Vegan diets that completely omit eggs and dairy products have to be extremely well planned and include vitamin B6 supplements to provide for children's nutritional needs. Eating a variety of foods is essential to good nutrition. The more foods or food groups you cut out of your child's diet, the greater the risk of nutritional deficiencies.

Know what you are doing if you want your child to be on a vegetarian diet. A major challenge is bulk. Unless the cook makes a special effort to include fat with the meals, the vegetarian diet tends to be so low in calories that it is hard for children to eat enough to satisfy their energy needs. Monica, a vegetarian, contacted me on Facebook, complaining that her two boys were always hungry and begging for food. She followed sDOR, had reliable meals and snacks, and her boys ate well at those times. But they were hungry soon after they ate. I wondered whether she was using enough fat. Casseroles need two or three tablespoons of fat per quart, and vegetables need to be seasoned with fat. She could also let her children have as much as they wanted of high-fat table spreads, sauces, gravies, dips, and salad dressings. That did the trick. With higher-fat menus, Monica's children were able to last comfortably from meal to snack and back to another meal.

Iron is another issue. About 3 to 8 percent of the iron in vegetables and grains is absorbed, compared to about 20 percent of the iron in meat, poultry, and fish. Without the well-absorbed iron and the meat factor from meat, poultry, and fish, getting enough iron will be more difficult for your child. You can partially solve that problem by being sure to include a source of vitamin C with each meal, because vitamin C enhances iron absorption from other foods. Broccoli with a bean and rice meal increases iron absorption, as does the tomato sauce in vegetarian lasagna.

BE WISE ABOUT MULTIVITAMIN-MINERAL SUPPLEMENTS

The Chapter 10 section, "Nutrients and your older baby," page 343, reviews specific nutrients. Your consistently following sDOR means your child does not need a multivitamin or mineral supplement, with the possible exception of fluoride if your drinking water is not fluoridated.

If you need to give your child a "vitamin" to feel comfortable, make it a multivitamin-mineral preparation. Use one of the standard brands—not a nutraceutical. Choose one that supplies a number of vitamins and minerals and check that it offers no greater than 100 percent of the DV—Daily Value—of each nutrient. Chewable Centrum for children has a number of vitamins and minerals in moderate quantities and also contains safe levels of trace elements such as copper, chromium, and selenium. Avoid toy-like supplements or supplements made to resemble gummy bears as they tempt children to sneak around and take too many. Avoid supplementing with single nutrients. Taking too much of one nutrient can impair the absorption or use of another. Taking too much iron, for instance, can impair the use of zinc and copper.

Trace elements

Chromium, copper, fluoride, iodine, manganese, molybdenum, selenium, and zinc are called trace elements because they're needed in very small amounts in the body. A varied diet is highly likely to provide enough trace elements. While an *adequate* level of trace elements is essential for good health, *too much* is dangerous for your child. The margin between *enough* and *too much* is very small, so don't take chances. Don't give individual trace-element supplements without specific recommendations from your health care provider.

The "health" food world picks on one nutrient and then another to be the star, the magic potion that will prevent disease and ensure health and vitality. Recently it was selenium, a trace element that, like other trace elements, has a very narrow margin of error between enough and too much. While selenium is an essential nutrient, if you or your child take too much, it can be downright toxic.

Nutrients as drugs

There will always be claims about the health benefits of taking a lot of one nutrient or another. Recently, a research report claimed that vitamin E, taken in large doses, could ward off heart attacks. Niacin (a B vitamin) taken in large doses supposedly lowers blood cholesterol. Vitamin C in large quantities may act as a decongestant. These are examples of nutrients being used as *medicines*, not for their nutritional effect.

As nutrients, vitamins are used in small amounts as essential ingredients in the body's structure and functioning. As medicines, vitamins are used in large amounts and do something to the body that has nothing to do with nutritional effects. Because high doses of vitamins can be toxic, use vitamins as medicines only under careful and ongoing medical supervision. Nutrients in natural supplements can also be toxic if levels are too high.

Natural supplements, nutraceuticals

Nutraceuticals are nutrients or other natural substances that are marketed for their supposed health or medicinal effects. Avoid nutraceuticals for your child. Because they are marketed as nutrients, not medications, they escape the scrutiny of the Food and Drug Administration and are subject to neither safety testing nor standards of purity and potency. People resort to nutraceuticals when they are suspicious of medicine or the food supply and seek do-it-yourself cures. These products have great potential for harm, both from the point of view of injury from taking in toxic levels of unknown substances and from the associated assumption that the food supply is lacking or even detrimental.

Whatever the source, a nutrient taken in large quantities is no longer a nutrient. It is a drug, and its effects are not nutrient effects, but drug effects.

HOW WILL THIS ALL WORK OUT?

"I wonder what will happen to resolve struggles like this," I mused as I watched my two-and-a-half-year-old granddaughter Emma face down her parents on the vital issue of who was to tie her shoelaces. She was determined but, of course, incapable, and they were frustrated because they knew she couldn't do it. Being in the enviable bystander position, almost as soon as I thought it, I had my answer. The struggle will resolve when Emma becomes capable. Right now, she has to get her helpful, concerned, and committed parents to back off to give her the chance to learn, try herself out, and become her own person. Emma's parents were changing right along with her. They were learning to let her be independent.

Someday, Emma would be able to tie her shoelaces. At that point, she would be a preschooler. The same is true for your child. Someday, you will call them to dinner, and they will come readily. Someday, you will introduce a new food and they may even eat it readily. Someday, you will be able to leave them in a room without having to worry that they will dismantle themself or the room. When that day comes, your toddler will have changed into a preschooler and peace, relatively speaking, will reign.

At this point, we have done most of the important work of establishing the behavioral and nutritional principles of feeding children. They are the same principles that you will use throughout your child's growing-up years. The next chapter demonstrates one more critical step, that of parenting the cooperative, thinking, independent child. That Norse god we talked about earlier could have gotten a preschooler to do his bidding. Therein lies the opportunity—and the hazard—of the preschool years.

REFERENCES

1. Tate AD. Association between parental resource depletion and parent use of specific food parenting practices: An ecological momentary assessment study. *Appetite*. 2024. doi:10.1016/j.appet.2024.107368

2. Alshamrani HA. Vitamin D intake, calcium intake and physical activity among children with wrist and ankle injuries and the association with fracture risk. *Nutrition and Health*. 2019;25:113–118.
3. Herdea A. Vitamin D—a risk factor for bone fractures in children: a population-based prospective case-control randomized cross-sectional study. *International Journal of Environmental Research and Public Health*. 2023. doi:10.3390/ijerph20043300
4. Goulding A. Children who avoid drinking cow's milk are at increased risk for prepubertal bone fractures. *Journal of the American Dietetic Association*. 2004;104:250–253.
5. U.S. Department of Health and Human Services. *Dietary Guidelines for Americans. 8th Edition*. 2020.
6. Fisher JO. Eating in the absence of hunger and overweight in girls from 5 to 7 y of age. *Am J Clin Nutr*. 2002;76:226–231.
7. Lohse B. Valid and reliable measure of adherence to Satter Division of Responsibility in Feeding. *J Nutr Educ Behav*. 2021;53:211–222.
8. Pelchat ML. Antecedents and correlates of feeding problems in young children. *J Nutr Educ*. 1986;18:23–28.
9. Monaghan M. Authoritative parenting, parenting stress, and self-care in pre-adolescents with type 1 diabetes. *J Clin Psychol Med Settings*. 2012;19:255–261.
10. Mariotti Zani E. Nutritional care in children with cystic fibrosis. *Nutrients*. 2023. doi:10.3390/nu15030479
11. Petropoulou A. Eating disorders and disordered eating behaviors in cystic fibrosis: a neglected issue. *Children*. 2022. doi:10.3390/children9060915
12. Satter Eating Competence Model (ecSatter): Evidence-based research. *https://www.needscenter.org/resources/satter-eating-competence-model-ecsatter/*
13. Neil CE. Food sources of energy and nutrients among adults in the US: NHANES 2003–2006. *Nutrients*. 2012;4:2097–2120. doi:10.3390/nu4122097
14. Bailey RL. Total usual nutrient intakes of US children (under 48 months): findings from the Feeding Infants and Toddlers Study (FITS) 2016. *J Nutr*. 2018;148:1557S–1566S.
15. Wolraich ML. The effect of sugar on behavior or cognition in children: a meta-analysis. *Journal of the American Medical Association*. 1995;274:1617–1621.
16. Wolraich ML. Effects of diets high in sucrose or aspartame on the behavior and cognitive performance of children. *New England Journal of Medicine*. 1994;330:301–307.

CHAPTER 12

Feeding Your Preschooler

After the commotion of raising a toddler, raising a preschooler feels like sailing into quiet waters. You are all set with feeding your preschooler when you provide the same routine plus trust that you provided when they were a toddler. However, not having to supervise your preschooler every single minute may make you feel less important than before. Not so. Your guidance and support are as important as ever—with feeding as with everything else in your preschooler's life. That guidance and support continue to be important, if in different ways, throughout your child's growing-up years.

What does love look like when parenting your preschooler? It looks like self-restraint. Your preschooler loves you, thinks you know everything, and wants to please you. You demonstrate your love by providing leadership and giving autonomy—with eating and with all other things. The autonomy part is trickier with preschoolers because their compliance can make you think it is okay to do their *how much* and *whether* with eating. Rather than immediately pushing back as they did when they were a toddler, your preschooler may go along with you. They don't like it, it takes a considerable toll on them, but they do it anyway. Even if they defy you, they feel bad about not pleasing you. In a child's mind, wanting something different from what you want means there is something wrong with *them*.

When your child was an infant, if you didn't read their signals right, they got fussy and kept fussing. When your child was a toddler, if you provided too little leadership or interfered with their autonomy, they became a tyrant on the one hand or dug in their heels on the other. The preschooler is less likely to put up a fuss but becomes disheartened. They lose confidence and gradually become less joyful and competent with eating.

Love with parenting your preschooler also means exposing them to the possibilities: showing them what there is to learn. Your preschooler takes an interest in a new vegetable—whether or not they eat it—because they see you enjoying it. They take an interest in using a fork and napkin because they see you using them. They take an interest in cooking because you cook—and because that is a way to be with you.

IN THIS CHAPTER

With respect to establishing and maintaining a positive feeding relationship with your child, this chapter discusses in more detail than before your tasks with feeding and your child's tasks with eating. Then it revisits patterns of parenting—again in more detail—and considers why authoritative parenting—the basis for sDOR—is best. The section "Understand established feeding problems," page 428, on solving feeding pulls together everything we have said on the subject. You might skip ahead to read it. Stories about when feeding goes poorly teach you as much, if not more, than advice about making feeding go right. Then we discuss nutrition-related odds and ends and sum up with helping protect you—once again—against interference.

THE PRESCHOOLER DIVISION OF RESPONSIBILITY

The Satter Division of Responsibility in Feeding (sDOR) that you established during the toddler years is still appropriate for your preschooler. It will, in fact, continue to be appropriate, with modest adjustments, throughout your child's growing-up years.

- You are responsible for the *what, when, where* of *feeding*.
- Your child is responsible for the *how much* and *whether* of *eating*.

Following sDOR raises your child to be Eating Competent: to enjoy family meals, to pick and choose from the foods you provide, and to eat as much or as little as they want. When your child is Eating Competent, your providing structure and repeated neutral exposure to food lets them eat the amount they need and learn to enjoy the variety of food that you and their other grown-ups eat.

More about a child's being a Competent Eater

It isn't easy to wean yourself from the expectation that you should try to get your child to eat certain amounts and types of food. But letting go of that expectation can make all the difference. Let me tell you two stories.

I was appalled when a father I had invited for dinner instructed Michael, his sullen five-year-old, in every bite Michael reluctantly ate. I was appalled by the father's behavior and felt so sorry for Michael. Altogether it was a *very* unpleasant meal.

Another set of parents whom I invited to dinner helped me to see the situation from the father's point of view. They thanked me for the invitation but confessed they were reluctant to accept it because they would be embarrassed if their child didn't eat what I had prepared. The situation put pressure on them, and it was my job to relieve that pressure. "Tell Elijah that he doesn't have to eat anything he doesn't want to," I suggested. I asked them if there was a food that Elijah generally ate when all else failed and they told me rice. That was easy. When we were sitting down to dinner, I said to Elijah, "We have rice and beans and pulled pork and fruit and bread. I hope you can find something you enjoy eating, but you don't have to eat anything if you don't want to. You will still get cake when we are ready to have it." When I entertained, I broke my own dessert rule, which is to put a serving at each place along with the meal. Elijah behaved nicely, his parents were relaxed, and we all enjoyed our meal.

Elijah was a Competent Eater, Michael wasn't. Elijah was learning to feel good about himself and about being with other people, Michael wasn't. They were both set up. Elijah was set up for success, Michael was set up for failure. Elijah ate fewer foods than Michael did, but Elijah enjoyed what he ate. Michael didn't.

Competent feeders raise Competent Eaters

Children are set up by their feeding situation to behave well—or poorly. When you feed well, your child learns positive attitudes and skills around eating. Sooner or later, Elijah will get around to sampling more and more foods—provided his *parents* eat and enjoy them. Michael will likely not—unless he is forced—and when he is no longer forced, he is unlikely to eat them. Your child is Eating Competent—and so are you—when you all behave nicely at meals, even though you eat only two or three vegetables total, or only parts of the family entrée.

The key for both you and your child with respect to increasing the variety in your diet is *repeated neutral exposure*. As I have said before, *repeated exposure* is having food show up from time to time at family meals. *Neutral* means *no pressure*: being absolutely willing to take no for an answer and reassuringly clear with your child that they don't have to eat anything they don't want to eat.

The Eating Competence definition lets both you and your child be successful. You are successful when the meal is ready and you keep it pleasant, whether or not your child eats. Your child is successful when they participate pleasantly in the meal, whether or not they eat. What children actually *eat* is a whole different matter. Some children readily eat almost everything, even if it is unfamiliar. Some are skeptical but gradually learn to eat new food as they go along. Others take *years* and are often entering or leaving their teens before they eat a greater variety of food. Even the most skeptical, slow-to-warm-up child can be successful with family meals.

Figure 1.1, "Children's Eating Competence," page 5, describes in more detail what it means to be a good eater. Consider the bullet point, "Can comfortably eat in other places besides home." John's mom described him as being picky, and, because she catered to his caution with eating new food, he actually *was* picky. She restricted family menus to foods John readily accepted and made substitutes if he didn't eat. In the process, John learned that his eating was desperately important—not eating was not an option. Mom was comfortable with catering to John until she got a job outside the home and it was time for John to go to child care. John was understandably nervous and downright afraid that he couldn't eat the food there. John, through no fault of his own, did not know how to be successful when somebody other than his mom was feeding him. He couldn't pick and choose from the available food, ignore it all if it didn't appeal, and eat as much or as little as he wanted. John's mother is to be forgiven: She had been forced to eat when she was little, and she was bending over backwards not to do that to John. She sought help to find a way to feed John where she neither catered nor forced.

Understand your preschooler

The preschooler's developmental task is *initiative.* Having begun to establish their own little self as a toddler, they are now on the move: trying things out, planning, experimenting. Play is their work, and they bring a lot of energy to learning, doing, experimenting with mastery, and figuring out and exploring in all areas of life—including eating. sDOR supports preschooler initiative by letting them look, touch, smell, taste, and talk about the food as well as eat as much or as little as they want.

Your preschooler learns from you whether or not their initiative is okay. They bring a lot of energy to their play and can recover from setbacks, provided they are allowed to hang on to the idea that their learning and doing is okay. That endorsement comes from you: They are aware of how you see and feel about them, so your reactions are powerful in a way that they weren't earlier. You support your preschooler's initiative by taking an interest, giving choices, allowing for mistakes, acknowledging their efforts, and supporting them in taking care of themself. Let yourself be surprised: Don't insist on a particular outcome. In fact, don't expect *any* outcome: Preschooler initiative is about *investigating*, not about *accomplishing*. Accomplishing comes in the next developmental stage with the school-age focus on industry. School-age children figure out how to make things work and apply themselves to getting better at the tasks and activities they consider important.

Your preschooler's self-centered way of looking at the world will give you some surprises. A preschooler will seriously ask, "Why do they put a pit in every cherry? We just have to throw it away." That same self-centered thinking can temporarily put a preschooler off beef or chicken when they discover where they come from. They think animals have the same thoughts, feelings, and fears as they do. They are not saying they want to be vegetarian, any more than the child in the previous example is saying they don't want to eat cherries. They are exploring.

The preschooler has a sense of self. After their struggles for autonomy as a toddler, they have emerged able to identify their own emotions, thoughts, and intentions and distinguish their own from those of others. Part of the preschooler's repeated neutral exposure to food is talking about it, cooking it, growing it, and studying it, and even discussing nutrition in simple terms. Such exposure can allow your child to be less skeptical of unfamiliar food and willing to taste it, provided you are *truly* neutral. By that I mean you talk, cook, grow, study, and discuss and even talk about nutrition for the enjoyment of sharing it with your child, not as a way to put leverage on them to eat. Such leverage destroys their initiative and slows down their food acceptance. Even without leverage, some children take a *lot* of exposures before they are ready to experiment with new food.

Play is your preschooler's work. Rather than approaching each experience as if it were new as they did when they were a toddler, your preschooler can remember and apply what they learned before, think ahead, and be deliberate about their actions. It is possible to discuss mealtime rules and expectations with them, but don't expect them to remember what you agree upon. It is your job to remember the rules and enforce them.

YOUR TASKS WITH FEEDING

Figure 11.2, "Your feeding jobs and your toddler's eating jobs," outlines sDOR for your preschooler and, essentially, for the growing-up years that follow. That figure, in turn, is copied from Figure 1.2, "The Satter

Division of Responsibility in Feeding," page 8. Your jobs with feeding are to provide the food for regular, sit-down family meals and snacks, being considerate of your child's still-limited food acceptance and ability to chew and swallow. You make eating times pleasant by being there yourself, sharing the same food, and not spoiling your own or your child's appetite by allowing between-times eating. During the process, you show your child what they have to learn and how to behave with respect to food and eating. Then you trust your child to eat what and as much as they need to be healthy and grow up to get the body that is right for them.

Your child depends on family mealtime to give reliable access to you and to the love and sociability of the family. Meals let your child learn social skills—how to behave, how to make conversation, how to be pleasant so other people are comfortable, how to pass and serve food, how to say, "Yes, please," and "No, thank you." Your preschooler loves you and wants to be with you. Certainly, they are hungry and need to eat, but they are far more interested in your attention and companionship than in the food. If their need for pleasant attention and companionship is satisfied, they will eat and eat well. Sooner or later.

Choose the foods for family meals

You are the menu planner and gatekeeper of the food that comes into your home. You know more than your child does about the food that is in the world, and while you consider your child's food preferences, you make the final decisions about family food. Your observing sDOR at home frees your child to experiment with food away from home. In the Chapter 11 section, "Celebrate food," page 395, I discussed food groups from the point of view of "it's all right to eat what you enjoy." I made more food-celebrating suggestions in my book *Secrets of Feeding a Healthy Family*, which also addresses time-saving ways to sharpen your cooking, planning, and shopping skills. Feeding a family goes easier when you can cook, and you may as well be efficient and effective at it.

Preschoolers are still inexperienced eaters, and they benefit from some meal-planning consideration. Your preschooler may prefer food to be lukewarm, benefit from a meal that offers some creamy foods that aid chewing and swallowing, and be likely to prefer eating salad without dressing with their fingers. Figure 11.9, "Make food easy to eat," page 394, applies to preschoolers as well as toddlers. In following those recommendations, just as when you are being considerate without catering with meal planning, you set up the meal to help your preschooler succeed. You are not limiting the menu to what they will eat, catering to them, or trying to get them to eat. Remember that the preschooler likes challenges, they just don't like being *defeated* by those challenges.

I fondly remember my mother asking, "Do your children like green beans?" I didn't know. Sometimes they *ate* green beans, and sometimes they didn't. One time they ate a whole can of green beans and looked around for more. Soon after, I made two cans of green beans, and they didn't touch them. I didn't do that again! Don't try to predict what your child will eat, and don't ask your child. They are too young to know, may experience your asking as pressure, and be less likely to eat whatever it is they choose. Your child may want a vegetable they had at child care or at a friend's house or a snack they saw in an advertisement. Honor these requests if you are comfortable with them, but not all the time. And don't expect your child to eat the food, even if they ask for it. The preschooler initiates the task, but they don't necessarily complete it.

Help, not harm, with nutrition lessons

Your preschooler will enjoy learning about food and nutrition, but they won't apply that learning to what they eat. While preschoolers and even children as old as ages 12 or 13 years can recite nutrition lessons about sugar and protein and vitamin C, they can't apply value judgments to choosing food. Making such value judgments requires abstract thinking, and that is beyond children's cognitive ability until they are well into their teen years. It puzzles me why professional nutrition educators, who by definition understand children's cognitive development, still expect children to eat "healthy" food as a result of being given lessons on nutrients, food requirements, food composition, planning "healthy" meals/snacks, and/or learning lists of good-food/bad-food and/or junk food [to avoid]. It doesn't work any better at school than it does at home and puts pressure on children's eating. Preschoolers don't go by the shoulds and oughts any more than adults do.

School nutrition programs are at their finest when they emphasize allowing children to be Competent Eaters. That is, they support children in enjoying food and let them say yes or no to eating it. At school, a child being a Competent Eater supports their food acceptance the same way it does at home. Adults provide repeated neutral exposure, being careful to reassure children—and reminding themselves—that children don't have to eat if they don't want to. That reassurance is *so* important in order to keep from slipping into being controlling, which would be presenting the food again and again in order to get children to give in and eat it.

Children can be trusted. They gradually learn to eat new food when they are given repeated opportunities, without pressure of any kind, to sort, study, touch, smell, prepare, and, eventually, taste. Preschoolers enjoy trying out gardening, cooking, and serving food. During the process, they get repeated exposure and likely increased food acceptance, but the exposure must be *neutral*. Pursuing any food activity to try to motivate a child to eat takes away their initiative and makes them less likely to eat the food, not more.

Do supportive serving

Your preschooler will enjoy putting food on their plate from serving dishes and pouring their own milk from a small pitcher. They may even be more experimental with eating when they serve themself, but that isn't the point. Supporting their initiative—letting them experiment with doing it—is the point.

Feeling in control supports preschooler initiative, as does your being willing to take no for an answer. Family-style meal service is tailor-made for preschooler initiative: Preschoolers love serving themselves. Giving them control over what and how much they take supports their eating what and as much as they need. *Family-style* means using serving bowls—of a size your child can manage—and letting them take their own helping. Don't expect your child to eat everything they take, or it will spoil the enjoyment of serving themself.

If you serve your child, ask if they want the food, and have them tell you how much. If you serve plates in the kitchen, reassure your child that they don't have to eat what you serve and that there is more of everything if they want more. Deliver on your promise.

Be prepared to serve dishes in parts. Your child is likely to eat only the spaghetti from the spaghetti and meat sauce or the rice from the stir-fry and rice, and that is fine. They may eat only the tater tots from the top of their serving of tater tot casserole, and that is fine. Eventually they will get around to eating the main dishes as a whole—provided you haven't made a fuss in the meantime. They may want to skim the tater tots off the top of the serving dish, and that is not fine. That is depriving someone else of enjoyment of their meal. Be sure to make enough spaghetti and rice and consider baking a separate batch of tater tots.

You may find you can't afford to serve enough expensive foods such as shrimp, asparagus, or fresh strawberries so everyone can eat their fill. Let your eaters know there is enough to go around one time and reassure them they can fill up on rice or noodles or bread. But don't "run out" of food on purpose. Some parents do that to put leverage on their child to eat less food in general or to eat smaller amounts of foods they want to limit. They aren't fooling anyone. Children experience the strategy as food scarcity and worry whether they will get enough to eat. And they eat more when food is available.

There is always waste when you share meals with children. To keep waste down as much as possible, encourage your child to take small helpings and more if they want more. It is fine if your child has several helpings of something they really enjoy as long as it doesn't deprive someone else of their share. Eating is a social activity, and sharing food is part of that sociability. At the same time, try not to run out of generally acceptable, filling foods. Serve enough food to go around more than once with some left over. Having leftover food is the only way you can tell if you have prepared enough for everyone.

Let your child help "cook"

Your child is likely to love being in the kitchen with you. At first, it is more work for you and the results are eccentric, but some day your child will have cooking skills that will impress and help you. In the meantime, use your ingenuity to come up with safe tasks that they can accomplish. The *Secrets of Feeding a Healthy Family* cooking chapters give "Involving your children" suggestions with each recipe. Suggestions include washing fruits and vegetables, opening packages, putting pickles in dishes, using a plastic picnic knife to cut up fruits and olives, measuring water and rice, and pushing buttons on the blender or the food processor. If you can live with a bit of mangling, let them crack eggs. Avoid sharp knives and don't let them scoop, pour, or dip anything hot. Let them set the table and go easy on the corrective feedback.

Do supportive restaurant ordering

You can still do your *what*, *when*, and *where* jobs in restaurants by making creative use of the menu. Your child gets to do more of the *what* than at home, but you don't have to let them have access to everything on the menu. Consider supportive ordering when you eat in restaurants. Most families eat out at least once a week. If you eat out only occasionally, eat what tastes good to you and let your child do the same. It will contribute to both of your nutritionally adequate diets. If you eat out often, still eat what tastes good to you! Also consider these strategies:

- Be considerate without catering by having the restaurant provide a basket of bread, so just like at home, your child can eat bread if all else fails.

- Offer your child meals that provide three or more food groups. That could be a hamburger, bun, and French fries; pizza (crust, cheese, and toppings); a salad, bread, and milk; a taco (tortilla, meat, lettuce, and tomatoes).
- Consider appetizers, children's menus, splitting an adult meal, and planning to take food home.
- Let your child have fried food if they enjoy it. Since many people don't fry at home, eating out is the only time they get to have it! Food that is fried is still food. The three-food-group guideline still applies.
- Apply the dessert guideline by limiting sweets to one per meal. A milkshake or soda counts as a sweet. To have dessert, have milk or water to drink. For more about sweets, see Figure 11.7, "Regularly offer 'forbidden' foods,'" page 366.
- Don't insist that your child eat what they ordered, and don't feel you have to share your food.

Tips for grandparents who pay the restaurant bill

Decide how much you are willing to spend on your grandchild's meal. Don't worry about being a cheapskate. Your grandchild will feel better knowing your limits whatever they are. Protect yourself from aggravation by assuming they won't eat it. Or maybe they will, but if you spend too much, they won't eat enough to make you feel the expenditure has been worthwhile. When your grandchild gets older, tell them how much they can spend and help them add it up. Do your best to ignore food waste. Do not feel obligated to order something different when they don't eat what they ordered. Make sure the waiter serves a bread basket so they won't have to go hungry unless they choose to. Don't worry if they eat nothing at all. They will last until snack time.

Be honest about your preferences

Don't make excuses for your food preferences but try not to be rigid. A friend fancied herself a gourmet cook and was committed to the use of all fresh ingredients and only the most respectful cooking techniques. She was appalled when her son came home from a play date, eager to introduce her to the delicious new food that his friend Chris's dad had made for lunch—boxed macaroni and cheese. She knew she was a food snob, and to her credit, she managed to squelch her negative reaction. "Good for you," she said. "It sounds like you found something new to eat!" When he later asked for boxed macaroni and cheese, she had her answer ready. "I like the macaroni and cheese I make myself better, but we can have it sometimes. It's fine if you eat it at Chris's house." How disrespectful and even shaming it would have been for her to say, "That stuff is awful, how can you even eat it?"

You do not have to buy your child sugar-coated cereals if you don't want to, even if they have seen them on their favorite TV program and are desperate to have them. You do not have to serve meat if you are a vegetarian. You do not have to serve vegetables you find unappealing. You must not, however, condemn those foods and your child for wanting them, and you must not try to keep your child from eating them at someone else's home or at child care. If you are ambivalent about saying no or if you try to talk your child out of those foods, they will feel guilty about wanting them.

You have made nutritional decisions and value judgments about the foods you serve, and you are entitled to those values and judgments. It is reasonable to hope and expect that your child will grow up to value and choose the foods that you do. But they might not.

Include everyone in mealtime conversation

Turn off the TV. Silence the cell phone and put away the tablet and computer. Family mealtime is for connecting with each other. If you allow electronics at mealtime, you won't connect. Certainly, a weekly meal in front of a video is a special treat that everyone can enjoy, but as a regular rule, electronic devices spoil meals. They are distracting so children don't eat as well, and they keep children from getting what they crave most of all—your attention.

Include your child in the mealtime conversation, but don't make them the center of attention. Ask about their day and make it a general, open-ended question. "What have you been up to today?" is better than "Did you have a good day?" "What went on in school today?" is better than "How was school today?" Take an interest when they tell you, as you do with anyone else. Conversation with your preschooler will give you a glimpse into their delightful thinking and surprising ways of looking at the world. Don't criticize or judge what they say, and don't seize the opportunity to give a lesson or try to fix their problems. Just accept what they tell you and find out how they feel about whatever happened. "Sounds like that really made you mad" will do, or "I would have felt the same way." You don't have to make your child feel better. Your understanding and accepting their feelings is supportive and helps them cope with whatever bothers them.

Bring a topic of conversation and be prepared to share it with your child at a level they can understand and be interested in, for instance, "I heard today that there's a new elephant at the zoo."

Expect your child to listen or at least not interfere with adult mealtime conversation. Ask them to wait if they interrupt and later ask them what they started to say. Include them when others are speaking by looking at them and smiling and perhaps throwing in a few words now and then to explain what's going on. "Daddy is having trouble with windows in that new building," or "Mommy's saying her new computer program really helps." I can remember as a child loving to listen to my parents and their guests make conversation.

Don't entertain your child, play games, or sing songs together as a way to make the table pleasant. That is you taking more responsibility for your child's mealtime behavior than they are, and it takes away their initiative.

Show your child how to behave at meals

Once you have satisfied yourself that you are making family mealtimes pleasant, show your child what they can do to contribute to that pleasure. They can eat or not eat, take part in conversation, sit more-or-less quietly, and not cause a commotion. Children eat with attention and focus when they are hungry. When they get full, they start to fool around and even misbehave. At that point, even if your child hasn't eaten much, excuse them from the table. Don't let them come back, and don't pack a doggie bag. You don't have to put up with whining, eating in provocative ways, crying, being sullen or belligerent, acting out physically, or (insert your child's negative behavior here).

Parents hesitate to discipline when it is about food and eating, but your child won't starve before snack time. Rather than being heartless, it says to the child, "You are important, and the way you behave affects everyone else." In fact, when your child settles down, you can put that message in words and have a little conversation with them. "Mealtime is special for all of us, and you are important for helping make it pleasant. When you [insert your child's misbehavior here], it makes it unpleasant for all of us." Have the conversation only once, expect your child to remember it, and use it as the basis for being firm and following through on your limit-setting.

Consider your own behavior

Make sure you aren't doing anything that contributes to your child's poor behavior. When you push food on your child and don't take no for an answer, they will be rude about refusing. When you limit the amount that your child can eat, they will beg for second and third helpings. When you say, "No dessert until you eat your vegetables," they will bargain with you. "How many bites? That's too many!" When you have an investment in getting food into your child, you will put up with negative behavior in hopes that they will eat, and their behavior will get worse and worse.

Solve ordinary feeding problems with sDOR

Up to half of typically developing children display ordinary food refusal, choosiness, seeming over- and undereating, and poor mealtime behavior. Those problems can be addressed by following sDOR and understanding normal child eating and growth. It is normal for children to be choosy and skeptical about unfamiliar food. It is normal for children to eat a lot one day and not much another. It is normal for children to behave poorly at mealtime if they are pressured to eat. It is normal for them to eat a lot if the food is particularly tasty to them or not eat much if it doesn't interest them. These normal behaviors turn into problems when parents *see* them as problems and try to get the child to eat more, less, or different food than they want to eat.

We all have to learn. Most parents give up on their efforts to change their child's eating when they observe those efforts don't work. They start following sDOR—or their own approximation of it—and the child goes back to eating in their own normally haphazard way. However, some parents can't or won't give up. The child might seem to be particularly vulnerable, or the parent might be particularly concerned about nutrition and wellness. Parents persist in their attempts at resolution, the child's eating behavior gets worse and worse, parents and child get more and more upset, and they are all caught in an established eating problem. The section starting in a few pages, "Understand established feeding problems," addresses those issues. I say "understand" rather than "solve" because those problems can be too complicated to solve on your own.

CHILDREN'S TASKS WITH EATING

Again copying directly from Figure 1.2, here are your child's tasks with eating. The distinction between your feeding and your child's eating is somewhat artificial because a critical element of your feeding tasks is giving your child autonomy with their eating. To do that, you have to trust them to determine whether and how much they will eat from the food that you provide and have the confidence that they will eat what they need and grow in the way nature intended for them. Put another way, children's being able to do their eating jobs depends both on your doing your feeding jobs *and* trusting them to do their eating jobs.

Your child's eating jobs

- Children will eat.
- They will eat the amount they need.
- They will learn to eat the food their parents eat.
- They will grow predictably.
- They will learn to behave well at mealtime.

In these controlling times, depending on your child to do their jobs with eating can seem all *wrong*. As I have said more than once before, following sDOR seems simple, but it does take a leap of faith that, once you do your jobs with feeding, you can trust your child to eat and grow well. Taking that leap can be difficult, especially if you don't trust yourself to eat as much as you want of food you enjoy. You will be doing both you and your child a service if, instead of managing what and how much you eat and how much you weigh, you "Discover the Joy of Eating," the topic of Chapter 5. Trusting yourself to eat as much as you want of food you enjoy lets you trust your child. As it says in Chapter 5, follow a division of responsibility with your own eating by feeding yourself faithfully and giving yourself permission to eat. Have meals made up of food you enjoy. Eat until you get enough and then stop, knowing another snack or meal is coming soon and you can do it again.

Preschooler mealtime behaviors

Your child will learn to behave nicely at mealtime. "Behave nicely" requires definition. Your preschooler will likely eat with their fingers or use their fingers to load the silverware, then eat with the silverware. Your preschooler will make mountains of mashed potatoes, create trails with green beans, and eat in otherwise quirky ways. Consider the boy I observed in a child care center who could drink his soup and spit out the celery at the same time. Your child's quirky behavior is not intended to get a rise out of you; they are just being themself.

Your preschooler's chewing and swallowing are still somewhat immature. As a consequence, they are vulnerable to losing control of a mouthful of food, letting it slip down to plug their windpipe, and choking. To be safe, they need to be seated, supervised, and calm while they eat. Instead of using an up-and-back motion of the tongue to propel food to the back of their mouth (try it), they use their cheeks as if they were drinking from a straw (try that, too). As a result, it is difficult for them to chew and swallow meat, and they are likely to take out a chewed wad of meat and slip it under the edge of their plate. Make the meat as juicy as you can and offer gravy or a sauce. Offer to cut up their meat. Now that they don't have to prove their independence in all ways as they did when they were a toddler, they will likely let you.

Your preschooler will squirm—soon if not already. Squirming seemed to strike each of my children when they were about six years old. They would be interested in the meal and the conversation and eat well, but back and forth on their chair they would go, side to side, leaning on the table, leaning back in the chair, doing pull-ups, first one arm and then the other, stretching first one leg and then the other. Amazing. As nearly as I could tell, it had to do with excess energy, and since they were doing their job with eating and not hurting anything, I didn't try to get them to sit still. When they got a bit older, the squirming went away—mostly.

The preschooler with functional needs

The Chapter 10 section, "Children with functional needs," page 330, applies to your preschooler who is tube-fed. After their medical issues are resolved, children who are tube-fed learn to eat. It takes time, repeated neutral exposure, and reassurance that they don't have to eat if they don't want to.

Whatever your child's issues, much about them is simply normal. Following sDOR from birth and therefore preserving your child's positive eating attitudes and behaviors is important and possible. They can have positive exposure to eating even if they are fully tube-fed. They can be included in family meals and allowed to finger and mouth food even if they can't swallow. When they are medically ready to eat by mouth, they can push themself along to learn when you include them in family meals, provide them with food they can comfortably eat, and follow sDOR.

Authoritative parenting is as important for the child who is vulnerable, ill, or has functional needs as it is for the child who doesn't have those challenges. In fact, in some ways, it is *more* important. Children with medical, physical, or cognitive challenges require emotional maturity and particularly good social skills to deal with the emotional and social challenges that are sure to come. It is natural to feel sorry for an ill child or one with functional needs and try to protect them. However, such protection doesn't really help, and it interferes with their need to learn, do, and experiment. To feel good about themselves, children need to feel they are capable, and authoritative parenting lets them do that. When you struggle to determine whether you are being realistic in your limits and expectations with your special child, ask yourself, "How would I handle this if they didn't have these issues?"

PARENTING PRESCHOOLERS

As I said earlier, the fact that preschoolers are easier to be with than younger children makes them, in some ways, more difficult to parent. It is so easy to take over, get them to do what you want, snuff out their drive to learn and grow, and make them feel bad about themselves.

The preschooler's developmental task is *initiative*. The preschooler wants to explore and try stuff out. Your job is to provide safe opportunities for your child to experiment and explore. Parenting a preschooler is formative and pivotal for you as well. Now that you have a breather from your toddler's unceasing demands, you can step back and consider your decisions about parenting. With feeding as with everything else, the task is to raise a child who is self-reliant, self-controlled, contented, and cooperative.

The Chapter 1 section, "Following sDOR teaches parenting," page 14, briefly outlines patterns of parenting: authoritative, authoritarian, and permissive. Consider those three patterns with respect to the preschooler's need to explore and try stuff out. Authoritative parents support preschooler exploration because they give autonomy—room to be and do—in a tuned-in and supportive fashion. At the same time, they provide guidance and the safety of clear limits. Both authoritarian and permissive parents undermine initiative, authoritarian parents by giving little or no room to be and do, permissive parents by giving *too much* room. Permissive parents provide little guidance and safety. Preschoolers need both the freedom to be and do and feedback about what is and isn't okay. Structure frees children. A fence around a playground frees children to run around and explore. When there is no fence, they are cautious and stay close to their teacher.

Child development specialist Diana Baumrind followed preschoolers through their pre-teen years and found that children of authoritative parents were most likely to become successful, happy with themselves, and generous with others. Children of authoritarian parents were likely to be obedient but unhappy. Children of permissive parents were cautious, fearful, and dependent.[1] sDOR is authoritative parenting.

Authoritative parenting

Baumrind found that authoritative parents held the middle ground between the extremes of being controlling on one hand and throwing away all control on the other. Authoritative parents were warm and nurturing, set limits and enforced rules, and supported their child's independence and individuality by listening respectfully to children's requests and questions and providing them with safety and well-being as they explored and mastered their world. Authoritative parents were good leaders. They were matter-of-fact and reasonable in enforcing their expectations. When children disobeyed, parents disciplined promptly, calmly, and matter-of-factly, and kept control of the situation.

Authoritarian parenting

Authoritarian parents were controlling and strict. They tended to be arbitrary in their expectations and enforced those expectations with guilt and/or fear. They were unclear about what behavior they expected and unpredictable about following through on their demands. They imposed haphazard and illogical expectations, expected immediate and unquestioning compliance, and punished for anything less. Children of authoritarian parents were likely to be obedient but unhappy.

"Eat that or you will get a spanking," threatened the authoritarian father I uncomfortably observed. "Finish your corn. You're not going to blow up, are you?" Bite after bite, food after food, the father persisted in his tyranny from the beginning to the end of the meal. His unhappy preschool daughter grudgingly, reluctantly, painfully pushed down each mouthful. Her distress and trauma were lost on him. At another meal, he ignored her eating. The father also ignored his two-year-old's eating, likely because he had tried to impose his will on his toddler's eating and had failed.

Permissive parenting

Permissive parents were warm and accepting of their child but considered having expectations to be hard-hearted. In reality, lack of expectations frightens children and undermines their growth and development. Preschoolers are in the business of learning, growing, and pleasing their grown-ups. They depend on parents to show them what they have to learn and to identify acceptable and unacceptable behavior. Baumrind's permissive parents were overly lenient, and offhand in their expectations and limits with respect to the child's mealtime, bedtime, and other behaviors, and they did not follow through to be sure the child did what they wished. Parents went along with children's demands until their patience was exhausted and then blamed and shamed children for their negative behavior, begged them to behave, or punished, sometimes harshly. Children were often aggressive, openly disobedient, or disrespectful.

Children play their part

We can't overlook the child's part in prompting a certain parenting style. Your child's willingness and ease in developing self-management and self-reliance may let you be a more effective, relaxed, and flexible parent than you otherwise would be. A child who comes readily to the table, takes an interest in the food there, and makes it their business to learn to eat will give you lots of reinforcement for being an authoritative parent with feeding. An aggressive child who constantly tests limits might make you more authoritarian than you really want to be—or give up on setting limits altogether. A cautious child who reacts negatively to new food experiences may make you feel like such a tyrant when you expect them to keep a grip and behave reasonably at the table that you become permissive and cater to them.

But what comes around goes around. You may have precipitated your child's extremes of behavior in the first place by being too permissive or too authoritarian. Often the original cause of parenting distortion appears to be a particular vulnerability of the child. Wherever the cycle starts, parents are the only ones who can stop it. And when they do, both parents and child behave better and feel better about themselves and each other.

Food-enticing is authoritarian—and permissive

Of course, parenting doesn't always fit into these neat categories and sorting it out is difficult. The conversation of concerned parents on a recent talk show demonstrates the complexities—and provides a springboard for addressing some common—and well-intended—errors with feeding. As you read, speculate about each person's upbringing with feeding.

> The show featured the author of a book of recipes promoted as "tempting even the pickiest child."
>
> *Choosing food to get children to eat is quite a different matter from helping children be successful with meals by being considerate without catering with meal planning.*

Callers were eager to tell what they did to get their child to eat.

When you hear the word "get" know that the parent is trying to control the child's eating. When that happens, children control their parents right back by being reluctant and incompetent with eating.

A mother said she would let her child have cereal or peanut butter bread if he wouldn't eat, but only plain, no jelly, no sugar.

Even without putting sugar on it, this is the catering part of being considerate without catering. Undoubtedly, she will find that there are more and more days when her child demands peanut butter or cereal and won't experiment with family food.

A father felt it was unfair to his children to expect them to eat what he picked out, so he let his children plan meals half the time.

Where to start? Investigating and mastering the world is children's work. It is not unfair to give them the opportunity to explore unfamiliar food. It is, however, unfair to expect them to eat it. It's okay for children to contribute menu ideas, but giving children parents' menu-planning jobs puts too much on them.

A mother said she had encouraged her son to try new foods by pointing out, "If you had never tried ice cream or corn on the cob, you wouldn't know how good it was. You might like this too."

Whether that approach was trusting or pressuring depends on whether the mother was willing to take no for an answer.

Another mother put a stop to her teenager saying, "Oh, yuck, that looks terrible!" "How would you feel," she asked, "if you had worked really hard on something and someone came along and said 'Oh, yuck, that looks terrible!'"

Good idea and trusting, provided she didn't expect her teenager to eat. Then, their "yuck" was a form of self-defense from being expected to eat it. I wondered, however, why she had waited so long to have that conversation when you can have it with a preschooler.

To wrap up our talk show discussion, what do you imagine about each person's upbringing with feeding? My thinking is that most of those parents had been pressured to eat when they were little, and they were trying to avoid doing that to children. Which leads me to the daunting conclusion that there is a *lot* of feeding pressure out there. Controlling attitudes and strategies are all around, and many of them seem plausible. How can you sort out what is useful from what is not?

I have suggested this handy tool before. Ask yourself what you intend to accomplish. Is it to get your child to eat? Or is it to make meals pleasant for you and your child so you can relax and trust your child to eat? The first is control, however cleverly disguised; the second is trust.

UNDERSTAND ESTABLISHED FEEDING PROBLEMS

I consider a child's feeding problem to be established when it has persisted for quite a while, when repeated attempts at resolution are unsuccessful, when parents and child are upset about family mealtimes and the child's eating, and/or when the child's nutritional status and/or growth are affected. The purpose of this section is to help you gain a greater understanding of the origin and complexity of those established feeding problems. While it is possible for parents to work their way out of stablished feeding problems on their own, the feelings and habit patterns that have built up around feeding can make it difficult to resolve them without outside support. To find someone well-versed in sDOR to help you, email *support@ellynsatterinstitute.org*.

It is normal for children to want to eat, to enjoy being with their family at mealtime, to take an interest in food, to sneak up on new food and learn to eat it (or ignore it), and to eat the amount they need in order to grow in the way that is right for them. In fact, that is how we have defined a good eater. What, then, is happening when preschoolers are consistently reluctant to join in with family meals, rudely reject new food, eat poorly, or whose growth abruptly diverges up or down from their usual pattern? What happened in the past that led to these feeding problems?

Solving feeding problems is a process

A feeding problem is made up of the parents' part and the child's part. It might start with the child, whose characteristics and/or medical condition have alarmed and overwhelmed parents, taken away their trust, and led them to feed in counterproductive ways. It might start with the parents, who didn't have trust in the first place and, indeed, had feeding agendas. They wanted their child to eat certain amounts or types of food and/or grow in certain ways. It might start with both of them. Each of them brought goals, characteristics, and behaviors that undermined feeding.

Wherever it started, solving a feeding problem requires restoring parents' trust in the child to do the *whether* and *how much* of eating. Establishing pleasant family meals and sit-down snacks is important, but restoration of trust is more difficult. To restore that trust, parents need to understand the backstory, what happened to take away their trust and therefore cause the problem in the first place. Understanding that allows them to be more receptive to insights about what they are doing now that continues to undermine that trust. To tease that out, my sDOR-committed colleagues and I start with an assessment that examines nutritional, medical, psychosocial, and feeding dynamics issues.[2]

We introduce parents to sDOR and reassure them that their child's eating attitudes and behaviors will recover when they follow sDOR. At first that is a leap of faith for them, and they need ongoing support to stay the course with sDOR. It takes time for parents to get the structure of meals and snacks reliably in place. It takes time for the parents to detect and address their tendencies to be controlling or neglectful with feeding. And it takes time for the child's eating to become more extreme before it moderates.

Mealtimes get better fast

Once sDOR is reliably in place, struggles around feeding quickly go away and meals quickly become pleasant. It takes longer for the child's eating attitudes and behaviors to recover. At first, children's eating becomes more extreme. That extreme eating is part of children's process of rediscovering their hunger, interest in food, and fullness. It also lets them test whether parents really mean they can eat—or not eat—what and as much as they want. During the extreme-eating stage, children seemingly confirm parents' worst fears of their eating if it wasn't controlled. Parents need support hanging in there with sDOR while they wait for their child's eating to moderate.

EXAMPLES OF FEEDING PROBLEMS

Let's take a look at some well-established feeding problems growing out of situations where parents have found it difficult to stick to their jobs with feeding and trust their child to do their jobs with eating. As you read these stories, think about what the feeding struggle did to the preschooler's developmental task of *initiative*, to their trying things out, planning, experimenting. Were they being allowed to investigate the food world: look, smell, touch, taste, and talk about the foods their parents provided and eat as much or as little as they wanted? Or did the expectation to eat in certain ways undermine their initiative?

The child who is cautious about food

Adrian's parents were very concerned that their four-year-old ate from a very short list of food and that he resisted joining the family at mealtime.

Even though Adrian's mother went through the cupboard with him before meals and let him pick out what he wanted to eat, Adrian generally consumed only milk. Between times, Adrian helped himself to the cupboards and refrigerator. Adrian's consistent growth indicated he was eating as much as he needed, although a four-year-old's self-selected diet is unlikely to be very well-balanced.

Adrian's parents complained that from the time they started him on solid food, he had been unwilling to try new food. Because they didn't want him to develop their own food selectivity, they encouraged and even forced him to eat. Adrian, the same as many children, could have been born with a particular sensitivity to food taste, texture, and smell and could have needed a long time to warm up to new food. Being so tuned-in can be positive or negative. Such children can enjoy food a lot, or they can be so upset by the appearance or smell of food that they can hardly bear to have it around.

However, as I also pointed out to them, the selective eater can be *created*. Parents pass along selective eating by pressuring their child to eat in the same way that they, themselves, were pressured. Despite parents' efforts to hide it, children pick up on their parents' aversion for certain foods. I reassured Adrian's parents that they didn't have to eat anything they didn't want to eat. They just had to be polite about refusing it. The same was true for Adrian. Being comfortable with unfamiliar food and able to behave well around it would allow Adrian to experiment with new food at family meals and with foods other families eat.

Summing up, it appeared the problem with Adrian was *both* limited food exposure and pressure to eat. Growing out of their concern for him, from the time he started his transition to solid food, his parents had bribed, over-encouraged, persuaded, and catered. The extended family even got into the act by doing all the above to Adrian and adding on pressuring tactics including weekends with them when they applied their own ways of trying to get him to eat. Through it all, Adrian held steadfast. He wouldn't eat anything he didn't want to eat.

I reassured Adrian's parents that when they followed sDOR they could trust Adrian to do his jobs with eating. Adrian could learn to behave nicely at family meals, eat what he could, and ignore or politely turn down the rest. They were to stop asking Adrian to choose what he wanted for meals, continue to choose food they enjoyed for family meals, and be considerate without catering at mealtime by including one or two of the foods he generally ate. Then they were to say to him, "You don't have to eat if you don't want to but keep us company for a bit while we eat." They delivered on their reassurance by letting him leave the meal when he was finished, whether or not he ate. That was a hard one because they felt they were making Adrian go hungry. Being able to say, "That's it for now. Snack time will be soon" made it easier. Being considerate without catering helped, too. They knew if Adrian didn't eat it was his choice, not their failure to provide for him.

At first, it was a big deal for Adrian to briefly stay at the table without making a fuss. He soon relaxed and enjoyed being there, and after two or three weeks, he even began to show signs of being interested in new food. He didn't want to eat spaghetti, but he did ask his parents to leave the spaghetti serving dish near his plate. Then he wanted a little spaghetti on his plate, and his mother was wise enough to reassure him, "You don't have to eat it if you don't want to." He didn't. By the fifth or sixth week, he occasionally tasted a mouthful of spaghetti, then took it out again. His parents continued to reassure him, "That's all right, you don't have to swallow it if you don't want to. Just put it in your napkin." Adrian made rapid progress because his parents really meant it when they told him, "It's up to you whether you eat."

At that point, Adrian and his parents were "cured." They were ready to continue on their own. The parents felt comfortable following sDOR, Adrian was confident he could behave nicely at meals, and his parents were proud of him—and of themselves.

The parents' remaining big challenge was in shutting down the interference from the extended family. They used the family therapy tactic of positive reframing: "We know you want the best for Adrian and have been worried about his eating. We have too. We found out, however, that trying to get him to eat makes his eating worse, not better. Instead, we have learned to follow a division of responsibility [explained]. Instead of trying to find food he would eat, we have a meal we enjoy and include one or two side dishes that he generally eats. After that, it is up to him. He can still leave the meal even if he doesn't eat. And . . . oh, yes . . . we also learned he needs a sit-down snack between meals, even if he doesn't eat at mealtime." The grandparents, aunts, and uncles weren't perfect or even very skillful in following sDOR, but Adrian seemed to overlook their feeding errors as long as his parents did well with feeding him.

As Adrian's parents continued to hold steady with sDOR, over the next couple of years that I knew them, he mastered a modest assortment of food. He will keep learning. Given his eating history and his cautious nature, he might not get to the point where he is a robust or enthusiastic eater, but he will get the job done. In my experience, when children have trouble with eating early on, their eating tends to be somewhat fragile and easily disrupted. When they are stressed or excited or preoccupied with some new life experience, they may not eat much for a while. When they are pressured in any way to eat, they revert back to being reluctant to eat. However, when the upset blows over, they go back to eating as well as ever and make up for lost time.

Parents who have been traumatized

Adrian's parents had been traumatized by their struggle with Adrian's eating. The trauma is even more severe when children have medical or other issues that complicate their eating. Layla is three years old. From age 12 weeks, she had trouble eating, her growth was faltering, and her parents felt she was starving. They had her evaluated by ENT and gastroenterology specialists as well as an occupational therapist and a speech-language pathologist. It was only when Layla was eight months old that they discovered that Layla had oversized adenoids. Those adenoids forced her to breathe through her mouth and made it difficult for her to close her mouth to eat or drink from a bottle. Until Layla's medical problem was addressed, her parents used a syringe to drop formula into Layla's mouth as they lived with the constant threat of her being hospitalized.

Layla's parents are currently trying to work their way out of their feeding problems. On their best days, they follow sDOR by making mealtimes as routine and enjoyable as possible. The family sits down together to eat, shares the same foods, and her parents try not to focus on what or how much Layla eats. When their courage starts to slip, they offer Layla foods that she's eaten in the past in hopes she will eat more. When they feel really desperate, they bribe and reward her for eating. They acknowledge, "I know this isn't right. It doesn't *ever* feel right. It certainly doesn't feel sustainable, but I still feel so worried about making sure she eats enough that backing off feels nearly impossible."

The parents' fear is understandable. When a child's very survival appears to be at stake, parents are likely to be too anxious to take the leap of faith that is necessary to allow the child to eat whether and as much as they need. It is a quandary, because children's eating doesn't improve until parents are able to consistently follow sDOR. Each time parents go back to their old ways with feeding, it reinforces the child's eating problems and increases the time it will take to resolve the problem.

Adopting the tactic of being considerate without catering with meal planning will address Layla's parents' need to offer Layla food she has eaten before. To help them keep their courage, they definitely need their physician's reassurance that Layla has the nutritional reserves to get safely through a period of poor eating. However, even with those elements in place, to hold steady they are likely to need several months' support from a trusted advisor who is thoroughly familiar with Layla's feeding issues.

The child who *loves* to eat

Parents prefer it when a child *loves* to eat. Well, they do, and they don't. The same as other extremes, a child's passion for food can make parents take evasive action. Given the normatively distorted—that is, generally warped—eating attitudes and behaviors in our culture, parents might assume that if a child loves to eat, they will eat too much and get "too fat." The reality is that children are such good regulators that if you truly maintain sDOR, even your passionate-about-food child will stop in the middle of a bowl of ice cream when they get enough. Such a child overeats only when parents are so alarmed by their gusto that they try to curb it. If you react to your child's passion for food by giving them only food that doesn't *inspire* passion, then they will be all the more ardent about the food you are trying to avoid.

Joshua *loved* to eat, and he couldn't wait for Friday night. His parents tried to tone down his food enthusiasm by following what they thought were healthy eating rules, but they kept getting ambushed by their own food cravings. Their solution was to plan for the ambush. They ate drab food all week, then took weekends off to eat what they enjoyed. For the parents, it seemed to work. They ate a few—well, all right, quite a few—foods they had been craving, then buckled down again on Monday.

Their strategy did not work for Joshua. During the week, he constantly begged for snacks. On Friday night, the family's food vacation started. When they went to the movies, Joshua was up and down all evening—visiting the snack bar to buy nachos, ice cream, buttered popcorn, and all the foods his parents wouldn't let him have during the week. At Sunday dinner at his grandmother's house, Joshua seemingly couldn't get enough fried chicken, mashed potatoes with gravy, and salad with blue cheese dressing.

I explained to Joshua's parents that their on-again-off-again strategy was creating the very problem with Joshua's eating they were trying to prevent. Joshua ate a lot of the food his parents considered against the food rules because he was being forced to go without. I encouraged them to lighten up. We did some menu planning that included their "weekend" foods during the week. I explained why eating those foods was all right and that if they began to feel the need for a food vacation, they were being too strict.

It worked. After a period of eating a *lot*, Joshua settled down with his eating. On Friday nights, he only wanted one treat at the movies. After all, now he could get those foods at home. His grandmother worried that he didn't like her fried chicken anymore, but he reassured her that now his dad made it, too.

Joshua's passion for good food was all right and, in fact, delightful. A child who enjoys eating—and feels positive about that enjoyment—is all set to be healthy and well-nourished and maintain a consistent weight. Being positive and trusting of their sensations and feelings about eating lets children tune-in accurately to their hunger, appetite, and satiety and eat the amount and type of food they need. All food is wonderful. Children can be passionate about vegetables only if they are allowed to be passionate about ice cream or boxed macaroni and cheese.

The child who eats for an audience

Don't deprive your child, but don't go off in the other direction either. Grayson's parents were truly following sDOR and neither restricting nor forcing, so I was stumped about why Grayson's weight was accelerating. With a bit of digging and watching a few mealtime videos, it emerged that Grayson was eating for his audience. His extended family gave him a lot of positive attention for being a hearty and robust eater. Grandparents and aunts and uncles and friends loved watching Grayson eat, exclaiming, "Grayson is such a good eater! I wish my child ate that well!" Grayson basked in the praise and attention, ate all the more, and in the process, lost track of his own feelings of hunger and fullness. Unless they are subjected to outside interference, even children who *love* to eat still have a reliable stopping place. Grayson's parents shut down his audience, and Grayson's eating moderated, and his weight leveled off.

The "obese" child

Four-year-old Toni couldn't get her mind off food, and that was new for her. In the past, she had eaten well but not a lot, at least compared with some of her thinner friends. Toni's parents had recently begun to follow a "healthy eating pattern" by pushing fruits and vegetables, limiting her meals to a single serving of each food, cutting way down on fats and sweets, and letting her have only an apple or some carrot sticks for snacks. Now Toni thought about food all the time, constantly pleaded for food handouts, sneaked into the kitchen to eat, and cried when her parents refused her. To their shame, they scolded her: "No, you have had enough—that's all for now. Why do you want to eat so much?" They could tell that Toni felt guilty about wanting to eat so much, but they didn't know what to do about it.

Toni's BMI had always been around the 95th percentile. While her parents were somewhat uneasy about her size, they had hung in there with sDOR, and the pediatrician had advised taking a wait-and-see approach. However, with the recent media attention on childhood "obesity," the parents had become alarmed and pressed their pediatrician to help them do something about Toni's weight. Toni's pediatrician was reluctant to go along with them, but he had pressures of his own. He was being told by his professional organization that "best practice" with children whose BMI was as high as Toni's was following the "healthy eating pattern."[3]

After a month of struggles around eating, Toni's parents came to see me, and we were able to get things straightened out. First of all, I told them that there was nothing wrong with Toni's size and shape. Her consistent weight and BMI indicated she was growing in the way that was normal for her and that she was a good regulator. She was capable of eating the amount she needed. Not only that, but it was apparent that they had given her the support she needed to do a good job with her eating. I advised them to go back to doing what they had done before. They had been feeding well and letting Toni develop the size and shape that was right for her. On their own, they had been following sDOR.

Toni's parents took my advice and told their daughter, "Toni, we talked with someone, and she told us that you know how much you need to eat. We have been trying to get you not to eat so much, but that was wrong. From now on, we will do it like we did before. We will have our meals and snacks, and you can eat as much as you want." Toni saw an opportunity. "Does that mean I can have all the cookies I want?" she asked. "No," said her parents. The answer was the same for Toni as for any other child. "What about dessert? Can I have more dessert?" "We'll do like we always did before. We'll put your dessert at your place, and you can eat it when you want it. You can't have seconds on dessert, but once in a while we will have cookies for snacks, and you can eat as many then as you want." After a week or two of eating quite a bit more than she had in the past, Toni's eating settled down to the way it had been before they started restricting her.

Toni's parents apologized to their pediatrician and explained their decision to go back to following sDOR. He was skeptical, so they gave him a copy of Chapter 3, Your Child Knows How Much to Eat. He was able to be supportive of what Toni's parents were doing and agreed to track her weight to see if it continued to be consistent. The parents were relieved. They liked him very much and respected his medical ability, but they were prepared to go elsewhere. You have my permission to copy that chapter for your pediatrician if you need to!

Toni's parents weren't alone in finding it difficult to hang in there on feeding their relatively large child. Mothers of higher-weight children say they feel guilty, sad, and responsible for their child's weight and that family members, children's physicians, and others blame them for letting their child get too heavy.[4] Taking Toni to the ice cream parlor required a thick skin, imagining that others were thinking, "Why are they letting that child have an ice cream cone? No wonder she is fat!" When Toni's grandfather confronted them about Toni's weight, they briefly revisited their anxieties, then explained their philosophy. He didn't accept it, but he agreed to stop making an issue of Toni's eating and weight. A news release from the Centers for Disease Control about the "alarming increase in childhood obesity" made them question what they were doing and decide again to follow sDOR. You are likely to find yourself doing the same. Whenever you are dealing with a chronic condition, you have to revisit it every so often to be sure you are on the right track.

"Are we supposed to put any limits on Toni at all?" asked the mother after they had been to a potluck. "All the kids lined up at the dessert table and filled their plates. Should I have made her stop?" "How would you have handled it if you hadn't been concerned about her weight?" I asked her. She thought a minute, then said, "I would have let it go. That seems to be pretty normal kid eating behavior. I remember doing the same thing when I was little and my parents trying to make me first eat something else. I took the other food, but I didn't eat it."

Resolve the weight dilemma for your child

Toni's parents were relieved about the feeding part but still concerned about her weight and health. What about all the research that says that obesity is unhealthy, they wondered. I reassured them that despite the media reports, and despite current public health recommendations, people who suffer negative health consequences associated with weight are those whose BMI is extremely high or extremely low.[5] Toni's weight was nowhere near being extreme. I discussed that extreme in the Chapter 4 section, "Consider an 'extremely obese' child," page 124.

Adults who have the most medical issues correlated with high body weight are those who show the typical consequences of weight-reduction dieting. They have gained weight as adults[6, 7] or their weight has fluctuated throughout life.[8, 9] The bottom line, however, was that even if Toni's size and shape persisted into her adult life and in the equally unlikely prospect that her adult weight was bad for her, there was *nothing they could do to change it.* Even intensive adolescent weight interventions with 50 to over 100 contact hours with a variety of professionals produced only a "small and highly variable" weight loss.[10]

Even without a weight reduction intervention, simply making an issue of Toni's weight increases her risk of weight acceleration. Children's weight accelerates when parents accept an "overweight/obese" diagnosis[11] or see their child as being "overweight" as opposed to being "about the right weight."[12] For more detail about that research, see the Chapter 4 section, "Parents are reluctant to accept diagnosis," page 122. Toni's parents understood the gist of that research very well. As they demonstrated with their brief food-restriction experiment, when they didn't let Toni eat as much as she wanted, she ate more, not less. For more support in holding steady with feeding and raising your large child, read my book *Your Child's Weight: Helping without Harming*.

A child who needed a lot of reassurance

Children who have been forced to go hungry, even briefly, need a lot of reassurance to trust that they will get enough to eat. If the trauma has gone on for a long time, it doesn't take much to scare them all over again. With Toni, it was a reasonably quick fix because her parents knew very soon that they were on the wrong track. With Lauren, it took considerably longer. I talked about Lauren in the Chapter 4 section, "Accept growth extremes," page 109. Lauren was the six-year-old whose food intake was restricted from birth. After she started following sDOR, Lauren's mother had to be absolutely consistent about offering Lauren meals and snacks and repeatedly reassure Lauren she could have as much as she wanted at those times.

Lauren's at-first-eating-a-lot stage made her mother so anxious she needed my support to let Lauren eat as much as she wanted. She had tried to do it on her own, but she simply could not, even though, logically, she knew how important it was for Lauren. "I start, and then stop, start, and then stop. That is worse for her than if I didn't do it at all," she said, and she was right. Her own long-term weight-reduction dieting made it seem all wrong for anyone to eat as much as they wanted. In order for Lauren's mother to be able to trust Lauren's eating, she had to trust her own. That, too, was part of the treatment.

Children who experience food insecurity

Restricted children grow up with food insecurity. Other children experience food insecurity when economic issues make it difficult for parents to provide enough for them to eat. Whether the food restriction is voluntary or driven by economic problems, the children all show the same preoccupation with food and tendency to overeat when they can.[13] Nutrition policy makers blame weight gain associated with food insecurity on inability to purchase fresh produce, lean meats, and low-fat dairy products. That doesn't make any more sense for low-income people than it does for people in any other income bracket. Eating low-calorie foods does not prevent weight acceleration. Eating *enough* food does.

Current nutrition policy condemns low-income people to a food restriction double whammy—not enough food and being expected to eat low-calorie food. Eating Competence based strategies would be far more responsive to the needs of the food insecure and are also nutritionally responsible. People who are confident of getting enough to eat naturally and gradually diversify their food selection.[14] Homemakers can manage the food budget and provide family members enough to eat by maintaining the structure of family meals and snacks and providing higher-calorie foods at those eating times. Higher calorie but equally nutritious forms of the usual foods include whole milk, fried chicken, and fruit canned in heavy syrup or baked in pie. Fatty foods can be offered as condiments, such as gravy and regular salad dressing at meals. Waste can be controlled by encouraging family members to take many small helpings. Random snacking can be discouraged by including "forbidden" food in meals and snacks. For more on this topic, see the Chapter 5 section, "Address food insecurity," page 142.

The vulnerable child

Children who are small, ill, or have medical, cognitive, neuromuscular, or developmental issues present particular challenges with feeding and parenting, and such children more frequently have mealtime difficulties. Such children scare parents and even health professionals, and the standard response is to become controlling with feeding. Negative mealtime interactions in response to illness tend to reflect overall negative patterns of family functioning.[15] The stress of having a child with functional needs can make families compensate in counterproductive ways. It is also difficult to adhere to clear limits and set firm expectations with a child who is seen as being fragile. Parents may show their concern through pressing food on the child, or by not providing structure and limits.

Ill children are children first and ill second. Being the resourceful little people that they are, even the ill child is not above using his parents' concern to his own advantage, as in, "If you don't let me do that, I won't eat." Then, of course, the parent is truly in a bind—how can you get angry at such a vulnerable child? The answer? Easily! You don't have to act on your anger, but it is a good guide that things are out of whack and need to be adjusted.

At times, parents' efforts to feed their vulnerable child can turn into force as they resort to increasingly desperate measures. The parents I met when giving a presentation in Louisiana were feeding their son in the bathtub. He was truly small, and the boy's doctor had reportedly advised the parents, "Feed him, I don't care how you do it." I can understand where a physician comes from in giving such advice. Their responsibility is to preserve life, and when your only tool is a hammer, everything looks like a nail. Practicing within the trust paradigm and following sDOR provide far more and better tools. If you are in this situation, feel free to give your child's doctor a copy of Chapter 3, Your Child Knows How Much to Eat. You can use their support, and they can use yours.

But I digress. Those Louisiana parents were pushing so hard to get food into their child, and he was fighting back so hard, that they made a terrible mess. Feeding him in the bathtub meant that they could rinse him down after meals. Such feeding is highly unusual, but it demonstrates just how frightened and desperate parents can become.

The situation nearly took my breath away, and no way was I going to be able to help them in five minutes after a talk. I offered to do a thorough evaluation with them and asked in passing if at any time their child willingly ate. "Yes," they said, "he eats his breakfast in front of the TV, and he eats well at child care." Clearly, their son ate when they backed off. However, in their desperation and, yes, anger, they had not recognized his capability and continued to torture their son and themselves with feeding. I had discussed sDOR in my talk, and I encouraged them to follow it and stop doing their son's jobs of what and how much he eats. I doubt if they were able to follow my advice because they were far too frightened for their child's welfare. In my experience, for such parents to have the courage to make such a drastic change, they have to be sure I clearly understand them, their child, and their situation, and they need step-by-step support as they work their way out of their difficulties with feeding.

Without examining the boy's growth records from birth, I don't know if he was just small or whether his growth was faltering. He may have been typical of other children whom I have evaluated whose growth started out relatively low—say around the 5th percentile—then diverged downward. Provided the child was well and neurotypical, the problem was feeding. The typical sequence of events was that the child's small size alarmed parents and health professionals and they tried to get them to eat more so they would grow faster, whereupon the child ate less and grew more slowly. The solution, of course, was maintaining sDOR, but that was unlikely to happen, at least initially. Instead, pressure gets piled on top of pressure and parents end up feeding a child in the bathtub. It is so difficult with relatively small children because their narrow margin for error makes it hard for both parents and professionals to take the chance of trusting the child to do their part with eating.

Children who *can't* eat enough

Feeding the ill child is the same as feeding any other child. You maintain sDOR. However, some children truly can't eat enough to keep themselves going and support growth. These include children whose neuromuscular difficulties are so severe they have trouble eating; children who have heart defects and are too worn out to eat enough; children who are in cancer treatment and don't have the appetite to maintain the nutrition they need to support therapy. In all cases, parents carry a tremendous burden. They feel they should and are often charged with doing what they simply can't do—get food into the child.

Children almost invariably eat more, not less, when you follow sDOR than when you try to get them to eat. However, the ill child may not be able to eat *enough*. Then, it is far better to tube-feed as an adjunct to family meals than to spoil the feeding relationship by pressuring the child to eat. The Chapter 11 section, "The toddler with cystic fibrosis," page 384, discusses routine use of tube-feedings to supplement oral intake when children can't eat enough. Dietitian Ellen O'Leary, who coordinated nutrition services in an Atlanta hospital pediatric oncology unit, was successful at routinely and matter-of-factly recommending tube-feeding for children in cancer treatment. Chemotherapy and radiation therapy distort children's hunger and fullness cues by making their mouths sore and slowing down the function of their stomach and intestines. As a consequence, the child on chemotherapy is often not hungry enough to eat as much as they need to keep their body strong. Forcing the not-hungry child to eat is miserable for both parents and children and can permanently spoil the way a child feels about eating. Supplemental tube-feedings—through either a nasogastric tube or gastrostomy tube (G-tube)—let the child eat as much as they want at family meals and snacks. Supplemental tube-feedings make it easier to follow sDOR by relieving pressure on parents to get their child to eat. When the child gets better and regains their appetite, the tube-feeding can taper off to nothing. When parents are comfortable that the child is capable of doing the *whether* and *how much* of eating, the tube can be removed.

I have said elsewhere that tube-fed children continue to have hunger and fullness cues and that you can use those cues to guide tube-feeding. That doesn't seem to work with children in cancer treatment. Cancer treatment spoils the child's appetite, so O'Leary encourages parents to tube-feed the child at night. She monitors the child's growth trajectory to guide what and how much goes into the tube-feeding.

Tube-feeding happens in a couple of ways. A nasogastric tube goes in through the nose, down the throat and esophagus, and into the stomach. A gastrostomy tube is placed directly into the stomach through the abdominal wall using a simple surgical procedure. For a young child whose chewing and swallowing are normal and who won't be self-conscious about having the tube coming out of their nose and taped to their cheek, O'Leary recommends a nasogastric tube. Her young patients say the small, soft feeding tubes are comfortable and don't complicate swallowing. She recommends a gastrostomy tube for older children, those whose chewing and swallowing are compromised, and when tube-feeding needs to last longer than a couple of months.

O'Leary says parents are greatly relieved to have lifted the terrible burden of getting food into their child. They can go back to enjoying pleasant family meals with their child without having to worry about how much their child eats. Her matter-of-fact approach is important, because tube-feeding can be viewed as negative and as a last resort. In fact, parents have told me they were warned, "If you don't get that child to eat, we will have to put in a tube." A father from New Orleans called me, desperately opposed to "letting them cut on my kid." I wasn't able to give him any specific advice, but I did reassure him that installing a feeding tube is not major surgery but a simple procedure. Temporarily having the tube-feeding to fall back on can help get things back on an even keel with feeding.

Colorado speech-language pathologist and swallowing therapist Gretchen Hanna has worked with children who have a disorder such as muscular dystrophy that impairs their chewing and swallowing. Hannah says it is all about supporting reasonable expectations. A child can enjoy the few bites of ice cream, soup, or food of whatever consistency they can manage, and both parents and child can focus on the pleasure of feeding. Then the child's nutritional needs can be satisfied with tube-feeding. She prefers a gastrostomy tube for children with swallowing difficulties because the nasogastric tube can further complicate their already-compromised swallowing.

The key consideration in using the tube-feeding is in *preserving*, *supporting*, and *restoring* the pleasure of normal feeding, rather than as an *alternative* to feeding. Of course, being able to use tube-feeding in a knowledgeable and skillful way requires careful guidance—for that, seek an experienced pediatric dietitian working with a team with a pediatric speech and language pathologist or occupational therapist.

Children with developmental disabilities

Salena had spina bifida, and after many surgeries was able to get around well using braces and crutches. She was plump and getting plumper, and her parents were concerned. Since she was born, they had been warned that children with spina bifida don't regulate their food intake and can get "too fat," and they had tried to be careful. They limited the amount she ate at meals, didn't let her have between-meal snacks, and strictly limited her fatty and sugary foods. But Salena was not willing to go with the program. She protested and complained at mealtime until they let her have a little more—and a little more after that. Between meals, she begged her parents for candy and potato chips, and if they wouldn't give them to her, she helped herself. The appeal of "forbidden food" aside, restricted children prefer candy and potato chips because they are high in calories and quickly satisfy their hunger. Salena's weight was accelerating, and she appeared to be the victim of a self-fulfilling prophecy. Predicting she would gain too much weight made her parents restrict her, she ate more, and she gained too much weight.

Children with developmental difficulties are often assumed to be incapable of knowing how much they need to eat. There is no evidence supporting that assumption, but there is considerable evidence that restricted children gain too much weight. Children with Prader-Willi syndrome do have a strong appetite combined with a thrifty metabolism. They can get by on very few calories. Once they get past their early-childhood medical fragility, almost all children with Prader-Willi syndrome are routinely and severely restricted to prevent typically rapid weight gain.

It is hard to know where that excessive eating—for them—and too-rapid weight gain comes from. Does it come from spoiling their regulatory ability with pressured feeding when they were infants? Does later restrained feeding make them eat too much and cause weight acceleration? Is it a true biologically mandated inability to regulate their food intake? Or is it a combination of all three? I wish I could tell you it is the first two and that following sDOR with your child who has Prader-Willi syndrome will allow them to follow a predictable growth trajectory, but I just do not know.

What I do know is that pressured feeding in infancy establishes negative patterns that cause feeding problems for years to come. Nurses doing follow-up with almost-toddlers and toddlers who had been born prematurely say those children are often heavier than appears normal for them. I absolutely acknowledge this is anecdotal information, but it also stands up to the logic of feeding dynamics. Parents of premature babies are all too often sent home with instructions to feed a set amount on an every-two-hour schedule. Being fed based on these external dictates makes babies lose sensitivity to their internal cues of hunger, appetite, and fullness and they make errors in food regulation. They eat based on the food available and what parents expect them to eat. That pattern persists when they join in with family meals. Such children can recover their internal-regulation ability, but it takes careful attention to sDOR and braving it out through the steps I described above in the section "Solving feeding problems is a process," page 428.

Preschoolers with food allergies

Pronounced food allergies can be serious and must be attended to medically and by an sDOR-expert dietitian who is experienced with the management of allergies. The Chapter 11 section, "The toddler who is allergic," page 380, gives more detail. There, I shared the advice of allergy specialist Alexia Beauregard, registered dietitian, to omit the toddler's food allergens from family menus so the whole family can eat the same food as the allergic child. Now that your child is a preschooler and can begin to distinguish between "okay" and "not okay" foods, you can gradually lighten up on those family food adaptations and begin to give your preschooler responsibility for avoiding foods that make them ill.

Allergic reactions include abdominal pain, nausea, vomiting and diarrhea; cough, runny nose, wheezing and pronounced breathing difficulties; skin rashes from mild to extreme; headache and irritability; and shock. Severe allergies are the exception. Don't put yourself through the stress of catering to a food allergy unless it is truly necessary.

The tendency with the allergic child is to hover and become a dietary policeman. Don't. You know after reading this far that if you hover with feeding, your child will not be capable with eating. Follow sDOR. Be matter of fact about telling your child what they can and can't eat. Be equally matter of fact about teaching them to be responsible for keeping their limitations in mind when they eat at friends' homes or at school. You can say, "You can't eat peanut butter, so when we have peanut butter, I will give you almond butter instead. But when you go to someone else's house and they have peanut butter and jelly sandwiches, they probably won't have almond butter. Just say, 'No, thank you,' and ask for plain bread and jelly. If your friend's parents insist, you can say you're allergic, but you don't have to make a big deal out of it."

Certainly, talk with the extended family, child care providers, school personnel, and friends' parents about your child's allergies, but you won't always be able to run interference. You can now treat severe allergic reactions with an EpiPen, but it wasn't always the case. My friend Rosie told me about a run to the emergency room with her severely citrus-allergic son when he ate a lemon drop at a neighbor's house. The neighbor felt terrible, but Rosie was philosophical about it. "I guess we all learned," she said. "One more thing he knows to look out for." Rosie didn't make it her life's work chasing around after her son to keep him safe or to try to purge his life of everything that might make him sick. That is, of course, far more easily said than done. Severe allergies can be a life-threatening condition, and it is entirely natural to be overprotective when a child is at such serious risk. Try to remember, however, that your child will be the safest in the long run if they learn to take responsibility for their own condition.

Preschoolers with diabetes

The Chapter 11 section, "The toddler with diabetes," page 382, talks about managing diabetes so you don't spoil your feeding relationship. It's a bit easier with preschoolers because they more readily comply with structure. Your preschooler with diabetes still can be trusted to do their part with *how much* and *whether.* Staying in your own lane of *what, when,* and *where* will provide your child with structure and support for managing their diabetes.

I won't advise you about medical management for your child's diabetes. However, if you find your current approach to managing your child's eating and diabetes is distorting your feeding relationship and making your child less capable with eating, talk with your health care team. They may be willing to modify your child's diabetes management regimen.

Explore creative ways to work with your school on behalf of your child with diabetes. Explain to your school your post-dosing approach to giving insulin, and if possible, use an insulin pump.

Preschoolers with cystic fibrosis

The Chapter 11 section, "The toddler with cystic fibrosis," page 384, discusses managing cystic fibrosis so it doesn't spoil your feeding relationship. You can follow sDOR in feeding your child with cystic fibrosis and raise your child to be Eating Competent.

Avoidant Restrictive Food Intake Disorder (ARFID)

You may be aware of ARFID, an increasingly used diagnosis generally reserved for the child who has a growth deficiency, relies on oral or tube-fed meal replacements, and/or whose restrictive eating has interfered with their social and emotional functioning.[16] Treatment of ARFID is beyond the scope of this book, but I will tell you that while sDOR forms the basis for treatment, parents of children diagnosed with ARFID can't simply be advised to follow sDOR. Such advice comes across as one of the many partial and piecemeal bits of instruction they have already been given. Feeding struggles that rise to the level of ARFID are complex, deep-rooted, and long-standing, and frightened parents need to be able to trust the intervention. Careful and individualized assessment and treatment-planning allows parents to feel that they, their child, and their situation are fully understood. Once sDOR is defined in individualized and achievable ways, parents need support for taking and maintaining the leap of faith necessary to let their child do the *how much* and *whether* of eating at the same time as they recognize the child's ways of gradually learning to eat. At times, a child's feeding/swallowing issues have to be addressed by an occupational therapist or speech/language pathologist.

NUTRITION-RELATED STUFF

Our discussion so far in *Ellyn Satter's Child of Mine* has woven together the themes of child development, parenting, and nutrition. There are still a few issues to consider, and this section pulls them together, in no particular order.

Activity

Activity relates to nutrition because we all need a minimum level of activity in order to accurately regulate food intake. I talked about this in the Chapter 3 section, "Respect your child's natural activity," page 86. While enjoyable family activities are wonderful, don't force activity, and don't feel you have to be your child's training coach or playmate. Don't try to make them physically fit, get them to be active to use up calories or to try to control their weight. Instead, follow Figure 3.2, "The Satter Division of Responsibility in activity," page 87. Provide your child with opportunities to be active and with a safe place to move and play. Then let them determine whether, how, and how much they move.

The small amount of research we have on children's physical activity usually shows up in the context of weight management interventions.

If we set aside the goal of slimming children down, those studies give us insight about what helps children be more active. Limiting children's sedentary activity has the greatest impact on their overall activity, more than when they were encouraged or even rewarded for being active.[17] Primarily, that means keeping control of your child's electronic media. Even if children turn to other seemingly sedentary activities such as reading or coloring, they are more active and not so sedated as when they watch TV. With respect to video games, the studies haven't been done, so I can only speculate. It certainly seems that children are more actively engaged and not as hypnotized by video games as they are by TV, but I could be wrong. I am on firmer ground in observing that setting limits on video games comes under the umbrella of good parenting. Keep them from taking over your child's life.

Don't worry if your child gets bored when you put controls on the electronic media, and don't try to rescue them from their boredom. It is lovely if you can spend time with your child, but your child also benefits from spending time alone and from being able to entertain themself. For children as for adults, boredom can stimulate creativity. Your child will come up with ways of being happily occupied if you aren't too quick to entertain them.

Some preschoolers get into sports, dance, and gymnastics, and that brings two main challenges: 1) Maintaining the meal and snack routine and 2) Being aware of and combatting negative body and weight comments and expectations that go along with particular sports. It might be assumed that your child will do better—or not as well—if they are bigger or smaller, more slender or muscular. Discuss this with your child's teacher or coach. At the same time as these attitudes are deeply embedded, the realization of their harmfulness is increasingly recognized. Your child's teacher or coach may be surprised and appalled that they are expressing them.

Provide sugary foods regularly

The word "moderation" may translate for you into "Don't eat so much; don't eat the food you enjoy." That's not where we are going. The issue with sugar is allowing your child to enjoy sweets without being preoccupied with them. We can do by not putting sweets on a "bad" list.

Children are born with a sweet tooth. Children's stomachs are small and their energy needs are high. Sweets in children's diets have a function with respect to helping them get the calories they need. But letting them have all they want will spoil their diet—and their teeth. Find the middle ground by following the forbidden food guidelines I gave you in the Chapter 11 section, "Include sweets," page 365.

The "healthy eating plan" advises keeping children's sugar consumption to a bare minimum. Nutritionists looking for ways to adhere to that advice may recommend "covert control," keeping sugar out of the house or avoiding settings where sweets are available. That plan might work when your child is small, but it will set them up for eating all the more when they are older and more out on their own. A study of over 600 two- to seven-year-olds found that greater "unhealthy" snack intake was associated with lower covert control by the parents, while greater "healthy" snack intake was associated with higher covert control.[18] Covert control *seemed* to work in the study—if you can call "working" depriving children and their parents of sweets and chips. But note the children were seven years old or younger. They were still mostly under the parents' influence. When they get older, those "covertly controlled" children are likely to sneak sweets and eat a lot of them when they can.

You don't have to worry about the sugar you use in cooking and what comes along with other nutritious foods, such as sugar syrup on canned fruit. The fact that a food contains sugar doesn't somehow negate the other nutrients it contains and make it a "bad food." Good cooks use a little sugar to make food taste better—not enough to disguise it, just to enhance it. A teaspoon of sugar in a tomato dish takes the harsh edge off the tomato taste and makes the dish more palatable, especially for younger taste buds. A teaspoon of sugar in the frozen peas gives them a "just picked" flavor. Some desserts and sweets are particularly nutritious. Custards, puddings, oatmeal or peanut butter cookies, and pumpkin pie are all nutritious choices. Let your child put sugar on their low-sugar breakfast cereal, enjoy flavoring in milk, and/or put jam on toast.

I object to sugar-coated cereals and their advertising because they teach kids that food has to be sweet to be good. Highly sweetened breakfast cereals dyed vivid colors disguise the delicious flavors of grains and promote substitute food that is more like candy than cereal. When my children were small, I would buy a few boxes of sugar-coated cereal to take on camping trips. The cereal was easy to pack and fun for our mini vacations. They thought it was a big treat, and they would wolf it down for snacks. They told me I was being too strict when I wouldn't buy it all the time. I told them it wouldn't be special if I bought it all the time.

The sticky topic of Halloween candy

Each year, at least one enterprising writer or reporter approaches me for my views on Halloween candy. One year, a local TV station made an emergency visit to my home to consider this critical issue. It was worth the trouble because the interview gave me my very first disclaimer. "The views of this interviewee are not necessarily those of the station management" the text read across the bottom of the screen as I was held forth. What had I said that was so alarming and revolutionary? Was it when I said that trick or treating and eating Halloween candy was a part of being a child and that children needed to be allowed to eat their candy without a lot of interference from their adults? Was it the routine I suggested when the child comes home from trick-or-treating: Let them lay out their booty, gloat over it, sort it, and eat as much of it as they want? Let them do the same the next day. Was it the advice I gave about managing candy even after *the day*, that is, have the child put it away and relegate it to snack time and mealtime? Let them have a couple of small pieces at meals for dessert and as much as they want at snack time along with a glass of milk?

The interviewer was appalled but gamely tried to herd me into what she considered safer territory. "That's pretty liberal advice," she skeptically pointed out. "Will something bad happen if parents follow that advice?"

After a moment's reflection, I said, "Well, I suppose if children were allowed to eat too much candy they would lose their taste for it, and I think that would be too bad. Candy eating is a wonderful part of being a child." Maybe that was what got the disclaimer, or maybe it was what I said next: "If parents do a good job with feeding, even a few days of candy eating won't impair a child's nutritional health. If they aren't, all the candy restriction in the world won't make any difference." I stand by my Halloween advice, but remember, those aren't the views of the station management!

Given regular opportunities to eat unlimited sweets, your child will develop the instinctive ability to keep sweets eating in proportion to the other food they eat. Halloween candy presents a learning opportunity. Work toward having your child be able to manage their own stash. Parents who have been following my Figure 11.7 advice, "Regularly offer 'forbidden' food," say they find dusty bags of Halloween candy in forgotten corners.

Sweets handouts at other times

That's all very well if it is only Halloween, say unconvinced parents. But what about sweets at all the other times? Children get sweets in school as rewards for doing well, at the deli counter in the grocery store, and from grandparents, aunts and uncles, and neighbors. Not to mention the ice cream truck and lollipops at the bank. In my experience, sweets handouts present a big problem only when children aren't allowed to have sweets in the first place. When parents follow the "forbidden food" routine, children are not particularly thrilled by sweets handouts. They eat them if they are hungry; not if they aren't. Also consider depending on structure. A grocery store cookie or ice cream truck popsicle can be a snack. I do not like the idea of sweets rewards in school—whatever happened to the child's achievement providing its own reward?

If you approach the teacher, consider the point of view of *timing*. Classroom food handouts of any type just before lunch can spoil children's lunch. Maybe the teacher can be interested in offering classroom treats at snack time to help tide children over for lunch. Managing timing is far more desirable than the good-food/bad-food strategy of banning sweets altogether used in many schools.

Let your child eat fat

Throughout this book I have encouraged you to use whole milk, include fat in cooking, offer high-fat condiments at mealtime, and let your child eat as much fat as they want. They will eat more fat when they need it, less fat when they don't.

Don't restrict your child's dietary fat in an attempt to get or keep them slim. It doesn't work and will make them overeat on high-fat food when they get the chance. Some health providers tell a child they need to eat less fat. That is a sneaky way of saying, "You're not all right the way you are" and makes a child feel just as bad as being told they are "too fat." Protect your child from such harm by asking your health professional to discuss your child's weight and/or eating only when your child is not around.

Children tend to have relatively high blood lipids when they are small and lower lipids as they get older. Some children have "familial hyperlipidemia," which is an inherited tendency toward highly elevated blood lipid levels and greater than usual susceptibility to heart disease. A modified fat diet appears to allow those children to have modest decreases in blood cholesterol and triglycerides, but it is unclear whether those decreases correlate with lower incidence of heart disease. A modified fat diet is not a low-fat diet, but rather a diet high in monounsaturated fat, moderate in polyunsaturated fat, and low in saturated fat. See the Chapter 11 section, "Enjoy fats and oils," page 400.

It won't hurt and it might help to follow a modified fat diet. If your physician determines that your child has familial hyperlipidemia and recommends a modified diet, see a dietitian who is well-versed in it. It is complicated, and you will likely be more rigid and avoidant than you have to be. Furthermore, you will need help maintaining sDOR. Whenever a child is on a restricted diet, it is far too easy to start making yourself responsible for whether and how much they eat. Struggles about your child's eating can cause eating problems that could worsen their condition.

Food and behavior

Food energy is the one nutritional factor that is likely to have a direct impact on your child's behavior. A child who is hungry is likely to be tired, irritable, and contrary. Sometimes a hungry child is too contrary to eat. The active, enthusiastic child will often get too busy and involved to be aware of being hungry until they run out of steam and have a behavioral meltdown. To head off such fusses, have sit-down meals and snacks at regular intervals and insist that your busy child take time to sit down. Once they get there, they may eat as enthusiastically as they play. To be filling and last a while, a snack needs two or three of the food groups—protein, grains or other starches, fruit or vegetables, whole milk. See the Chapter 11 section, "Have sit-down snacks," page 370.

Pseudo-scientists promote books saying eating certain foods can cause behavioral problems such as irritability, contrariness, sleeplessness, rebelliousness, and general nastiness. For the embattled parent, it is tempting to believe that some external, definable force can be responsible for all these maddening traits. Allergies can impact behavior, not because particular foods directly affect the nervous system but because particular foods can precipitate allergic reactions that, in turn, make a child miserable and crabby. A child with severe dermatitis, stomachaches, intestinal cramps, and headaches is likely to be an irritable child and may also have trouble sleeping, which further exacerbates their negative behavior.

A related scam is promoting nutritional supplements to address hyperactivity, cognitive deficits, and learning disabilities. They do not work. To have a nutritional solution, you must have a nutritional problem. *Deficiency* of almost any vitamin or mineral is likely to make someone behave differently because they will be physically weak and susceptible to disease. However, these scam supplements aren't talking about addressing deficiency, they are talking about nutrients used as drugs.

Nutritional *deficiencies* that impact behavior include iron deficiency. Anemia can cause listlessness and irritability. B vitamins such as niacin and thiamine are particularly important for a steady and well-functioning nervous system. But if you are following sDOR your child will eat the variety of foods they need to have a nutritionally adequate diet.

Can sugar restriction and avoidance of artificial colors and flavors help control hyperactivity in children? Perhaps, but only for a few. Carefully-controlled studies have shown that a fraction of 1 percent of young children with hyperactivity show a mild decrease in hyperactive behavior as the result of dietary modifications.[19] Those studies are rarely repeated because they are so fiendishly difficult and expensive to do.

Vitamins and minerals

The two Chapter 10 sections starting on page 333, "Choosing food" and "Nutrients and your older baby," addresses food sources of vitamins and minerals and the nutrients themselves. If your drinking water is inadequately fluoridated, your child may need to take a fluoride supplement. Beyond that, if you are successfully following sDOR, your child will not need to take vitamin and/or mineral supplements. However, if you need to give your child a "vitamin" in order to feel comfortable, make it a multivitamin-mineral preparation. The Chapter 11 section, "Be wise about mutivitamin-mineral supplements," page 404, outlines recommendations for choosing a supplement.

While some nutrients are of particular concern, you can easily provide them for your child with regular meals and sit-down snacks. Don't make yourself crazy by keeping track of what your child eats—it will be erratic. Instead, pay attention to what you *offer* over a week or two at meals and snacks—and the way you offer it. Having pleasant family meals with a variety of food that you enjoy will predict your child's nutritional status much more clearly than any analysis of what they happen to eat on a particular day or even over a few days. Offer your child whole milk at most meals and some snacks. Too many children don't get enough calcium because they drink juice and soda rather than milk.

Lactose intolerance

Lactose is milk sugar. People who can't digest lactose don't make lactase in their small intestine and have lactose intolerance. Within 12 hours after they drink milk, they get intestinal gas, loose stools, or explosive diarrhea accompanied by gas from drinking milk, and they may have stomach cramps. Lactose intolerance affects about 70 percent of the world's population. If your ancestors came from Northern Europe, you probably digest lactose. If you're of African, Asian, Mediterranean, Hispanic, or Native American ancestry, your chances of being lactose-intolerant are greater. Lactose intolerance generally doesn't appear before ages five or six, and even lactose-intolerant people make some lactase.

Even if your child is beginning to show inherited lactose intolerance, they likely can still comfortably drink a small glass of whole milk with meals or snacks. If not, consider offering lactose-free milk or soy milk enriched with calcium and vitamin D. Because it is made from the high-protein, high-vitamin-and-mineral soybean, soy milk is far more nutritious than other non-dairy milk, such as oat, almond, hemp, or cashew milk. Even milks made from cashews and almonds don't have that much protein.

It is likely still possible for the child who is feeling well to drink a few ounces of milk at any one time. It won't harm them and it provides them with calcium and vitamin D. How much milk they can drink depends both on their individual sensitivity to lactose and on what other foods they eat along with the milk. Drinking whole milk helps. So does drinking milk along with a meal or snack containing fat. Fat slows down the emptying time of the stomach, so the lactose gets to the intestine more slowly and doesn't cause an overload.

SUSPECT CURRENT PRACTICE

I already addressed this theme with my talk-show story, so forgive me for being repetitive. There is just *so much* misinformation about feeding! Consider these ridiculous statements:

FROM A POPULAR BLOG:

Make a list of the foods your child is willing to eat. If the number of foods is less than 20, your child may be a problem feeder.

> *Particularly cautious children go for years eating from a short list of food, then make up for lost time in their teens. As long as the child has positive eating attitudes and behaviors, they are learning to be comfortable with new food so, eventually, they can eat it. Keep their eating from being a problem by not pressuring them in any way to eat and being considerate without catering with menu planning. Eventually, your giving them repeated neutral exposure to the foods you eat will support them in learning to eat a greater variety.*

FROM A PEDIATRIC DIETITIAN:

When parents complain to me about their picky kids, I give them the standard advice about removing junk food from their child's diet. I say their child will eat when they get hungry, and I reassure them that there is no need to worry unless the child loses weight or stops growing.

What cruel advice, given without understanding the child or the situation! How is removing "junk food" supposed to address the child's food selectivity? Instead, reassure parents that it is normal for kids to be skeptical of new food and slow to learn to eat it. Instead of worrying about what the child eats, put the emphasis on letting them be Eating Competent: enjoy family meals, pick and choose from the food there, and eat as much or as little as they want. Teach parents sDOR and emphasize being considerate without catering with meal planning.

FROM A LEADING MEDICAL CENTER:

Following a healthy diet as a family can help children reach and stay at a healthy weight.

This, too, is cruel advice that ignores the data. Poor food selection does not make children fat, and "following a healthy diet" food does not make them achieve a "healthy weight." sDOR supports children in growing in the way that is right for them.

Feeding norms can trip you up

You wouldn't deliberately take away your preschooler's curiosity and good feelings about themself. However, feeding norms do exactly that. Parents of preschoolers observed at mealtime say their primary goal is getting children to eat more during meals. Three quarters serve their child without input from the child. Eighty-five percent reward, praise, and threaten children to get them to eat more, and an equal percentage of children give in and keep eating after they say they are finished.[20] Parents in focus groups endorse good nutrition, but over 90 percent bribe, pressure, cater, limit menus to foods their child eats, don't believe their child when they say they are full, and encourage their child to eat more.[21] Think of it! Almost all parents have a basic misunderstanding about feeding! It is little wonder that up to half of typically developing children have feeding problems such as food refusal, disruptive mealtime behavior, rigid food preferences, failure to master eating skills, growth faltering, or growth acceleration.[22]

Those parents were laboring under the maddening and "impossible expectation of getting their child to eat certain foods and grow in certain ways" that I opened with in Chapter 1. Following sDOR frees you of those expectations. It does, however, put you out of step with common practice, and that can make you feel there is something wrong with what you are doing. Reassure yourself by tuning in on your child. How do they feel when you follow sDOR? Alternatively, how do they react when they are forced to eat food they don't want? Keep in mind this isn't just about the child's eating or not eating, but about the way the child feels about *themself*. A video of a four-year-old whose parents interfere provides just such reassurance. Adam is in the preschooler segment of my earlier video, *Feeding with Love and Good Sense*. I know today's parents are skeptical of older media, but these demonstrations of positive and negative feeding dynamics remain as fresh and pertinent as when they were first captured.

Adam is eating his spaghetti in first-rate preschooler fashion—spearing his spaghetti with his fork and slurping it into his mouth, helping it along with his fingers. Meanwhile he is clearly enjoying telling his parents about the day's events. He runs out of spaghetti and asks for more. In the grand tradition of generations of parents, his parents respond, "yes, but first you have to eat the rest of your food." Adam is a typically compliant preschooler—he bravely eats his way through his peas and grapes and drinks his milk. He even manages to choke down two slices of the hated cucumbers, although we notice his difficulty swallowing and wonder if he will throw up on his plate.

Since we have no responsibility for Adam, we can feel for him. The longer he eats, the more dejected he becomes. He loses interest in the mealtime conversation, leans back in his chair, pulls his knees up to his chest, and watches his fist as he throws it into the air. His father scolds him, "Sit up straight, Adam." Words couldn't say it more clearly. As far as Adam is concerned, this meal is a real bust. Moreover, so is he. What he wants is *definitely* not okay with his parents. Finally, his father gives him more spaghetti. Adam perks up and undergoes a complete personality transplant. He sprinkles Parmesan cheese on his spaghetti and licks off the top of the can, which makes his parents smile at each other, but they don't say anything. He goes back to being a happy, companionable boy who enjoys being with his family. Adam's parents have gotten so caught up in getting him to eat a variety of food that they have nearly spoiled their time together. It's clear they have what it takes to overlook Adam's preschooler awkwardness, but their sense of nutritional obligation takes precedence over their sensitivity.

Adam's parents didn't enjoy making him miserable, but they felt obligated to make him jump over his fruit and vegetable hurdles before they could let him eat what he wanted. They are not alone. Parents worry, and they ask, often in an exasperated how-can-you-let-that-kid-get-away-with-that voice, "Well, what would *you* do? Just let him have more spaghetti?" My answer? Yes. Adam's eating is not a chore that he has to do. It is a pleasant and rewarding activity that he *gets* to do. Moreover, it is an activity that he can be *successful* doing. From a preschooler perspective, that has everything to do with how he feels about eating—and about himself.

Sooner or later—if not this spaghetti meal then the next or the 5 or 40 or 80 times after that—Adam will get filled up on spaghetti and take an interest in peas. Or grapes. But maybe not cucumbers. We all are entitled to some likes and dislikes, and it appears that Adam and cucumbers will never be close. It takes a long time to learn to eat a variety of food, and if Adam's parents back off, he will make it his business to push himself along and learn. If his parents continue to force him to eat, they will take away his initiative and he will eat vegetables because his parents *make* him. When they stop pushing him, Adam will stop eating them altogether—or eat them out of obligation, not because he enjoys them.

Adam's parents are already doing a great job! They have prepared an attractive, varied meal and are eating together as a family. They include Adam in conversation. They don't badger him about table manners. They ignore his sloppy spaghetti-eating and Parmesan-can-licking. Why in the world do they take it upon themselves to do Adam's jobs with eating?

I suspect they were being controlling because they thought they should, and I expect you understand where they are coming from.

Taking leadership—or not

The most well-intended, caring, committed parents can get derailed with feeding, as demonstrated by the mothers in a small and devoted parenting support group who invited me to speak with them. I went through my schtick about sDOR, and that went down all right. I talked about letting the child be responsible for what and how much they eat. Ditto. But when I got to the part about providing regular meals and snacks and not allowing the child to eat between times, they began avoiding my eyes.

Suspecting something was afoot, I opened the topic for discussion. One brave woman shared her objections, saying, "I don't think they should have to sit at the table for a long time. I had to do that when I was little, and it was awful. If I try that with my child, he has such a fit that I don't enjoy my meal." It hadn't occurred to her that she could let him leave the meal when he finished eating. She had been traumatized with feeding and that made it hard for her to find a solution that meshed with authoritative parenting.

Another said, "My four-year-old gets so busy playing, and it is so much trouble to get her to come for meals, that I just don't bother. I remember meals when I was little as being really unpleasant. Meals are more pleasant when she isn't around." That one required some unpacking. To include her child at mealtime, that mom would have to stop giving food handouts, help her daughter settle down and refocus on eating, and make sure mealtimes were pleasant. Again, it is difficult when you have had an unpleasant upbringing with eating.

Even the group leader—regarded as the parenting expert—waffled on her earlier statement that children need clear limits. "I make meals, but I let my four-year-old come to the meal if he wants to and he can take something from the meal and eat it somewhere else. It seems to me that it is cruel to make him sit there while he eats." I asked why she felt limits were necessary in one area and not in the other, and she became tearful. "My mother shamed me when I was little and didn't eat and said I was an ungrateful girl who was lucky to have such nice food," she said. "I don't want to do that to my son." It hadn't occurred to her that she could follow sDOR and not manipulate and belittle her son as her mother had her.

The mothers in the group were attempting to resolve their feeding issues by feeding in ways that were the opposite of the authoritarian tactics they had grown up with. For them, the structure and predictability of sit-down meals and snacks was negative and rigid. They were missing the point that preschoolers need structure, and that they challenge themselves to live up to their parents' expectations—when those expectations are realistic.

The mothers are not the only ones whose parenting logic breaks down when it comes to feeding. Attachment parenting advocate Dr. William Sears describes his methods as being authoritative parenting. However, with respect to feeding, he becomes permissive. He argues against expecting young children to participate in family meals and, instead, advocates feeding them on the run.

Finding the middle ground

The Chapter 11 section, "Sort out control issues," page 357, discusses what crossing the lines of sDOR looks like. Western Massachusetts Growth Study researchers found parents did both: theydid their jobs *and* intruded on their child's jobs. They did the *what*, *when*, and *where* of providing meals, then crossed over into doing their child's jobs by trying to get them to eat certain types and amounts of food. Between meals, parents gave children their own jobs by letting them eat whatever and whenever they wanted from the refrigerator and cupboards.[23] This muddled approach is hard on children. Children love their parents, want them around, and do more and dare more when their parents are nearby. However, when the Massachusetts parents were around, they spoiled their child's eating by being controlling. The only way children could eat whether and as much as they wanted was by going off on their own to do it. Learning that lesson is grave and goes far beyond feeding. The children were learning that to be their own person they had to be by themselves! Being given autonomy with eating when parents are around powerfully reinforces to the child that they—and what they want—are okay.

IT'S TIME TO SAY GOODBYE

Our work in *Ellyn Satter's Child of Mine* is finished. Thank you for taking this journey with me and best wishes to you and your child as you continue on your way. You now have the information you need to finish raising your child with food and feeding: sDOR, basic information about family food selection and meal planning, a clear sense of your own importance, and a thinking approach to parenting. As your child gets older, these tools will continue to be important. Your school-age child and teenager will still depend on you to maintain the structure of family meals and give them autonomy with their eating and growth. As they get older, your child will do more and more of their own food selection outside the home, but you will still be the gatekeeper and the one who takes responsibility for family food preparation and nurturing. Continue to have pleasant family meals and expect your older child and teenager to show up for meals on time and hungry. If your child is a Competent Eater, they have earned the privilege of making suggestions for family meals, can participate in planning the family menus, and can even cook once in a while.

Your child has a very good chance of carrying into older life the positive eating attitudes and behaviors they have gained from you in these early years. Certainly, during their teen years they will experiment and even be rebellious with food selection, the same as with everything else. But they will settle down. You have started them in the right direction, and sooner or later, they will return to what you have taught in these first few years. For more about parenting with food during the school-age and teen years, read the booklets *Feeding with Love and Good Sense: 6 through 13 Years* and *Feeding with Love and Good Sense: 12 through 18 Years.* You can find them on the Ellyn Satter Institute website. Also consider reading the chapters on the school-age child and adolescent in *Your Child's Weight: Helping without Harming.*

For now, I hope you have learned to lighten up at the same time as you take good care of yourself and your child with food. Eating well is one of life's great pleasures. It is too important to turn it into a hassle. Enjoy your child and celebrate eating.

REFERENCES

1. Baumrind D. Current patterns of parental authority. *Developmental Psychology Monograph.* 1971;4:1–103.
2. Davies WH. Reconceptualizing feeding and feeding disorders in interpersonal context: the case for a relational disorder. *J Fam Psychol.* 2006;20:409–417.
3. Hample SE. Executive Summary: clinical practice guideline for the evaluation and treatment of children and adolescents with obesity. *Pediatrics.* 2023. doi:e2022060641
4. Gorlick JC. "I feel like less of a mom:" experiences of weight stigma by association among mothers of children with overweight and obesity. *Childhood Obesity.* 2020;17:68–75.
5. Flegal KM. Association of all-cause mortality with overweight and obesity using standard body mass index categories: a systematic review and meta-analysis. *JAMA.* 2013;309:71–82.
6. Abraham S. Relationship of childhood weight status to morbidity in adults. *Int J Epidemiol.* 2016;45:1020–1031.
7. Llewellyn A. Childhood obesity as a predictor of morbidity in adulthood: a systematic review and meta-analysis. *Obes Rev.* 2016;17:56–67.
8. Park SY. Weight change in older adults and mortality: the Multiethnic Cohort Study. *Int J Obes (Lond).* 2018;42:205–212.
9. Diaz VA. The association between weight fluctuation and mortality: results from a population-based cohort study. *J Community Health.* 2005;30:153–65.
10. O'Connor EA. Screening for obesity and intervention for weight management in children and adolescents: evidence report and systematic review for the US Preventive Services Task Force. *JAMA.* 2017;317:2427–2444.
11. Gerards SM. Parental perception of child's weight status and subsequent BMIz change: the KOALA birth cohort study. *BMC public health.* 2014. doi:10.1186/1471-2458-14-291
12. Robinson E. Parental perception of weight status and weight gain across childhood. *Pediatrics.* 2016. doi:10.1542/peds.2015-3957
13. Tester JM. Disordered eating behaviours and food insecurity: A qualitative study about children with obesity in low-income households. *Obes Res Clin Pract.* 2016;10:544–552.
14. Satter E. Hierarchy of food needs. *J Nutr Educ Behav.* 2007;39:S187–S188.
15. Davies HW. Mealtime interactions and family characteristics in CF. *Eighth Annual North American Cystic Fibrosis Conference.* 1994.
16. Zimmerman J. Avoidant/Restrictive Food Intake Disorder (ARFID). *Curr Probl Pediatr Adolesc Health Care.* 2017;47:95–103.
17. Epstein L. Effects of manipulating sedentary behavior on physical activity and food intake. *Journal of Pediatrics.* 2002;140:334–339.

18. Boots SB. Managing young children's snack food intake. The role of parenting style and feeding strategies. *Appetite*. 2015;92:94–101.
19. Rowe K. Synthetic food coloring and behavior: a dose-response effect in double-blind, placebo-controlled, repeated measures study. *Journal of Pediatrics*. 1994;125:691–698.
20. Orrell-Valente JK. "Just three more bites": an observational analysis of parents' socialization of children's eating at mealtime. *Appetite*. 2007;48:37–45.
21. Sherry B. Attitudes, practices, and concerns about child feeding and child weight status among socioeconomically diverse white, Hispanic, and African-American mothers. *J Am Diet Assoc*. 2004;104:215–221.
22. Silverman AH. Feeding and vomiting problems in pediatric populations. In: Roberts MC, Steele RC, eds. *Handbook of Pediatric Psychology*. Guilford Publications; 2017:402–416.
23. Anliker JA. Mothers' reports of their three-year-old children's control over foods and involvement in food-related activities. *Journal of Nutrition Education*. 1992;24:285–291.

INDEX

F

G

H

O

www.ingramcontent.com/pod-product-compliance
Lightning Source LLC
Jackson TN
JSHW070032101125
93871JS00003B/4

* 9 7 8 0 9 9 0 8 9 7 5 4 5 *